Granade

HANDBOOK OF PAEDIATRICS

SEVENTH EDITION

Disclaimer
While every effort has been made to check drug dosages in this handbook, it is still possible that errors have been overlooked. Dosages continue to be revised and new side effects recognized. Oxford University Press makes no representation, express or implied, that the drug dosages in this book are correct. For these reasons, the reader is strongly urged to consult the *South African Medicines Formulary* or the drug manufacturer's printed instructions before administering any of the drugs recommended in this clinical handbook. The authors and the publishers do not accept responsibility or legal liability for any errors in the text or for the misuse or misapplication of material in this work.

The authors and the publishers gratefully acknowledge permission to reproduce material in this book. Every effort has been made to trace copyright holders, but where this has proved impossible, the publishers would be grateful for information which would enable them to amend any omissions in future editions.

HANDBOOK OF PAEDIATRICS

SEVENTH EDITION

Content editor
Cassim Motala

Section editors
Alan Davidson
Anthony Figaji
Michael Levin

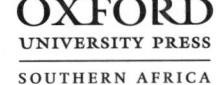

OXFORD
UNIVERSITY PRESS
SOUTHERN AFRICA

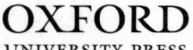

OXFORD
UNIVERSITY PRESS

Oxford University Press is a department of the University of Oxford.
It furthers the University's objective of excellence in research, scholarship,
and education by publishing worldwide. Oxford is a registered trade mark of
Oxford University Press in the UK and in certain other countries

Published in South Africa by
Oxford University Press Southern Africa (Pty) Limited

Vasco Boulevard, Goodwood, N1 City, Cape Town, South Africa, 7460
P O Box 12119, N1 City, Cape Town, South Africa, 7463

© University of Cape Town 2010

The moral rights of the author have been asserted

First edition published 1975 by the Department of Paediatrics and Child Health, University of Cape Town
Second edition published 1989 by Haum Educational Publishers, Pretoria.
Subsequent editions published by Oxford University Press Southern Africa

Third edition published 1992
Fourth edition published 1995
Fourth revised edition published 1997
Fifth edition published 1998
Sixth edition published 2004
Seventh edition, second impression published 2011

All rights reserved. No part of this publication may be reproduced, stored in a retrieval system, or transmitted,
in any form or by any means, without the prior permission in writing of Oxford University Press Southern
Africa (Pty) Ltd, or as expressly permitted by law, by licence, or under terms agreed with the appropriate
reprographic rights organisation, DALRO, The Dramatic, Artistic and Literary Rights Organisation atdalro@
dalro.co.za. Enquiries concerning reproduction outside the scope of the above should be sent to the Rights
Department, Oxford University Press Southern Africa (Pty) Ltd, at the above address.

You must not circulate this work in any other form
and you must impose this same condition on any acquirer.

Handbook of Paediatrics

ISBN 978 0 19 599117 8

Third impression 2014

Typeset in Utopia 8pt on 10pt
Printed on 75 gsm woodfree paper

Acknowledgements
Publishing manager: Alida Terblanche
Commissioning editor: Marisa Montemarano
Managing editor: Lisa Andrews
Editor: Dr Bridget Farham
Specialist proofreaders: Prof David Beatty and Prof Maurice Kibel
Designer: Judith Cross
Typesetter: Elbert Visser
Indexer: Adrienne Pretorius
Printed and bound by: ABC Press, Cape Town
121527

The authors and publisher gratefully acknowledge permission to reproduce copyright material in this book.
Every effort has been made to trace copyright holders, but if any copyright infringements have been made,
the publisher would be grateful for information that would enable any omissions or errors to be corrected in
subsequent impressions.

Links to third party websites are provided by Oxford in good faith and for information only. Oxford disclaims
any responsibility for the materials contained in any third party website referenced in this work.

Abridged table of contents

Chapter 1	Emergencies and trauma	1
Chapter 2	Neonatal problems	44
Chapter 3	Respiratory problems	88
Chapter 4	Gastrointestinal problems	121
Chapter 5	Growth and nutrition	153
Chapter 6	Cardiovascular problems	167
Chapter 7	Nervous system and neuromuscular problems	183
Chapter 8	Renal system problems	218
Chapter 9	Immunization and infections	247
Chapter 10	HIV infection	295
Chapter 11	Asthma, allergic problems and immunodeficiency	319
Chapter 12	Development	338
Chapter 13	Child psychiatry	353
Chapter 14	Endocrinology	363
Chapter 15	Haematology and oncology	394
Chapter 16	Dermatology	409
Chapter 17	Bone and joint problems	425
Chapter 18	Eyes and vision	439
Chapter 19	Ear, nose and throat problems	448
Chapter 20	Fluids, electrolytes and acid base	461
Chapter 21	Surgical problems	487
Chapter 22	Palliative care and pain management	508
Chapter 23	Procedures	521
Chapter 24	Burns	544

Contents

List of contributors	xiii
List of reviewers	xvii
An evidence-based red Book?	xxi
Preface	xxiii
Foreword	xxv

1 Emergencies and trauma — 1
- The critically ill child — 1
- Clinical priorities — 6
- Drugs — 19
- Fluid administration in the critically ill — 19
- The injured child — 20
- Primary survey and resuscitation — 21
- Secondary survey and management — 23
- Management of minor injuries — 27
- Child abuse — 29
- Childhood poisoning — 38

2 Neonatal problems — 44
- Resuscitation at birth — 44
- Hypoxic ischaemic encephalopathy (HIE) — 48
- Neonatal seizures — 52
- The low birthweight infant — 53
- Hypoglycaemia — 57
- Hypothermia — 60
- Infection in the newborn — 61
- Respiratory diseases of the newborn — 68
- Neonatal jaundice — 74
- Breastfeeding – getting the right start — 82

3 Respiratory problems — 88
- An approach to cough — 88
- An approach to fast breathing — 89
- An approach to noisy breathing — 89
- An approach to peripheral airway obstruction (PAO) — 92
- Laryngomalacia — 95
- Bronchiolitis — 96
- Croup — 99

	Febrile dysphagia syndrome	102
	Pneumonia	104
	Sleep-disordered breathing (SDB)	107
	Aspiration lung disease	110
	Bronchiectasis	112
	Cystic fibrosis (CF)	113
	Choking and foreign body (FB) inhalation	114
	Pleural collections	115
	Respiratory muscle dysfunction	118
	Tracheo-bronchial obstruction	119
4	**Gastrointestinal problems**	**121**
	Gastroenteritis	121
	Persistent diarrhoea	126
	Approach to blood in stool	130
	An approach to jaundice	132
	Hepatitis	134
	Acute liver failure (ALF)	137
	Chronic hepatic disease	140
	Cystic fibrosis	140
	The approach to a child with hepatosplenomegaly	142
	Infantile colic	145
	Functional gastrointestinal disorders	146
	Constipation and faecal impaction	147
	An approach to vomiting	149
	Gastro-oesophageal reflux	151
5	**Growth and nutrition**	**153**
	Malnutrition	153
	Nutrient deficiencies	161
	An approach to failure to thrive	162
6	**Cardiovascular problems**	**167**
	An initial approach to the diagnosis of congenital heart disease	167
	Common symptom complexes	169
	Acquired heart disease	175
	Disorders of cardiac rhythm	180
7	**Nervous system and neuromuscular problems**	**183**
	Clinical diagnosis	183
	Problems with the head	184
	Problems with the neck	185
	Problems with the back	186

	Raised intracranial pressure	187
	Headache	189
	Migraine headache	190
	Altered states of consciousness	191
	Seizures and epilepsy	192
	Epilepsy	194
	Paroxysms	200
	Movement disorders	201
	Hemiplegia	203
	The floppy infant	205
	The weak child	206
	Chronic weakness: proximal	208
	Chronic weakness: distal	209
	Loss of skills: neuro-regression	210
	Acute disseminated encephalomyelitis (ADEM)	210
	Infections of the CNS	210
8	**Renal system problems**	**218**
	Urinary incontinence in children	218
	Urinary tract infection (UTI)	224
	An approach to haematuria	227
	Acute post-streptococcal glomerulonephritis (APSGN)	230
	Nephrotic syndrome	232
	Acute renal failure	236
	Chronic renal failure	241
	Hypertension	242
9	**Immunization and infections**	**247**
	Immunization	247
	Bacterial and viral infections	254
	Common parasitic diseases	278
	Protozoa	278
	Metazoa	289
	Statutory notifiable diseases	293
10	**HIV infection**	**295**
	Prevention of vertical transmission	295
	Diagnosis	296
	Selected clinical problems	301
	Prophylaxis	303
	Clinical staging and immunological assessment	306
	Antiretroviral therapy	307
	Post exposure prophylaxis (PEP)	316

11	**Asthma, allergic problems and immunodeficiency**	**319**
	Asthma	319
	Allergic disorders	325
	Immunology	334
12	**Development**	**338**
	An approach to developmental disabilities	338
	An approach to intellectual disability	339
	Approach to a child with developmental delay	341
	Cerebral palsy	341
	Approach to management of a child with cerebral palsy	343
	Developmental milestones and warning signs	344
13	**Child psychiatry**	**353**
	Autistic-like conditions and autism	353
	Attention deficit hyperactivity disorder	354
	Conversion disorder	357
	Delirium	358
	Major depressive disorder	360
	Traumatic stress	361
14	**Endocrinology**	**363**
	Diabetic emergencies	363
	Endocrine emergencies	371
	Growth and development	375
	Disorders of the thyroid gland	385
	Rickets	389
	Problems with calcium and parathyroid hormone	391
15	**Haematology and oncology**	**394**
	Haematology	394
	Anaemia	394
	Congenital haemolytic anaemias	398
	Bleeding disorders	400
	Acquired bleeding disorders	402
	Inherited bleeding disorders	403
	Oncology	404
	Warning signs in childhood cancer	404
	Approach to a suspected malignancy in children	405
16	**Dermatology**	**408**
	Acne	408
	Birthmarks	409

	Eczema (or dermatitis)	410
	Drug reactions	413
	Fungal infections of the skin	413
	Ichthyosis	417
	Molluscum contagiosum	417
	Papular urticaria	418
	Pediculosis	418
	Pityriasis rosea	419
	Psoriasis	419
	Scabies	420
	Streptococcal and staphylococcal infections	421
	Warts	422
17	**Bone and joint problems**	**425**
	An approach to a child with arthritis	425
	Acute haematogenous osteomyelitis (AHO) and septic arthritis (SA)	431
	Transient synovitis of the hip	432
	Skeletal tuberculosis	433
	Congenital deformities	434
	Developmental dysplasia of the hip (DDH)	434
	Rotational variations in children: intoeing and outtoeing	435
	Genu varum and genu valgum	435
	Perthes' disease	436
	Slipped upper femoral epiphysis (SUFE)	437
	Flexible or postural flat foot	438
18	**Eyes and vision**	**439**
	Visual assessment	439
	Amblyopia (lazy eye)	440
	External abnormalities	441
	Red eyes with purulent discharge	443
	Red eyes with watery discharge	444
	Red itchy eyes	444
	The unilateral red eye	445
	The white pupil (leucocoria)	445
	The injured eye	446
19	**Ear, nose and throat problems**	**448**
	The ear	448
	The nose	454
	The throat	458

20	**Fluids, electrolytes and acid base**	**461**
	Maintenance fluids	461
	Replacement fluids	463
	Acid-base disturbances	468
	Hypoglycaemia	473
	Electrolyte abnormalities	474
21	**Surgical problems**	**487**
	Problems of the newborn	487
	Diaphragmatic hernia (congenital)	488
	Exomphalos (unruptured)	488
	Gastroschisis and ruptured exomphalos	489
	Intestinal obstruction	489
	Oesophageal atresia	490
	Duodenal atresia	491
	Malrotation	491
	Proximal small-bowel obstruction	491
	Distal small-bowel obstruction	491
	Meconium ileus	492
	Hirschsprung's disease	492
	Meconium plug syndrome	493
	Ano-rectal malformations/imperforate anus	493
	Cleft lip and palate	494
	Abscess	494
	Peri-anal abscess	496
	Anal fissure	496
	Appendicitis	496
	Ascariasis	496
	Biliary atresia	497
	Branchial arch and cleft remnants	498
	Cervical lymphadenopathy	498
	Circumcision	498
	Cystic hygroma	499
	Ectopia vesicae (bladder exstrophy)	499
	Fused labia	499
	Cutaneous vascular lesions	500
	Hernia	501
	Hypospadias and chordee	502
	Intussusception	502
	Macroglossia (enlarged tongue)	503
	Meatal stenosis	503
	Parotid enlargement	504

	Pyloric stenosis	504
	Sublingual cysts	505
	Rectal prolapse	505
	Acute scrotum	506
	Sternomastoid tumour	506
	Tongue tie	506
	Undescended testis	507
	Umbilicus	507
22	**Palliative care and pain management**	**508**
	Palliative care	508
	Practical management of pain in children	512
	Conclusion	518
23	**Procedures**	**521**
	General principles	521
	Abdominal paracentesis (e.g. ascitic tap)	522
	Intravenous (IV) line placement	526
	Injections	529
	Lumbar puncture	532
	Nasogastric intubation	534
	Pleural drainage	535
	Fine needle aspiration biopsy	535
	Thoracentesis	537
	Urine collection	538
	Endotracheal intubation	539
	TecÙique and principles of acute peritoneal dialysis	542
24	**Burns**	**544**
	Appendix A (WHO charts)	**555**
	Index	**573**

List of Contributors

A. Argent
Division of Critical Care and
Children's Heart Disease
Department of Paediatrics and
Child Health
University of Cape Town
Cape Town

K. I. Barnes
Division of Clinical
Pharmacology
Department of Medicine
University of Cape Town
Cape Town

H. Buys
Division of Ambulatory
and Emergency Paediatrics
Department of Paediatrics and
Child Health
University of Cape Town
Cape Town

M. Carrihill
Division of Paediatric
Endocrinology
Department of Paediatrics and
Child Health
University of Cape Town
Cape Town

M. L. Cooke
Division of Ambulatory
Paediatrics
Department of Paediatrics
Stellenbosch University
Stellenbosch

G. Copley
Division of Otorhinolaryngology
Department of Surgery
University of Cape Town
Cape Town

S. Cox
Division of Paediatric Surgery
Department of Surgery
University of Cape Town
Cape Town

R. De Decker
Paediatric Cardiology Service
of Western Cape
Department of Paediatrics
and Child Health
University of Cape Town
Cape Town

R. De Lacy
Division of Paediatric
Gastroenterology
Department of Paediatrics
and Child Health
University of Cape Town
Cape Town

S. V. Delport
Division of Paediatric
Endocrinology
Department of Paediatrics
and Child Health
University of Cape Town
Cape Town

F. Desai
Division of Paediatric
Haematology/Oncology
Department of Paediatrics
and Child Health
University of Cape Town
Cape Town

R. Diedericks
Division of Ambulatory and
Emergency Paediatrics
Department of Paediatrics
and Child Health
University of Cape Town
Cape Town

K. Donald
Division of Child Development and Neurosciences
Department of Paediatrics and Child Health
University of Cape Town
Cape Town

B. Eley
Division of Infectious Disease and Immunology
Department of Paediatrics and Child Health
University of Cape Town
Cape Town

G. Fieggen
Division of Neurosurgery
Department of Surgery
University of Cape Town
Cape Town

A. Flisher (deceased)
Division of Child and Adolescent Psychiatry
Department of Psychiatry
University of Cape Town
Cape Town

P. Gajjar
Division of Paediatric Nephrology
Department of Paediatrics and Child Health
University of Cape Town
Cape Town

L. J. Glynn
Division of Neonatal Medicine
Department of Paediatrics and Child Health
University of Cape Town
Cape Town

L. Goddard
Division of Paediatric Gastroenterology
Department of Paediatrics and Child Health
University of Cape Town
Cape Town

R. Grotte
Division of Ophthalmology
Department of Surgery
University of Cape Town
Cape Town

M. C. Harrison
Division of Neonatal Medicine
Department of Paediatrics and Child Health
University of Cape Town
Cape Town

Marc Hendricks
Division of Haematology/Oncology
Department of Paediatrics and Child Health
University of Cape Town
Cape Town

Michael Hendricks
Division of Child Health Unit
Department of Paediatrics and Child Health
University of Cape Town
Cape Town

T. Hoffman
Division of Orthopaedics
Department of Surgery
University of Cape Town
Cape Town

A. R. Horn
Division of Neonatal Medicine
Department of Paediatrics and Child Health
University of Cape Town
Cape Town

G. Hussey
 Institute of Infectious
 Diseases and Molecular
 Medicine
 University of Cape Town
 Cape Town

J. Karpelowsky
 Division of Paediatric Surgery
 Department of Surgery
 University of Cape Town
 Cape Town

M. Klein
 Emeritus Professor
 Division of Paediatric
 Pulmonology
 Department of Paediatrics
 and Child Health
 University of Cape Town
 Cape Town

J. Lawrenson
 Paediatric Cardiology Service
 of Western Cape
 Department of Paediatrics
 and Child Health
 Stellenbosch University
 Stellenbosch

L. L. Linley
 Division of Neonatal
 Medicine
 Department of Paediatrics
 and Child Health
 University of Cape Town
 Cape Town

M. McCulloch
 Department of Paediatric
 Nephrology
 Evelina Children's Hospital
 Guy's and St. Thomas'
 Foundation Trust
 London U.K.

A. Millar
 Division of Paediatric Surgery
 Department of Surgery
 University of Cape Town
 Cape Town

C. Motala (deceased)
 Division of Allergy Department
 of Paediatrics and Child Health
 University of Cape Town
 Cape Town

E. Nel
 Division of Paediatric
 Gastroenterology
 Department of Paediatrics
 Stellenbosch University
 Stellenbosch

P. Nourse
 Division of Paediatric
 Nephrology
 Department of Paediatrics and
 Child Health
 University of Cape Town
 Cape Town

J. Nuttall
 Division of Infectious Disease
 and Immunology
 Department of Paediatrics and
 Child Health
 University of Cape Town
 Cape Town

C. H. Pieper
 Division of Neonatal Medicine
 Department of Paediatrics and
 Child Health
 University of Cape Town
 Cape Town

H. Pribut
 Paediatric Cardiology Service of
 Western Cape
 Department of Paediatrics and
 Child Health
 University of Cape Town
 Cape Town

V. Ramanjam
  Division of Child Development and Neurosciences
  Department of Paediatrics and Child Health
  University of Cape Town and 2 Military Hospital
  Cape Town

L. G. Reynolds
  Division of Ambulatory and Emergency Paediatrics
  Department of Paediatrics and Child Health
  University of Cape Town
  Cape Town

G. Riordan
  Division of Child Development and Neurosciences
  Department of Paediatrics and Child Health
  University of Cape Town
  Cape Town

H. Rode
  Division of Paediatric Surgery
  Department of Surgery
  University of Cape Town
  Cape Town

P. Roux
  Department of Paediatrics and Child Health
  University of Cape Town
  Cape Town

A. Spitaels
  Division of Paediatric Endocrinology
  Department of Paediatrics and Child Health
  University of Cape Town
  Cape Town

J. Thomas
  Division of Paediatric Anaesthesia
  Department of Anaesthesiology
  University of Cape Town
  Cape Town

G. Todd
  Department of Dermatology
  University of Cape Town
  Cape Town

A. B. (Sebastian) Van As
  Trauma Unit of Paediatric Surgery
  University of Cape Town
  Cape Town

J. Wilmshurst
  Division of Child Development and Neurosciences
  Department of Paediatrics and Child Health
  University of Cape Town
  Cape Town

H. J. Zar
  Head of Department of Paediatrics and Child Health
  Division of Paediatric Pulmonology
  University of Cape Town
  Cape Town

L. Zühlke
  Paediatric Cardiology Service of Western Cape
  Department of Paediatrics and Child Health
  University of Cape Town
  Cape Town

List of Reviewers

A. Argent
  Division of Critical Care &
  Children's Heart Disease
  Department of Paediatrics
  and Child Health
  Faculty of Health Sciences
  University of Cape Town
  Cape Town

D. Ballot
  Division of Neonatology
  Department of Paediatrics &
  Child Health
  Faculty of Health Sciences
  University of Witwatersrand
  Johannesburg

G. Boon,
  Department of Paediatrics
  East London Hospital
  Complex
  East London

A. Cilliers
  Division of Paediatric
  Cardiology
  Department of Paediatrics &
  Child Health
  Faculty of Health Sciences
  University of Witwatersrand
  Johannesburg

M. Cotton
  Paediatric Infectious Diseases
  Unit
  Department of Paediatrics &
  Child Health
  Faculty of Health Sciences
  Stellenbosch University
  Tygerberg

M. Esser
  Division of Medical
  Microbiology
  NHLS & Faculty of Health
  Sciences
  Stellenbosch University
  Tygerberg

G. Faller
  Division of Rheumatology
  Department of Paediatrics &
  Child Health
  Faculty of Health Sciences
  University of Witwatersrand
  Johannesburg

R. Green,
  Chair of Department of
  Paediatrics and Child Health
  Division of Paediatric
  Pulmonology
  Faculty of Health Sciences
  University of Pretoria.
  Pretoria

V.C. Harrison
  Emeritus Professor
  Division of Neonatal
  Medicine
  Department of Paediatrics &
  Child Health
  Faculty of Health Sciences
  University of Cape Town
  Cape Town

M. Hatherill,
  Institute of Infectious
  Diseases and Molecular
  Medicine
  Faculty of Health Sciences
  University of Cape Town
  Cape Town

L. Jacklin
Division of Child Psychiatry
Department of Psychiatry and Mental Health
Faculty of Health Sciences
University of Witwatersrand
Johannesburg

N. Kalis
Consultant Cardiologist & Lecturer/Tutor
Mohamed Al-Khalifa Cardiac Centre and AGU Medical University
Kingdom of Bahrain

U. Kalla
Division of Paediatric Nephrology
Department of Paediatrics & Child Health
Faculty of Health Sciences
University of Witwatersrand
Johannesburg

C. Lazarus
Department of Paediatric Surgery
East London Hospital Complex
East London

S. Madhi
Professor of Vaccinology
University of Witwatersrand
Johannesburg

I. Mayet
Division of Ophthalmology
Department of Surgery
Faculty of Health Sciences
University of Witwatersrand
Johannesburg

M. Meiring
Paediatric Palliative Care Consultant
Hospice & Palliative Care Association of South Africa
and University of Cape Town
Cape Town

D. Modi
Department of Dermatology
Faculty of Health Sciences
University of Witwatersrand
Johannesburg

S. Moore
Head: Paediatric Surgery
Division of Paediatric Surgery
Faculty of Health Sciences
Stellenbosch University
Tygerberg

A.D.N. Murray
Emeritus Professor
Division of Ophthalmology
Department of Surgery
Faculty of Health Sciences
University of Cape Town
Cape Town

P. Nourse
Division of Paediatric Nephrology
Department of Paediatrics and Child Health
Faculty of Health Sciences
University of Cape Town
Cape Town

J. Poole
Haematologist
Department of Paediatrics & Child Health
Faculty of Health Sciences
University of Witwatersrand
Johannesburg

C. Prescott
  Division of Otorhinolaryngology
  Department of Surgery
  Faculty of Health Sciences
  University of Cape Town
  Cape Town

J. Rodda
  Paediatric Neurologist
  Department of Paediatrics &
  Child Health
  Faculty of Health Sciences
  University of Witwatersrand
  Johannesburg

S. Schaaf
  Department of Paediatrics &
  Child Health
  Faculty of Health Sciences
  Stellenbosch University
  Tygerberg

R.Y. Seedat
  Department of
  Otorhinolarongoly
  Faculty of Health Sciences
  University of Free State
  Bloemfontein

W. Sinclair
  Department of Dermatology
  Faculty of Health Sciences
  University of Free State
  Bloemfontein

P. Thomson
  Paediatric Nephrologist
  Donald Gordon Medical Centre
  Johannesburg

R. Van Toorn
  Paediatric Neurologist
  Department of Paediatrics &
  Child Health
  Faculty of Health Sciences
  Stellenbosch University
  Tygerberg

A. Venter
  Paediatric Neurologist
  Department of Paediatrics &
  Child Health
  Faculty of Health Sciences
  University of Free State
  Bloemfontein

L. Wallis
  Head: Emergency Medicine
  Faculty of Health Sciences
  Stellenbosch University and
  University of Cape Town
  Cape Town

E.G. Weinberg
  Emeritus Professor
  Division of Allergology
  Department of Paediatrics &
  Child Health
  Faculty of Health Sciences
  University of Cape Town
  Cape Town

D.F. Wittenberg
  Emeritus Professor
  Department of Paediatrics &
  Child Health
  Faculty of Health Sciences
  University of Pretoria
  Pretoria

M. Zuckerman
  Paediatric Gastroenterologist
  Department of Child Health
  The Royal Victoria Infirmary
  & University of Newcastle
  upon Tyne
  Newcastle upon Tyne
  United Kingdom

Specialist proofreaders

D.W. Beatty
 Emeritus Professor
 Department of Paediatrics
 and Child Health
 University of Cape Town
 Cape Town

M.A. Kibel
 Emeritus Professor of
 Child Health
 School of Child and
 Adolescent Health
 University of Cape Town
 Cape Town

An evidence-based Handbook?

We have taken some simple steps to make the new edition of the Handbook as evidence based as possible. We have done this by being as explicit as possible about the basis for our recommendations. The internationally recognized GRADE system rates 2 components of recommendation:

A The *quality of the evidence* (how believable it is) rated using 1 to 4 ☆ symbols:
   - *High quality*– further research *is very unlikely to change what we know* about whether something works, or how much it works
   - *Moderate quality* – further research *may change what we know* about whether something works, or how much it works
   - *Low quality* – further research *is likely to change what we know* about whether something works, or how much it works
   - *Very low quality* – *we don't really know*
B The overall strength of the recommendation (how good an idea it is) rated using ☝ or ☟ or ☺ symbols.
   This takes into account the quality of the evidence (above), trade-offs between benefits and harms, the target population, the values and preferences of the target population (not of the doctors), and the availability of resources.
   - *Strong* – the desirable effects of an intervention clearly outweigh the undesirable effects ☝: A 'good' intervention – or clearly do not ☟: A 'bad' intervention.
   - *Weak/conditional/discretionary* – the trade-offs are less certain— either because of low quality evidence or the desirable and undesirable effects appear closely balanced ☺

These examples show how the symbols are used:

☝ ☆☆☆	Moderate quality evidence of an important beneficial effect
☟ ☆☆☆☆	High quality evidence of a clear harmful effect
☺ ☆	Very low quality evidence
☺	Grading of this recommendation not attempted

Where Red Cross War Memorial Children's Hospital follows a practice not widely followed elsewhere we have used the following symbol: ✢

Preface

The primary aim of *The Handbook of Paediatrics* is to provide undergraduate students and health professionals with practical guidelines for the diagnosis, management and prevention of common childhood conditions. There are, of course, many textbooks in this field, mainly from developed countries. This book, however, has a distinctly African flavour, particularly with regard to common diseases and their management in resource-limited settings. It is intended to serve as a quick reference and to complement standard clinical textbooks.

The new edition of this book benefits from a new infusion of contributors and ideas. Chapters have been revised and several have been restructured. Broad practical guidelines are included, as well as more in-depth information about selected topics such as nutrition, immunization, tuberculosis, HIV/AIDS, palliative care and pain management. Recommendations are evidence-based or consistent with best practice standards. A list of useful recommended resources appears at the end of most chapters and on the companion web site.

Producing a book of this nature has been an enormous task. I have been very fortunate to have worked with a team of talented and highly enthusiastic section editors, Alan Davidson, Michael Levin and Anthony Figaji. I owe a special debt of thanks to members of our own department (both past and present) for their excellent contributions and to the many reviewers for painstakingly going through all of the chapters in detail. Their critical comments and constructive suggestions are much appreciated. In particular, I wish to acknowledge Professor George Swingler's contribution to implementing an evidence-based approach in this edition of *The Handbook of Paediatrics*. I am also most grateful to Professor Heather Zar for dignifying this book with a Foreword. She has been fully supportive.

Oxford University Press have given constant help and reassurance throughout these proceedings and for this I would like to thank Ms Marisa Montemarano and Ms Lisa Andrews (project co-ordinators). The editorial aspects of the work have been truly monumental and no praise can be high enough for the untiring efforts of the section editors, for their management and attention to detail. I am also appreciative of Bridget Farham's editorial skills, her sound advice and invaluable assistance at the many stages of the editorial process. Above all, I am indebted to my administrative assistant, Ms Deborah Paulse for tecÿical support and her ever willingness to help.

Content Editor:
C. Motala

Foreword

It is a great pleasure to contribute this foreword to *The Handbook of Paediatrics* 7th Edition. The *Handbook* has become a flagship publication from the Department of Paediatrics and Child Health and the School of Child and Adolescent Health at the University of Cape Town, South Africa. The first edition was produced in 1975. Oxford University Press has published the Handbook since the 3rd edition in 1992. The emergence of new diseases, such as paediatric HIV and increasing and new knowledge have necessitated this new, revised edition. This recent edition represents an updated, evidenced based, practical manual on the management and prevention of common childhood illnesses. The *Handbook* also represents the collective expertise of our highly skilled staff in paediatrics and paediatric sub-specialties.

Production of the new edition of the *Handbook* has been led by Professor Cassim Motala, as the Content Editor, together with the section editors Dr Alan Davidson, Dr Michael Levin and Prof Anthony Figaji. They have done an outstanding job in producing a very handy, practical book for use by health professionals working in South Africa and the rest of Africa. In addition to the editors, I wish to thank all the members of the department who have provided contributions to this edition. This publication is a tribute to the expertise and commitment of our exceptional staff who strive to provide the highest standards of clinical care for children.

The *Handbook* is intended for use by health care professionals working in facilities of all levels of care, medical practitioners, paediatricians and undergraduate students. I hope that you will find this *Handbook* of value in managing sick children and in preventing childhood illness and that it will ultimately benefit children in your care, so promoting child health.

Heather Zar
Professor and Head of the Department of Paediatrics and Child Health
University of Cape Town
April 2010

Dedication

The recent passing of Prof Cas Motala has been a great loss for so many people and especially for paediatrics and for paediatric allergology. Cas was a pillar of Red Cross Children's Hospital, an outstanding doctor, a driver of paediatric allergy in South Africa, nationally and internationally recognised for his contributions. He spent more than 30 years working at Red Cross Children's Hospital, contributing immensely to the development of the institution, to the training and mentorship of countless doctors and nurses and to the academic growth especially of paediatric allergology. He was a major leader of the Department of Paediatrics and Child Health at the University of Cape Town – Director of clinical services, Head of Paediatric Allergology, content editor of the Department's recently published *Handbook of Paediatrics* 7e, leading many initiatives for upgrading the hospital and its facilities and representing the department in many structures and committees. In recognition of his outstanding contribution he was recently promoted to full Professor at the University of Cape Town. His wisdom and guidance, his gentle way of resolving conflict and his insights made him an invaluable member of the Department. Cas's deep sense of humanity touched so many people's lives – he will be remembered for his compassion, his generosity, the wonderful care and respect that he showed everyone.

1 Emergencies and trauma

A. Argent, R. Diedericks, A.B. Van As

The critically ill child

Introduction

Definition: the child with a life-threatening illness or injury. Management priorities are to:
- Recognize the severity of the illness or injury.
- Identify immediately life-threatening issues.
- Provide an immediate therapeutic response.
- Identify underlying problems and consider the aetiology.
- Move on to definitive therapy.

After immediate resuscitation, aim to maintain 'adequate physiology' and support the patient during the ongoing illness and recovery period, always maintaining (A)irway, (B)reathing, (C)irculation and so on.

What kills children?

Commonly: poorer communities – infections and trauma; in wealthier communities – congenital disorders and abnormalities.

The pathways to death include the following (either alone or in combination):
- Airway obstruction
- Hypoxaemia, usually related to
  - Respiratory disease
  - Cardiac disease
  - Trauma
  - Neurological/neuromuscular disease with inadequate respiratory effort (uncommon).
- Shock. Probably < 15% of cardiac arrest episodes in children are related to cardiac arrhythmias.
- Neurological:
  - Trauma (head and spinal cord)
  - Infections (particularly meningitis and meningo-encephalitis)
  - Intoxications
  - Weakness including Guillain-Barrè syndrome and severe hypokalaemia.

The prognosis for children who suffer cardiac arrest episodes is poor, while most who suffer a respiratory arrest will recover normally if adequately treated.

The approach to the critically ill child

It is impossible to resuscitate adequately as an individual – a coordinated team is essential.

The context

Organization:
- Requires an environment specifically geared for the needs of children. The following improves mortality:
  - Acutely ill or injured children are seen in an appropriate dedicated emergency area
  - Experienced staff with triage and resuscitation training
  - Paediatric resuscitation equipment.
- Encourage parents or caregivers to remain with their children, where possible.
- Requires infection control to avoid nosocomial infection in emergency departments.

Triage systems

These are useful and effective. They are required to:
- Identify children at risk of dying.
- Streamline the care of sick children.
- Provide a tool to measure and assess the adequacy of the system to provide care.

Early warning systems

Many institutions have instituted early warning systems (see below), whereby resuscitation teams MUST be called. This may significantly reduce 'unexpected' collapse episodes with improvements in outcomes.

Table 1.1 Early warning criteria for hospital wards

Hospital emergency team to be contacted if any ONE or more of:		
1 Staff member or parent worried about clinical state		
2 Airway threat		
3 Hypoxaemia:		SpO_2
		< 90% in any amount of oxygen
		< 60% in any amount of oxygen (cyanotic heart disease)
4 Severe respiratory distress, apnoea or cyanosis		

5 Tachypnoea		
	Age	**Respiratory rate/min**
	Term–3 months	> 60
	4–12 months	> 50
	1–4 years	> 40
	5–12 years	> 30
	12 years +	> 30

6 Bradycardia or tachycardia:			
	Age	**Bradycardia (beats/min)**	**Tachycardia (beats/min)**
	Term–3 months	< 100	> 180
	4–12 months	< 100	> 180
	1–4 years	< 90	> 160
	5–12 years	< 80	> 140
	12 years +	< 60	> 130

7 Hypotension:		
	Age	**BP (systolic mmHg)**
	12 years+	< 90
	5–12 years	< 80
	1–4 years	< 70
	4–12 months	< 60
	Term–3 months	< 50

8 Acute change in neurological status or convulsion
9 Cardiac or respiratory arrest

- Report if a child fulfils any of these criteria or has worsening trends in vital signs.
- Notify the treating medical team and the Medical Emergency Team service

—*Modified from Tibballs, J. et al Ped Crit Care Med 2009;10:306–312*

Equipment

This need not be extensive. Relatively few specialized diagnostic equipment items are required.

Table 1.2 Monitoring equipment for resuscitation areas

Airway	End-tidal CO_2 monitor*	Valuable to confirm endotracheal intubation (not in cardiac arrest) and for monitoring adequacy of ventilation
	Radiology services	For confirming ETT position, diagnostic views of the chest, trauma

Breathing	Saturation monitors*	Wide range available
	Blood gas analyzer	To get rapid results of blood gas analysis
Circulation	Cardiac monitor*	Essential monitoring
	Automated blood pressure measurement*	May be very useful, but may not be accurate or reliable in the setting of severe shock
	Invasive pressure monitoring facility	Not required generally, useful in more complex and critically ill
Disability	Brain activity monitoring	Possible convulsions and subclinical status epilepticus
	Glucometer	

*This is best mounted around the resuscitation area, and for patient transport.

Resuscitation equipment: to ensure an airway; provide oxygen or ventilatory support; achieve vascular access and treat shock, following which more sophisticated equipment may be required to deal with more complex problems.

Table 1.3 Resuscitation equipment

Note: ranges of sizes are required for most of these

Airway	Guedel airways	To maintain and support airway in unresponsive patients.
	McGill's forceps	
	Laryngoscopes	Also requires spare batteries and bulbs (or spare handles), and range of shapes
	Endotracheal tubes	
	Suctioning equipment	Must have Yankauer suckers, appropriate tubing and effective suction sources available
	Equipment for surgical airway	
	Hard collar for neck and cervical spine	Different sizes available and required
	Spinal boards and head locks	Must be compatible with neck immobilization system and preferably interchangeable with emergency medical system equipment

Breathing	Tubing and connections	Ensure that the appropriate connections and adequate length tubing are available to connect gas systems to the patient safely
	Facemasks	To give oxygen safely and at a range of concentrations. Non-rebreathing masks for shocked and hypoxic patients
	Head boxes	Must accommodate infants of < 6–12 months comfortably (NB: adequate gas flow is ALWAYS required)
	Nasal cannulae	
	Equipment for bag-mask ventilation	Self-inflating ventilatory bag; masks; connections for gas flow. Ventilators for ongoing ventilatory support
Circulation	Intravenous cannulae	
	Intra-osseous needles	Specific sets, or any needle with trochar and adequate rigidity
	Drip tubing and administration sets	Microdroppers are useful for limiting the amount of fluid, but not for rapid resuscitation
	Buretrols	Potentially very dangerous to connect large volumes of fluid (500 ml or 1 l) directly to small children
	Three-way taps and syringes	Facilitates rapid administration of fluids and medication
	Resuscitation fluid	Alternatives included: Ringer's lactate, 0.9% saline, Plasmalyte B. 10% glucose should be available.
	Refrigerator with O –ve blood	Essential, especially where trauma or major bleeding may be seen regularly
Neurological	Opthalmoscope	Very useful for assessment of pupillary size as well as fundoscopy

Highlighted items relate to areas that will be used in paediatric trauma

When paediatric resuscitation or critical care is not a regular occurrence, it may be helpful to have all basic paediatric resuscitation equipment stored in sealed boxes, which can then be opened at the time of need. This helps to ensure that all the correct equipment is in the right place at the right time.

Documentation and information

Document:
- On systematically structured forms
- All clinical features, particularly at time of presentation
- Changes in vital signs
- Procedures and therapeutic interventions.

Information required for staff who are prescribing therapy must be readily available, including:
- Systems for estimating patient weight
- Emergency drug dosages
- Information for endotracheal tube size; gastric tube size; urinary catheter size etc.

Clinical priorities

A structured approach to clinical assessment and management is provided by:
- **A**(irway and cervical spine management)
- **B**(reathing)
- **C**(irculation and control of ongoing bleeding)
- **D**(isability).

This algorithm can also be extended to include
- **D**(on't) **E**(ver) **F**(orget) the **G**(lucose) or **H**(ypotension).

Always beware of causing harm in children by excessive intervention.

There is, however, increasing evidence that the following interventions may be associated with significantly improved patient outcome:
- Early administration of appropriate antibiotics. ☆☆☆◍
- Goal-directed treatment of shock, using goals such as mixed venous saturation, lactate levels etc. ☆☆☆◍

Airway (and cervical spine)

If the child has suddenly collapsed:
- Assess whether there is an adequate airway, or whether there is some obstruction to breathing.

A full description of medical conditions affecting the airway is available in Chapter 3, Respiratory problems. In trauma, see p. 21.

Assessment

If unconscious and unable to defend the airway adequately, secure the airway to ensure that aspiration does not occur.

Clinical signs of airway obstruction include:
- Absence of air movement (assessed by: 'look – for chest movement, listen – for breath sounds either at the mouth and nose or in the chest, and feel – for air movement at the mouth and nose')
- Abnormal sounds, particularly in association with recession of parts of the chest wall and use of accessory muscles of ventilation:
  — Stridor (see Chapter 3, Respiratory problems)
  — Stertor
  — Wheeze.

> ***Practice point:***
>
> There is a tendency for noises in the airway to become quieter as patients get worse.

Consider cervical spine injury and assume unstable neck in:
- Trauma (including drowning)
- Pain on movement or palpation of the cervical spine
- Local crepitus or distortion on palpation of neck
- Limitation of movement (only appropriate in conscious patient)
- Unconscious patient with any suggestion of trauma.

Treatment

- If obstruction to the airway is above the level of the larynx, use an appropriately sized Guedel airway or possibly nasopharyngeal airway. If this is inadequate, or difficult to maintain, then use a laryngeal mask. This may be difficult to use in small infants, and training is required.
- If obstruction to the airway is at the laryngeal level or below, endotracheal intubation may be required to maintain a patent airway, and if that is not possible then surgical interventions such as cricothyroidotomy or tracheostomy are possible. Securing a surgical airway in small infants may be very difficult, particularly in environments with limited resources. However, these manoeuvres may also be life saving.
- Unless patients are unresponsive, anaesthesia must be provided for endotracheal intubation. Where at all possible the most senior clinician available should be present throughout the procedure. If airway obstruction at the pharynx or below is the indication for intubation resources for management of the difficult airway MUST be instantly available.

Table 1.4 Indications for endotracheal intubation

Inadequate airway	*A high risk indication for intubation. Needs experience. If there are problems with the airway, this is also the ideal opportunity to clearly visualize the airway and establish the exact problem*
Inadequate oxygenation and/or ventilation	*Intubation of a hypoxaemic patient is a very high risk procedure – needs experience*
Airway protection	When the patient has lost the capacity to maintain patency of their own airway. Concerns: maintain spinal stability; prevent intracranial hypertension

Table 1.5 Anaesthesia for endotracheal intubation

Drug	Comment
Ketamine	Anaesthesia, analgesia and amnesia. Has some myocardial depressant action, but maintains vascular tone and blood pressure does not usually drop unless there is a failing heart. Does not depress respiratory drive, but may be associated with increased respiratory secretions. May be associated with increased intracranial pressure
Etomidate	Very stable cardiovascularly. Does not increase intracranial pressure. Burns on injection. Has adrenal suppressive activity
Diazepam	Provides sedation, but does not blunt the responses to endotracheal intubation. May be associated with drop in blood pressure
Midazolam	Provides sedation, but does not blunt the responses to endotracheal intubation. May have unpredictable effects. Blood pressure drops in shocked patients
Propofol	Provides excellent conditions for intubation. Blood pressure tends to drop. Burns on injection
Thiopentone	Blood pressure may drop
Paralysis	Muscle paralysis does make intubation easier, however it should only be given if the operator is confident that they can either intubate the patient successfully or at least maintain ventilation until an airway can be secured

If there is any reason to suspect cervical spine injury:
- In-line stabilization of the neck must continue at all times:
  - If the patient is restless and agitated, this may best be done by a person holding the head in a neutral position with both hands and reassuring the child as much as possible.
  - If the patient will tolerate application of an appropriately sized hard collar this will free up assistants for other duties in resuscitation.
  - After application of the collar, the head must be held in place with head-blocks or sand-bags, using a securing system.
- Normal X-rays do not exclude cervical spine injury.

Breathing

Oxygen should be provided to any child who is either shocked or has evidence of hypoxaemia. *Clinical assessment of hypoxaemia is poor and pulse oximetry is an essential tool.* ☆☆☆☆☘

Assessment

Consider the:
- Effort of breathing (respiratory rate, use of accessory muscles, chest wall recession) – be aware that the effort of breathing may be very difficult to assess in patients with:
  - Exhaustion
  - Poor respiratory drive, and
  - Weakness.
- Effectiveness of efforts:
  - Chest wall movement relative to apparent effort
  - Breath sounds
  - Oxygen saturation
  - Blood gas analysis.

It is particularly important to monitor and document trends (particularly respiratory rate and oxygen saturation – both with and without oxygen therapy).

Therapy

In general, patients with any reason for poor tissue delivery of oxygen should be given supplementary oxygen.

There is some debate about the indications for oxygen therapy. However if the saturation in room air is < 88% (or < 85% at high altitude) oxygen therapy should be provided if at all possible. Different delivery methods for oxygen therapy are shown in Table 1.6.

Table 1.6 Oxygen therapy

Technique	Oxygen flow required	Comment
1 Nasal catheter	2–3 l/min	The concentration of inspired oxygen that can be achieved is variable (as high as 70% in very small infants, less than 30% in adolescents)
2 Nasal cannula	1–2 l/min	Concerns are: possible inflation of the stomach, blocking of the catheter in the nose related to dry secretions
3 Face mask oxygen	5–6 l/pm (need bottled gas or central supply system)	Variety available, with non-rebreathing masks high concentrations can be achieved. Often not well tolerated by infants and small children
4 Head box oxygen	> 8 l/min (need bottled gas or central supply system)	In infants this technique can achieve high concentrations of inspired oxygen. Either Venturi systems or oxygen blenders are required to vary the oxygen concentration that is delivered. Monitor oxygen concentration in the head box. Ensure adequate gas flow into the system to avoid CO_2 accumulation
5 Bag mask ventilation using a self-inflating bag (with reservoir bag)	10–15 l/min (need bottled gas or central supply system)	High concentrations of oxygen can be achieved if there is a reservoir bag in the system. Positive end expiratory pressure can also be provided depending on the details of the system. Ventilation can be continued even if the gas supply fails
6 T-piece ventilation	10–15 l/m (need bottled gas or central supply system)	Requires training and experience, but can be particularly effective in patients requiring positive end expiratory pressure. Utterly dependant on a constant flow of gas

Technique	Oxygen flow required	Comment
7 Positive pressure ventilation – non-invasive	Wall oxygen and air required to drive some ventilators, other ventilators have compressor to provide air and require oxygen from a gas source	Variety of systems available, providing: face masks, nasal masks, head masks connected to ventilators that are able to provide ventilatory support without the need for endotracheal intubation. There is limited data available on these systems and their particular optimal uses are still being elucidated
8 Positive pressure ventilation – invasive	Wall gas sources	Wide range of ventilators available with varying degrees of sophistication
9 Advanced ventilatory strategies	Wall gas sources	

Note: options 1–2 can be provided from an oxygen concentrator, 3–6 need bottled gas or central supply, and 7–9 need wall oxygen

Monitoring

- *Monitor saturation.* Continuous saturation monitoring is mandatory in any child who requires either high concentrations of inspired oxygen or ventilatory support.
- *Blood gas analysis* is required to provide at least some baseline assessment of ventilation and oxygenation. For severe burns, co-oximetry also allows the diagnosis of carbon monoxide poisoning and methaemoglobinaemia.
- *End-tidal pCO_2 monitoring* is extremely useful for: endotracheal intubation, transportation (particularly by vehicle), special clinical conditions (e.g. severe weakness, intracranial hypertension).

What are acceptable saturations? These depend on the clinical condition. If cardiac output is poor or haemoglobin is low, it may be essential to maintain saturations in the high 90 percents. However, if there is good cardiac output and a relatively high haemoglobin, then adequate oxygen delivery can be achieved with saturations as low as 70%.

- The risks of inadequate oxygen delivery to tissues have to be balanced against the risks associated with the techniques that are used to achieve higher blood oxygen content.

— High inspired oxygen concentrations and high ventilator pressures can damage the lung. Therefore, benefits must be balanced against risks.
- In general tissues are receiving adequate oxygen delivery when: the organs such as the gut, kidneys or brain are functioning normally and when lactate levels are not rising in the blood.
- In the context of pulmonary or intracranial hypertension, it is safer to aim at high saturations.

What is an acceptable pCO_2? Normalize if possible. However in difficult situations the ventilator support required to do this may damage the lung. Thus, in general pCO_2 in the ventilated patient can be allowed to rise as long as the pH is ≥ 7.25 and as long as:
- There is a complete understanding of the reason for the high pCO_2.
- There is not a specific contra-indication such as intracranial hypertension or pulmonary hypertension.
- The patient is not having to make excessive respiratory effort to maintain that pCO_2 level.

Ventilation

Indicated for:
- Inadequate respiratory effort
- Hypoxaemia unresponsive to simple oxygen administration
- Respiratory distress manifest in high effort with high respiratory rates, recession of parts of the chest wall, flaring, etc that is deteriorating despite appropriate therapy
- Hypercapnoea despite appropriate respiratory effort
- Depressed level of consciousness
- Need for transport when their condition may deteriorate *en route* and where intervention *en route* may be difficult.

Ventilatory support can be provided using: non-invasive positive pressure support via a mask, invasive positive pressure support, negative pressure ventilatory devices, or a combination of such techniques.

The major challenges of ventilation are to:
- Avoid patient injury (local and distal)
- Maintain airway patency
- Optimize patient comfort
- Avoid harmful cardiopulmonary interactions
- Continue appropriate nutrition
- Prevent nosocomial infection.

Nasal CPAP has been widely utilized in neonatal and now increasingly in infant ventilatory support. Particular problems include:
- Selection of appropriately-sized nasal prongs maintaining pressure in the system without causing damage to the nose or nasal structures
- Humidification of gases
- Appropriate monitoring.

If ongoing ventilatory support is required, the child must be transferred to an appropriate paediatric ICU.

Circulation (and control of haemorrhage)

Shock is an important cause of death, and requires rapid and effective management.

Table 1.7 Types and causes of shock

Type	Group	Causes	Therapy required
Hypo-volaemia	Hypovolaemic	Haemorrhage, fluid losses	Fluids
Cardiogenic	Cardiogenic	Poor cardiac function related to anatomy (congenital cardiac lesions), function (cardiomyopathy, myocarditis)	Inotropic support and correct underlying anatomical defects if present
Septic	Combination	Infections	Treat infection, fluid administration, possibly inotropes
Anaphylactic	Combination	Vasodilatation, fluid leak, cardiac dysfunction	Adrenaline, fluids, subsequently steroids and possibly antihistamines
Neurogenic (e.g. spinal shock)	Hypovolaemia	Following spinal cord transection	Fluids, possibly chronotropes if bradycardic
Obstructive		Tension pneumothorax	Drain pneumothorax
Dissociative		Carbon monoxide poisoning, cyanide poisoning	Will require high concentrations of inspired oxygen

Assessment

Cardiovascular signs of shock:
- Heart rate
- Pulse volume
- Capillary refill
- Temperature gradients
- BP.

Evidence of ongoing bleeding may be obvious or hidden. Turn over to check:
- Bleeding must be controlled.
- If shock persists despite apparently adequate fluid resuscitation in the context of trauma, consider ongoing bleeding, especially abdominal, thoracic and fracture sites

Note: Ongoing bleeding must be controlled and may need surgery.

Table 1.8 Clinical signs of shock

Clinical sign	Objectivity and reproducibility	Confounding factors	Comment
Heart rate			
Tachycardia	+++	Pain, anxiety, pyrexia, anaemia	Extreme tachycardia (> 200/min) – consider cardiac arrhythmia
Bradycardia	+++	Unusual except in pre-terminal situation	Occasionally, occurs with congenital heart block. In general the smaller the child the worse bradycardia is tolerated
Pulse volume	+		Issues of where pulse can be felt (peripheral, central)
Blood pressure	+++		BP only falls very late in shock
Capillary refill	+–	Environmental temperature	Capillary refill may be difficult to assess, correlates poorly with shock
Temperature gradients	+–	Environmental temperature	

Clinical sign	Objectivity and reproducibility	Confounding factors	Comment
Mixed venous saturation	+++	Respiratory function	Trend is more important than absolute number. May be difficult to measure true mixed venous saturation in paediatric patients
Lactate levels	+++	Liver function	Hyperlactataemia is a feature of shock. Rising levels of lactate is a particularly worrying feature

Features of organ dysfunction:
- Depressed level of consciousness
- Poor urine output
- Ileus or poor gut function.

Specific tests:
- Mixed (or central) venous saturation
- Lactic acid levels.

Monitoring

Cardiac monitors are required in any patient who has cardiac arrhythmias. Start non-invasive blood pressure monitoring as soon as possible. Saturation monitoring is useful, but it may be difficult to obtain an accurate reading. Do not reduce oxygen therapy just because oxygen saturation is high.

Invasive arterial pressure monitoring is controversial, but important if shock is not rapidly responsive, or if considering vasoactive drugs. Complications of intra-arterial lines include:
- Damage to the vessel, with threatened circulation
- Infection
- Thrombosis and embolization.

Balance *the relative risks and benefits*.

Central venous pressure monitoring is also controversial. Can provide:
- Secure vascular access
- Access for CVP and saturation monitoring
- Access for certain infusions.

Complications:
- On insertion (bleeding, damage to vessels, pneumothorax, etc)
- While in situ (venous thrombosis, sepsis) and
- On removal (bleeding, embolization).

Thus *there must be a clear indication for insertion*. Remove as soon as possible.

CVP is not particularly helpful in predicting whether or not a patient would improve with administration of a fluid bolus. However, central venous saturations are closely related to adequacy of cardiac output and oxygen delivery to tissues.

Acid base monitoring is an insensitive measure of the adequacy of tissue perfusion. Changes in lactate may be better.

Treatment

Shock requires immediate and effective treatment.

The priorities in the management of shock are to:
- Diagnose:
  - Establish baseline observations
- Ensure patent airway, provide oxygen
- Establish vascular access:
  - If unable to establish peripheral vascular access within 90 seconds, then use intra-osseous route
  - Use central vascular access if there is a specific indication (see below) and when an appropriately qualified person is present.
- Collect blood for testing (glucose, culture, cross-match, depending on the specific situation)
- Treat hypovolaemia
- Provide additional support as required
- If sepsis is considered give an appropriate broad spectrum antibiotic intravenously as soon as possible.

The purpose of circulatory support is to optimize cardiac output and tissue perfusion without placing undue demands on the circulatory system.

Volume administration

If hypovolaemic, rapidly administer intravenous fluid according to the following protocol:

1. Start with 20 ml/kg of fluid as a bolus intravenously (in trauma use 10 ml/kg boluses):

- Monitor response.
- Repeat as necessary. Once 40–60 ml/kg have been administered without resolution of inadequate circulation, consider:
  - Additional inotropic support
  - Blood products or colloids (gel, starch or albumen containing resuscitation fluids).
2. Selection of fluid:
   - If blood loss is the cause of hypovolaemia, then administer blood, especially if poorly responsive.
   - For all other causes of hypovolaemia, start with crystalloids. The electrolyte content of the crystalloid used should be close to that of plasma, e.g. 0.9% saline, Ringers lactate and plasmalyte B.

Vaso-active drugs

In general vaso-active drugs should not be administered without the capacity to monitor the effects of the drugs, and this requires an intensive care unit.

Table 1.9 Vaso-active drugs

Drug	Dose and mode of administration	Comment
Inotropic drugs		
Adrenaline	0.01–2 µg/kg/min as continuous infusion	Low doses – predominantly inotropic; higher doses – more vasoconstrictive
Dopamine	2–15 µg/kg/min as continuous infusion	As above for dose effect. Concerns about effects on immune system
Dobutamine	2–15 µg/kg/min as continuous infusion	Predominantly inotropic, perhaps some vasodilation. Often associated with tachycardia. May be better inotrope in young infants
Milrinone	0.25–1 µg/kg/min as continuous infusion	Much slower onset and offset of action. Can be given via peripheral line. Inotropic, lusitropic and vasodilator effects. May need combination with vasoconstrictor

Drug	Dose and mode of administration	Comment
Vasodilator drugs		
Sodium nitroprusside	0.3 – 4 µg/kg/min	Potent systemic vasodilator. Very rapid onset and offset of action. Toxic in higher doses and longer duration
Nitroglycerine	0.5 – 5 µg/kg/min	More effective pulmonary vasodilator, less effect as systemic vasodilator

Disability/neurological

Goals: prevent ongoing damage from seizure activity, limit secondary brain injury, ensure adequate delivery of oxygen to the brain without causing problems in other parts of the body.

Assessment

Rapid clinical assessment of level of consciousness can be performed using the AVPU score:
- Alert and responsive
- Voice – not fully alert, but responds to voice
- Pain – not fully alert, does not respond to voice, but does respond to painful stimulus
- Unresponsive.

Ongoing assessment of level of consciousness (LOC) should be carried out using the Glasgow Coma scale.

Be aware of the contribution of drugs to changes in level of consciousness.

Document seizure activity including:
- Duration
- Exact nature
- Treatment given.

Monitoring

- Always monitor cardiovascular parameters, respiratory rate, and LOC (see above).
- Ensure child is well oxygenated with adequate circulation.
- Always get a CT to diagnose aetiology and neurological/neurosurgical management input.

Management
- Maintain excellent oxygenation and brain perfusion.
- Optimal positioning:
  - The head is slightly elevated relative to the body
  - The neck is in a neutral position (ensures venous drainage, stabilizes potentially injured neck).
- Close observation for and control of any seizures (requires monitoring).

Drugs

Important issues:
- Sick children often have high water content following resuscitation and this may decrease drug levels achieved.
- Take care to limit the amount of fluid administered with drugs. Include volumes used for drug administration in calculations and estimates of fluid balance.
- Don't assume that tissue perfusion is normal; drugs should very rarely be administered intramuscularly.
- Renal function is often abnormal, thus drugs that are excreted renally may be excreted very slowly with subsequent toxic effects.
- Multiple drugs are often administered; take care to minimize drug interactions.
- In the presence of circulatory or respiratory problems it is often appropriate to carefully titrate drug administration to required effect, rather than to give standard therapeutic doses.

In the setting of possible infection, it is essential that antibiotics are given intravenously as soon as possible. Always:
- Give intravenously
- Give immediately
- Give broadly enough to cover setting; narrow later
- Give dosage for severe infection, likely to dilute with resuscitation
- Be very cautious of potentially nephrotoxic agents.

Fluid administration in the critically ill

Maintenance of fluid and electrolyte homeostasis in critically ill or injured children may be difficult because:
- Large volumes and leaky capillaries leads to tissue oedema
- Renal function is limited
- High levels of antidiuretic hormone are common

- Multiple medications often used
- Immobility predisposes to oedema.

Thus conventional 'maintenance fluid requirements' may actually be excessive. Monitor closely. See also Chapter 20, Fluids, electrolytes and acid-base.

The injured child

Background, classification and statistics

Injuries are a common cause of death in children globally and the injury rate in South Africa is more than double the global rate. Injuries are the leading cause of death in children between the age of 1 and 18 years. The 2 leading causes of child and adolescent injury deaths are road traffic accidents and drowning. Children in poor families are at higher risk of injuries. Many injuries occur in or around the home. Most injuries are preventable and safety education is crucial. The WHO has classified injuries according to the ICD 10.

Table 1.10 The WHO classification of injuries

UNINTENTIONAL INJURIES:
Road traffic accidents
Falls
Burns
Flame
Scalds
Drowning
Poisoning
Animal bites
INTENTIONAL INJURIES
Interpersonal violence
Homicide
Sexual violence
Self-harm (attempted suicide)
Self-mutilation
Legal interventions
War

A review by the World Health Organization indicates the following causes for child and adolescent death due to injuries (Table 1.11).

Table 1.11 Causes of child and adolescent death due to injuries

Road traffic accidents	26%
Drowning	20%
Burns	10%
Falls	5%
Poisons	5%
Violence	4%
Self-inflicted	2%
Others (choking, animal stings and bites, electrocution, fire-arm injuries and conflicts)	28%

Management of childhood injuries

Successful management of an injured child requires:
- An organized approach that combines diagnosis and treatment.
- A designated team leader.
- Frequent review and documentation of the patient's response to treatment.

The treatment of major injuries involves:
- Primary survey and resuscitation:
  - Restore and stabilize vital functions.
  - Identify and correct life-threatening abnormalities, e.g. tension pneumothorax.
- Secondary survey and definitive management:
  - Determine the full extent of all injuries.
  - Treat injuries in order of priority.

Primary survey and resuscitation

Airway and breathing

Impaired ventilation may be due to:
- Aspiration, e.g. vomitus or foreign body
- Brain or spinal cord injury
- Chest injury, e.g. tension pneumothorax, flail segment
- Distension of the stomach, causing elevation and splinting of the diaphragm.

> **Warning:**
>
> Before moving the head ensure that the neck has not been injured (remember SCIWORA (spinal cord injury w/o radiographic abnormality)).

Circulation

As soon as venous access is obtained, draw blood for:
- Crossmatching, full blood count, urea and electrolytes, serum amylase (pancreatic injury)
- Arterial blood gases.

Treatment
- Limit blood loss.
- Splint fractures.
- Elevate a bleeding limb.
- Apply pressure directly to a bleeding point with a clean dressing (do not use a tourniquet or compress a pressure point).

Circulatory shock following injury

Possible causes are:
- Concealed haemorrhage – usually abdominal, pelvic or from multiple fractures
- Blunt chest injury – cardiac contusion, tension pneumothorax
- Spinal cord injury – presents with a low blood pressure and warm peripheries
- Brainstem injury – usually a terminal event.

Note: A considerable amount of blood can be lost into the peritoneal cavity without causing significant abdominal distension.

Failure to respond to fluid resuscitation

Consider:
- Non-haemorrhagic chest injury (tension pneumothorax, cardiac contusion)
- Exsanguinating intra-abdominal haemorrhage requiring urgent laparotomy.

Aerophagia and acute gastric dilatation

This is common in head, abdominal, and multiple injuries and is caused by aerophagia (swallowing of air). It is aggravated by assisted ventilation and causes respiratory decompensation by elevating and splinting the diaphragm. Aspiration of gastric contents is a resultant hazard.

Management:
- Insert a nasogastric tube (p. 534) as soon as possible (Figure 1.1).
- Decompress the stomach.

Figure 1.1 Aerophagia and gastric dilatation

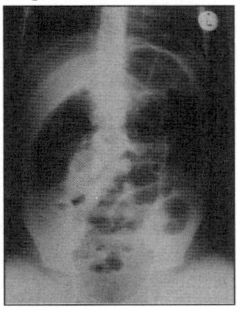

Secondary survey and management

Management involves:
- Remove all clothing.
- Avoid excessive heat loss.
- Monitor vital signs.
- Provide adequate analgesia (p. 515).
- **AMPLE** – Obtain a brief history from a guardian or ambulance staff concerning **a**llergies, **m**edication (past and present), **p**ast medical history, **l**ast meal (time of), and **e**vents surrounding the injury.

Head and neck injuries

Determine:
- Soft-tissue injuries to face and scalp
- Cerebrospinal fluid (CSF) leak or bleeding from nose or ears
- Level of consciousness
- Pupils – size and reaction to light
- Limbs – movement, sensation, and reflexes.

Urgent investigations
- Arterial blood gases if the level of consciousness (LOC) is decreased
- X-ray cervical spine if unconscious or if there is a limited range of movement. A normal X-ray does not exclude spinal cord injury
- Skull X-rays if fractures are suspected clinically.

Ominous features

Indications for a computerised tomography (CT) brain scan include (but are not limited to):
- Glasgow coma score of 12 or less
- Generalized or focal seizures
- Any focal neurological deficit
- Progressive irritability or restlessness
- Decreasing LOC or failure to improve over 24 hours
- Spinal shock manifested by low blood pressure, warm peripheries and absent anal sphincter tone
- Skull fracture
- Fractures of the occiput or skull base (50% of children with a skull fracture have intra-cranial pathology)
- Children under the age of 2 with large scalp haematoma (50% have intra-cranial pathology)
- Suspected child abuse (p. 29).

If neurological signs are localized and progressive, assume that there is a space-occupying mass, e.g. blood.

Treatment
- Ensure adequate ventilation and perfusion.
- Obtain a CT brain scan if any ominous features are noted.
- Abort seizures with lorazepam 0.1 mg/kg IV given rectally.
- Consider intubation if the Glasgow coma scale is less than 8. If not, keep on nasal prong oxygen
- Early craniotomy or craniectomy is indicated only for intracranial haematoma or compound depressed skull fractures.
- Spinal cord injury: decompress stomach and bladder. Institute assisted ventilation if the chest is involved. When turning the patient, ensure that the head and neck do not move relative to the trunk ('log-roll').

Injuries to the thorax

Extensive injuries of internal organs are possible without rib fractures.
Examine for:
- Visible rib-cage injuries, contusions, abrasions
- Difficulty with respiration – cyanosis, dyspnoea, tachypnoea
- Abnormal movement of chest wall
- Unilateral dullness or decreased air entry
- The position of mediastinum by palpating the trachea and the apex beat

- The presence and quality of the heart sounds. Dull or muffled sounds indicate myocardial contusion or pericardial tamponade.

Urgent investigations
- Arterial blood gases
- Antero-posterior chest X-ray to exclude collections and contusions and to determine the position and contour of the diaphragm
- ECG and cardiac iso-enzymes.

Ominous features
- Progressive dyspnoea and mediastinal shift from a tension pneumothorax or ruptured diaphragm
- Subcutaneous emphysema caused by rupture of bronchus, trachea or oesophagus
- Circulatory shock resistant to resuscitation due to cardiac injury or tamponade.

Treatment
- Adequate oxygenation and oxygen saturation monitoring
- Urgent drainage of large intrapleural collections
- Adequate analgesia for multiple rib fractures, e.g. IV morphine infusion. Ventilation for flail segment and respiratory failure
- Urgent surgical repair of a ruptured diaphragm
- Frequent chest physiotherapy for atelectasis.

Note: A child's trachea is short (approximately 5 cm) so ensure that during intubation the endotracheal tube is not inserted too far (Figure 1.2).

The child with a chest injury who needs assisted ventilation may require a prophylactic intercostal drain on the side of the injury.

Figure 1.2 Endotracheal tube in the right main bronchus with collapse of the left lung

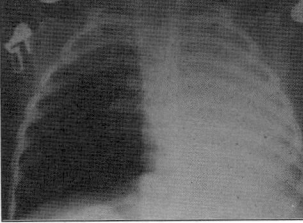

Abdomen

Distension: Nearly always due to aerophagia rather than intra-abdominal bleeding. The latter causes severe shock at an early stage. Remember to deflate the stomach!

Check the following:
- Haemodynamic status, e.g. shock, anaemia
- Abdominal wall bruising, abrasions, distension
- Focal or generalized guarding, tenderness
- Presence or absence of bowel sounds
- Microscopic or macroscopic haematuria
- Pelvic tenderness, induration or rectal bleeding.

Urgent investigations
- Full blood count, serum amylase (pancreatic injury).
- Chest X-ray, abdominal X-ray (erect or shoot-through)
- Intravenous pyelography (IVP) and urethrogram for a suspected urinary tract injury.

Ominous features
- Hypotension and abdominal distension: *haemorrhage from liver, spleen*
- Increasing tenderness and/or peritonism: *perforated viscus*
- Persistent macroscopic haematuria: *renal injury*
- Failure to pass urine despite adequate resuscitation: *injury to bladder, urethra*.

Indications for laparotomy
- Peritonitis or pneumo-peritoneum (ruptured hollow viscus)
- Hemodynamic instability in spite of resuscitation
- Massive or ongoing haemorrhage requiring more than 40 ml/kg blood transfusion within 24 hours.

Limb and bone injuries

Examine for:
- Pain, deformity, swelling
- Limitation of movement
- Signs of congenital bone disease, e.g. osteogenesis imperfecta (blue sclerae, wormian bones)
- Distal neurovascular status, i.e. perfusion (capillary refill and pulse, temperature), muscular movements and sensation
- Related soft-tissue wounds indicating compound fractures.

Urgent investigations

- X-ray of the affected limb in two planes. Always include joints above and below the fracture
- If in doubt, X-ray the healthy side too for comparison
- Full blood count and erythrocyte sedimentation rate (ESR) for suspected non-traumatic conditions such as osteitis and septic arthritis.

Ominous features

- Signs of ischaemia distal to the fracture
- Pain, swelling, pain on passive extension distal to the fracture (consider a compartment syndrome)
- Unstable pelvic fracture: exclude bladder, urethral, or rectal injury by cysto-urethrogram and sigmoidoscopy.

Treatment

- Early reduction and immobilisation of fractures
- Early debridement of soft-tissue wound with IV antibiotic cover, e.g. cefoxitin, in compound fractures
- On-table angiography for suspected vascular injury, reduction and immobilization of bony fracture followed by vascular repair
- Urgent fasciotomy of all affected muscular compartments in suspected compartment syndrome.

The child and family

- Communicate openly and frequently.
- Avoid ill-founded optimism or prognoses.
- Provide the best emotional support possible.

Management of minor injuries

Simple lacerations

- Clean and debride meticulously.
- Use tissue glue (Dermabond®, Histoacryl®) when possible.
- Before suturing, provide adequate local anaesthesia, e.g TAC (cocaine, adrenaline, lignocaine) can be dripped on the wound, less painful and frightening or lignocaine 1–2% is injected around the wound.
- Close in layers without tension.
- Use interrupted monofilament sutures for the skin.
- Give anti-tetanus prophylaxis: tetanus toxoid 0.5 ml IM.

Fingertip injuries

- Preserve maximum possible length.
- Follow same principles as for simple lacerations:
  - Avulsed fingertip: clean, dress with paraffin gauze, and allow to granulate
  - Exposed bone: cut back to allow soft-tissue coverage.

Tongue lacerations

Repair under general anaesthetic if there is profuse bleeding, if the full thickness of the tongue is involved or if the child is unable to suck, drink or eat. Use absorbable sutures and bury the knot.

Bites

- Clean and suture recent animal bites
- Neglected bites or those below the knee should be debrided and allowed to granulate
- Consider the possibility of rabies and vaccinate if appropriate (p. 265)
- Indications for antibiotics, e.g. penicillin, if clinical evidence of sepsis, animal bites in hands and feet, human bites and immuno-compromised patients
- Tetanus toxoid 0.5 ml IM.

Foreign bodies

- *Soft tissues:* remove wherever possible.
- *Inhaled:* remove with bronchoscope.
- *Ingested*: remove if lodged in the oesophagus, otherwise allow to pass per rectum. Intervene only if there are symptoms and signs of obstruction or perforation.
- *Alkaline disc batteries:* remove if in oesophagus. If in stomach or beyond, monitor progress by daily X-ray. Evacuation from stomach may be encouraged by oral magnesium sulphate and metoclopramide.

Figure 1.3 The most common ingested foreign body (a coin) lodged in the oesophagus at the typical place (between the aortic arch and the trachea)

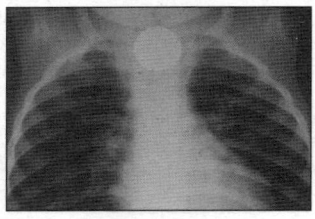

Corrosive oesophageal burns

The first essential is to identify those who have actually swallowed a corrosive that has burned the pharyngeal, oesophageal or gastric mucosa. The history is often unreliable but indicators of significant injury are reluctance to swallow and drooling of saliva. Adequate examination of the pharynx is difficult and requires endoscopy with either a rigid or a flexible scope. Children with significant symptoms must be referred urgently to an ENT or paediatric surgery unit.

Minimal burns: The child is able to swallow and does not drool saliva.
Significant burns: The child cannot swallow and drools saliva.

Management

- *Emergency treatment*: urgently contact a poison information centre (see page 43 for a list of numbers).
- *Minimal burns*: observe for 24 hours and then discharge if swallowing is unimpaired. Follow up at 2 weeks to check that swallowing is normal.
- *Severe burns*: refer urgently to a centre with facilities for endoscopy.

Further management

Severe burns:
- Pass a naso-gastric tube to maintain a patent oesophagus and to provide a channel for nutrition. Once saliva can be swallowed, encourage fluids by mouth but keep the naso-gastric tube in place and thereafter introduce solids. Give nystatin drops to prevent thrush.
- Reduce factors that exacerbate the formation of strictures as the oesophageal mucosa heals. This requires IV antibiotics, e.g. ampicillin and antacids, e.g. sucralfate via the naso-gastric tube.
- High-dose steroids may be of benefit but careful selection is needed.
- Re-examination and dilatation of the oesophagus is done 2-weekly until mucosal healing has taken place.
- A delay in healing is indicative of deep burns and stricture formation can be expected. This will require long-term hospitalization and repeated dilatation of the oesophagus. An oesophageal bypass by colon transposition may eventually be necessary should the stricturing be severe.

Child abuse

Child abuse and neglect refers to the interaction between individuals or institutions and children that result in non-accidental harm to the physical, emotional or developmental state of the child or adolescent. The actual incidence is hard to ascertain and figures depend on rates of reporting and recognition of the problem.

A high degree of vigilance and awareness is necessary in all aspects of caring for children. Small children are particularly vulnerable and are at greater risk of fatal outcome. The long term effects of abuse are difficult to assess and manage. Abuse patterns tend to be repetitive with a likelihood of being passed from generation to generation.

Predisposing factors

More than 90% of perpetrators have no psychological problems or criminal nature. They tend to be lonely, unhappy and angry adults under tremendous stress.

Additional factors are:
- Parents or caretakers who were themselves abused as children
- Severe psychiatric problems in up to 10%
- Social isolation
- Poverty
- Unemployment
- Alcoholism and drug abuse.

Types of abuse

- *Physical abuse* refers to non-accidental injuries inflicted by the caretaker.
- *Sexual abuse* is the use of a child for sexual gratification. Besides sexual intercourse it includes:
  - Touching, fondling or licking of genitals or breasts
  - Masturbation of a child by an adult or vice versa and adult masturbation in the presence of a child
  - Body contact with adult genitals
  - Exhibitionism
  - Pornography.
- *Failure to thrive* due to nutritional deprivation is common in the first 2 years of life. Approximately 50% of 'failure to thrive' at this age is due to maternal neglect.
- *Intentional drugging* or poisoning occurs when parents give a prescribed drug, which is harmful and not intended for the child.
- *Medical care neglect* occurs when a child with a (chronic) disease worsens because parents ignore the condition.
- *Safety neglect* implies a gross lack of supervision especially in younger age categories.

- *Emotional abuse* is the repeated blaming of a child for incidents, or the rejection of a child by its carers and includes severe verbal abuse.
- *Organized abuse* is a form of crime, and often involves multiple victims and perpetrators, who may include paedophilic and pornographic rings.

Physical abuse

The Red Cross Children's Hospital trauma unit treats about 500 cases of abuse annually and approximately 100 are sexually-related. A third of physical abuse occurs under the age of 6 months, a third under 3 years and a third over 3 years of age. At particular risk are males, those born prematurely and step-children.

Presentation

- A child may readily indicate that a particular adult has inflicted the injury. Take this seriously as children rarely lie about such conditions.
- An unexplained injury is always suspicious, especially when parents are reluctant to clarify the accident. They often state that the child was 'just found like that' or 'might have fallen' or might have been 'hit by someone else'.
- A discrepancy in the history given by parents is also suggestive. It may differ in time, date and cause.
- The severity of an injury may be out of proportion to the attributed cause, e.g. a child covered in bruises may have 'fallen off a bed'.
- Improbable self-inflicted trauma, e.g. the baby rolled over and 'broke an arm'.
- A third party may be accused of having caused the injury.
- A delay in seeking medical help: rarely do parents bring their injured child more than 24 hours after the event.
- Repetitive injuries are suspicious.

Types of injuries

- *Head*: fractures, intra-cranial injuries
- *Trunk*: fractured ribs, spinal cord and internal organ injuries
- *Limbs*: single fracture with multiple bruises, multiple fractures of different stages, possibly no bruise or soft tissue injury, metaphyseal or epiphyseal injuries, often multiple
- *Superficial*: cuts, bruises, burns, scalds, signs of hypothermia and frostbite
- *Suffocation*
- *Poisoning.*

Notes on injury types

Skin

- Lesions can occur anywhere. Bruises on the buttocks and lower back are often related to punishment, those on the cheek are usually from slapping (Figure 1.4).
- Other typical findings are grip marks, pinch marks and circumferential bruises.
- Defining the age of the injuries is difficult. Initially most lesions are red and turn reddish-purple within 24 hours. Over the next week they become purple and within 3 weeks may be yellow, green or brown from degradation of haemoglobin.

Figure 1.4 Extensive skin lesions and conjunctival bleeding after assault

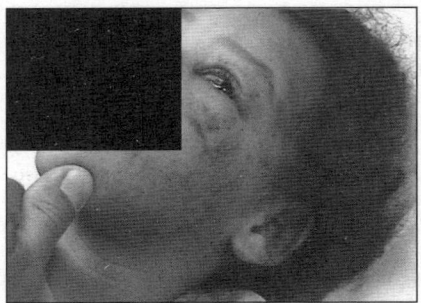

Burns

Approximately 10% of physical abuse involves burns (Figure 1.5) Typical lesions are cigarette burns and stocking/glove injuries in toddlers from immersion in hot water.

Figure 1.5 Partial thickness burns around the perineum due to hot water enema

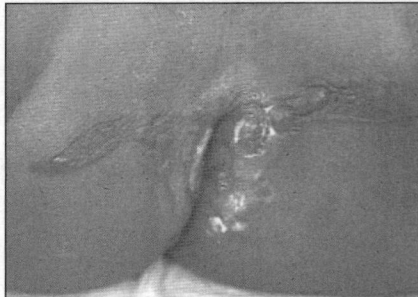

Head injuries

The spectrum ranges from mild trauma to severe lethal extra-dural and sub-dural haematomas. (Figures 1.6, 1.7) Skull fractures are common and may be associated with subdural haematomas. These may also result from shaking. The rapid acceleration and deceleration of the head tears bridging veins and causes bleeding, often bilaterally, in the subdural space. Retinal haemorrhages are nearly always present.

Figure 1.6 A CT-scan of a severely injured brain of a 1-year-old child. The scan shows the 'white cerebellum' sign, a diffuse oedema of both cerebral hemispheres

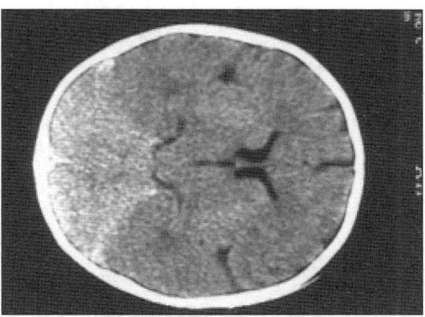

Figure 1.7 A CT-scan of the child, 3 months later. There is extensive and diffuse atrophy

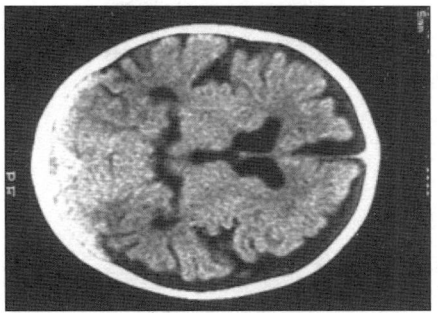

Skeletal injuries

Approximately a quarter of cases have skeletal lesions. Fractures rarely occur under 3 years of age and when present without an adequate explanation, are likely to be due to abuse. Two-thirds of fractures involve long bones and are spiral or transverse. A chip fracture (*corner fracture*) is almost pathognomonic. The corner of the metaphysis is usually torn from the periostium during a wrenching injury to a long bone (Figures 1.8, 1.9 and 1.10). Approximately 10 days after the injury, calcification of sub-periostal bleeding gives a classical double-cortex line.

Figure 1.8 Corner fracture of the metaphysis. This is typical and results from violent wrenching and shaking of the extremity.

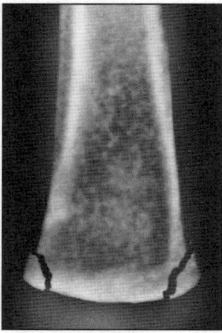

Figure 1.9 Bucket handle fracture of the metaphysis. This is also a typical fracture from violent wrenching and shaking of the extremity.

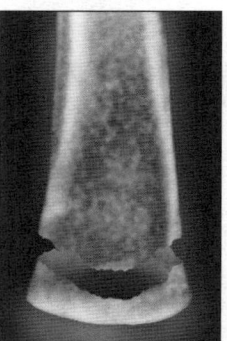

Figure 1.10 Bucket handle fracture of the tibial metaphysis. The child was picked up by the feet and shaken.

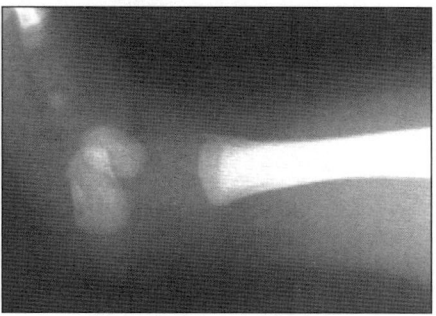

Investigations

Table 1.12 Evaluation of child abuse

History	Obtain a detailed history of the alleged assault. This includes informants, dates, time, place, sequence of events, people present, etc. Also interview the child and document the psychological state (distressed, crying, withdrawn etc)
Physical examination	It is essential to undress and examine the whole child. Do not omit the oral cavity and genitals. Record the size, shape, position, colour and age of bruises, strap and grip marks etc *Sexual abuse:* in a first-time case examine the child under general anaesthesia. An accurate examination might be painful and very difficult if the child is frightened, distressed and un-cooperative. If lesions are found, surgical treatment can be performed immediately
Imaging	Every child under 5 years should have a skeletal survey, consisting of an AP skull, AP chest, AP pelvis, AP spine and AP arms and legs. A radio-nuclear bone scan is more sensitive for old injuries, but is unreliable under 1 year of age. If a head injury is suspected, a CT-scan is performed for medico-legal purposes as well as to screen for injuries. Refer the child for retinoscopy. (Flame-shaped retinal haematomas are typical in child abuse)

Bleeding disorder screen	Platelet count, bleeding time, partial thromboplastin time, prothrombin time and thrombin time are done for bruising that parents deny having inflicted or when there is a history of alleged easy bruising
Photographs	Formal pictures should be taken of severe injuries as many physical signs disappear rapidly. This is best delegated to a particular person. Digital photographs are acceptable as long as they are printed immediately and signed by the person who took them
Examination of siblings	This may be necessary as 20% will be abused at some stage
Medical reporting	The doctor who *initially* examines the child must provide adequate and complete medical reports, including a social work referral form and a police form if indicated
Behavioural assessment	An abused child is likely to have behavioural problems and must be observed closely in the ward by experienced people. Behaviour often reveals important clues as to the nature of the abuse

Sexual assault

- This is common in all societies. Many studies quote 1 in 4 girls being abused before 18 years and 1 in 10 boys. Most perpetrators (70%) are either family members or are well known to the family (friends or neighbours).
- Any child with perineal injuries or infection should be suspected of being a victim. Sexual abuse can be chronic (without signs of fresh injuries, but absent hymen) or acute (often with fresh physical injuries). Small children often present with a bruised perineum.
- Because of the discrepancy in sexual organ size, penetration is infrequent. However lack of penetration doesn't imply absence of abuse. According to the South African legal definition there can be penetration without physical injuries (hymen intact) and in a local study, one-third of the victims had no physical injuries. Nevertheless forced penetration can cause mutilating injuries in a small child.

Classification of perineal injuries

- Inflammation, discharge
- Bruising, erythema
- First degree tear: skin laceration only
- Second degree tear: muscle involved, but anal sphincter intact
- Third degree tear: anal sphincter involved, recto-vaginal injury.

Investigations

- A police Crime Kit should be used to collect medico-legal samples. After taking the evidence, the box is sealed and kept in a safe place until it is collected by the police Child Protection Unit.
- Pus swabs, blood and other samples can be taken under general anaesthesia while the child is undergoing examination.
- Injuries should be graded at this time.

Treatment

- Bruises and first and second-degree tears can usually be repaired primarily.
- When the anal sphincter is disrupted or the recto-vaginal septum is involved, a diverting colostomy and washout is necessary. A secondary repair is performed once all signs of infection have settled (usually between 6 weeks and 3 months).
- Check for syphilis (VDRL) and HIV/AIDS.
- Antibiotic therapy can be deferred until culture results are available.
- Antiretroviral therapy: this should be offered to those who are HIV-negative if they present within 72 hours of exposure (p. 318). Those who have been chronically abused are not treated as exposure usually exceeds 72 hours.

General management

- Take a comprehensive history, document accurately the clinical findings and extent of the injuries and provide appropriate treatment. This may vary from analgesics to extensive surgical procedures. A distinction between accidental and non-accidental injury may be very difficult and the physician must bear in mind that playing detective is not the primary objective.
- Abuse is a family problem and involves a multi-disciplinary team from the child protection services, the courts, the police department, the rape crises centres, the hospitals and the mental health services. Avoid making the child repeat statements to different agencies. Management of the child by a social worker and a child psychologist is highly recommended. The task of the social worker is not only to interview the child but also to reunify the family.
- In exceptional states the child may have to be removed from home. This invariably causes severe psychological damage as the child perceives it to be punishment. Specific reactions such as guilt, anxiety, phobia, anger and depression should be appropriately addressed.
- The management of the abusing parents is extremely difficult and often involves issues of their own childhood. The perpetrators

must accept responsibility for their behaviour. A rebuke or a harsh or condescending lecture is rarely effective. In case of alcoholism, referral to Alcoholics Anonymous (AA) may be helpful.

Reporting suspected abuse and court testimony

- Parents or caretakers regularly threaten legal action if accused. However the law protects anyone who, in good faith, reports a possible case of child abuse.
- It is of utmost importance to the judicial process that medical staff should complete a written affidavit within 24 hours that can be presented in court.
- All sexual abuse cases should be investigated by the Child Protection Unit. Very few cases are successfully prosecuted. Sexual abuse cases cannot be withdrawn (as in adult cases) when the victim changes her/his mind.
- It is a *criminal offence* for medical staff not to report child abuse. Under South African law, doctors who are aware of child abuse and do not report it (to the Child Protection Unit of the police and/or social worker), can be prosecuted under the Prevention of Family Violence Act of 1993.

Childhood poisoning

The Red Cross Children's Hospital Poisons Information Centre documented that, for the 5 year period 2003 to 2007, just over 2 400 cases of known or suspected poisonings were seen at the hospital.

The majority of poisoning episodes occur from accidental ingestion by children in the first 5 years of life. Accidental single substance ingestion is common in young children between 2–3 years. Intentional ingestion of 1 or more drugs is more likely in older children and may require psychological or psychiatric intervention.

The commonest poisons are:
- Paraffin
- Organophosphates
- Medications – tricyclic antidepressants and so on
- Atropine-like substances
- Ethanol
- Houshold cleaning agents.

Repeated episodes of poisoning or inconsistent histories should raise the possibility of child abuse or neglect.

> ***Practice point:***
>
> All cases of poisoning should be investigated by the social worker or Child Protection Team.

Management

Supportive management

- Initial resuscitation should always pay attention to assessment of the airway, breathing and circulation. It is essential to maintain an adequate airway and provide oxygen if necessary to prevent hypoxia. Toxins may induce CNS depression or seizures with the risk of airway compromise, respiratory failure or aspiration. Intubation may be required.
- Fluid replacement: losses from vomiting, diarrhoea or urine may need rapid replacement. Intravenous lines should be secured early and dehydration and shock should be aggressively managed (see Chapter 20, Fluids, electrolytes, and acid-base). Shock should be treated with fluid boluses and inotropes should be avoided if possible. The combination of an inotrope with a toxin may produce arrhythmias.
- Control and prevent hypoglycaemia. Always check the blood glucose level early in the assessment of the patient and correct hypoglycaemia with IV glucose infusions. Give 5 ml/kg of 10% dextrose.
- Convulsions: IV lorazepam and phenobarbitone are the drugs of choice.
- Sedation and pain relief: use IV morphine 50–100 mcg/kg for severe pain.
- Decontamination: remove contaminated clothing, wash the child thoroughly to eliminate contact with corrosives and reduce absorption of toxins (especially important in organophosphate poisoning).
- Blood pressure and ECG monitoring is essential for cardiovascular symptoms and to monitor the effects of tricyclic antidepressants, calcium channel blockers, organophosphates and arrhythmogenic medications, e.g. antihistamines, anti arrhythmic drugs, theophylline and atropine.
- Electrolytes and acid-base disturbances should be anticipated and treated appropriately.

Identifying the poison

Always try to identify the substance ingested and its constituents. Take a full history and attempt to recover any undigested medications or toxins.

Where possible the exact dosage per kilogram of body weight should be determined as accurately as possible.

Table 1.13 Recognisable poison syndromes and clinical clues

Poison syndrome	Associated signs	Possible toxins
Increased sympathetic nervous system activity (these features are common in disease generally)	Pyrexia Flushing Tachycardia Hypertension Pupillary constriction Sweating	Cough and decongestant preparations Amphetamines Cocaine Ecstasy Theophylline

Anticholinergic activity	Similar clinical picture to sympathomimetics
	Clinical differences include:
	    Pupillary dilatation
	    Dry mouth
	    Hot dry skin
		Tricyclic antidepressants
		Antiparkinsonian drugs
		Antihistamines
		Atropine and nightshade
		Antispasmodics
		Phenothiazines
		Mushroom poisoning (*Amanita* species)
		Cyclopentolate eye drops

Increased parasympathetic nervous system activity	Pupillary constriction Diarrhoea Urinary incontinence Sweating Excessive salivation Muscle weakness Fasciculation Paralysis	Organophosphate insecticides Drugs for myasthenia gravis, e.g. pyridostigmine
Metabolic acidosis	Tachypnoea Kussmaul breathing (sighing respiration)	Ethanol Carbon monoxide Antifreeze Iron Diabetic medication Tricyclic antidepressants Salicylates Ecstasy
Chemical pneumonitis	Cough Respiratory distress Central nervous system depression A history of vomiting following ingestion need not be a feature	White spirit Turpentine Essential oils

Poison syndrome	Associated signs	Possible toxins
Acute ataxia or nystagmus		Antihistamines Alcohol Anticonvulsants (especially phenytoin and carbamazepine) Piperazine Diphenylhydantoin Barbiturates Carbon monoxide Organic solvents Bromides
Methaemoglobinaemia	Cyanosis resistant to oxygen therapy	Alanine dyes Nitrates Benzocaine Phenacetin Nitrobenzene Chlorates Sulphonamides and metoclopramide (in neonates)
Renal failure	Oliguria or anuria Haematuria Myoglobinuria	Carbon tetrachloride Ethylene glycol Methanol Mushrooms Oxalates
Violent emesis		Aspirin Theophylline Corrosives Fluoride Boric acid Iron

Corrosive injury:
- Alkalis tend to cause more damage than acids. Batteries and dishwasher tablets may become trapped in the oesophagus causing local tissue destruction.
- Attempts to empty the stomach are contraindicated. Activated charcoal should not be given.
- Use water or milk orally in an attempt to dilute the effect of the corrosive agent and thereafter keep nil per mouth. Oesophagoscopy may be indicated for more severe injury. Persistent drooling and dysphagia are markers of oesophageal scar formation.

Dystonic reactions:
- Seen with metoclopramide, phenothiazines, haloperidol, phenytoin, tricyclic antidepressants
- The features can be rapidly reversed with biperiden 2.5–5 mg IV.

Drug elimination procedures

- Activated charcoal is best given if ingestion has occurred within 2 hours, but may be given even if ingestion exceeds 2 hours. The dose is 1 g/kg in 50–100 ml water every 2–4 hours. It is often not swallowed by children and should be given by nasogastric tube.
- Activated charcoal is contraindicated in ingestion of corrosive agents and paraffin ingestion. Activated charcoal is proven to be ineffective in poisoning by alcohols (ethanol and methanol), iron, lithium, bleach, boric acid, DDT, cyanide.
- Gastric lavage is best indicated within 1 hour of ingestion. Intubation with a cuffed endotracheal tube is indicated for children with a depressed level of consciousness who cannot protect the airway.
- Gut irrigation. Enteral administration of electrolyte-balanced polyethylene glycol can increase gut transit time and eliminate toxins not absorbed by activated charcoal. 30 ml/kg/hour is given until rectal effluent clears. May be useful for ingestion of iron and enteric coated preparations.
- Diuresis: forced diuresis is generally not recommended.
- Ringers lactate or isotonic normal saline is administered for volume expansion to maintain urine flow at 1–2 ml/kg/hr. Excessive fluid volumes should be avoided, especially in patients at risk of pulmonary or cerebral oedema.
- Haemodialysis
- In cases of severe toxicity consult the Poison Centre or a paediatric nephrology service.

Specific antidotes

- Flumazenil 0.02 mg/kg IV as 1% solution for benzodiazepine overdosage. This may produce seizures in patients on long term treatment with benzodiazepines for epilepsy and in concomitant tricyclic antidepressant overdose and so is contraindicated in these situations
- Naloxone 0.1 mg/kg IV for narcotics
- Atropine for organophosphate poisoning
- Obidoxime for confirmed organophosphate poisoning
- Desferoxamine for iron poisoning
- Vitamin K for warfarin and coumarins
- N-acetyl-cysteine for paracetamol intoxication

- Methylene blue for methaemoglobinaemia
- Pyridoxine, sodium bicarbonate for INH
- Biperiden for dystonic reactions from phenothiazines and metoclopramide.

Laboratory support

- Where the poison is not known, samples of urine and blood may be sent for toxicology screening. The clinical picture should act as a guide to specific toxicology testing. The tests usually do not provide immediate results but may have importance later when treatment is reviewed and for medico-legal purposes.
- Blood tests for electrolytes, estimation of renal function, acid base status and screening for sepsis (FBC, ESR and blood culture) may be very useful depending on the clinical picture.
- Markedly decreased serum cholinesterase levels will confirm the clinical suspicion of organophosphate or carbamate poisoning.
- Chest X-rays are necessary when respiratory symptoms are present and for suspected aspiration. Abdominal X-rays may be useful for radiopaque substances, e.g. iron.
- For more detailed treatment regimes for specific toxins consult the Poisons Information Centres.

Poisons information centres

Tygerberg Hospital: 021 938 6084 (office hours)
021 931 6129 (24 hours)
Red Cross Children's Hospital: 021 689 5227 (24 hours)

Recommended reading

1 *Paediatric Trauma and Child Abuse.* Van As, S and Naidoo, S (Eds). Oxford University Press. Cape Town. 2006.
2 *World Report on Child Injury Prevention.* Peden, M et al. (Eds). World Health Organization & UNICEF, Geneva. Switzerland. 2008.
3 *Handbook of Trauma.* Nicol, A and Steyn, E (Eds). Oxford University Press. Cape Town. 2004.
4 *Child and adolescent injury prevention.* A WHO plan of action. World Health Organization, Geneva. Switzerland. 2006.
5 *Health for all children.* (4e) Hall, DMB and Elliman, D (Eds). Oxford University Press. Cape Town. 2003.
6 Subhi R, Smith K, Duke T. When should oxygen be given to children at high altitude? A systematic review to define altitude-specific hypoxaemia. *Arch Dis Child* 2009; 94(1): 6–10.

2 Neonatal problems

L.J. Glynn, M.C. Harrison, A.R. Horn, L.L. Linley, C.H. Pieper

This chapter focuses on the optimal management of neonatal problems that will ensure the best possible outcome for every newborn infant. The problems addressed are birth asphyxia and resuscitation, hypoxic ischaemic encephalopathy, seizures, neonatal hypoglycaemia, hypothermia, infection, respiratory disease and jaundice. The chapter also discusses care of the low birthweight infant, breastfeeding and highly effective kangaroo mother care for small babies.

Resuscitation at birth

Resuscitation may be required to assist the transition from intra-uterine to extra-uterine life. It should be anticipated in the presence of any abnormal delivery: instrumental delivery, preterm delivery, intrapartum hypoxia, congenital sepsis/anomaly, meconium stained liquor and maternal sedation.

Birth asphyxia

The World Health Organization defines birth asphyxia as the failure to initiate and sustain breathing after birth. Other authorities interpret the term to mean impaired fetal gas exchange during labour (intrapartum fetal hypoxia).

The following details will assist in determining the potential contribution of intrapartum fetal hypoxia:
- A time-based description of the resuscitation and the infant's responses
- Gestational age and clinical examination of the infant *and the placenta*
- Arterial cord blood gas or infant blood gas as soon as possible after birth
- History suggesting fetal hypoxia or other abnormalities
- Subsequent presence or absence of neonatal encephalopathy
- Subsequent diagnostic tests, *including placental histology if available*.

Intrapartum fetal hypoxia

Definition:
- A base deficit > 10 mmol/l from arterial blood (umbilical artery or infant) in the first hour of life suggests intrapartum hypoxia, but does not indicate its severity.
- Resuscitation is often required after intrapartum hypoxia, but significant cerebral ischaemia is only suspected if seizures or encephalopathy occur.

The Apgar score

Diagnosis:
- This indicates the infant's condition and response to resuscitation.
- Record the score at 1, 5 and 10 minutes, and at 20 minutes if still abnormal.
- A score below 7 at any stage indicates the need for ongoing intervention.
- A heart rate persistently < 100 bpm and/or cyanosis usually indicates inadequate ventilation.

Table 2.1 The Apgar score

	0	1	2
Heart rate	Absent	Under 100/min	Over 100/min
Respiratory effort	Absent	Weak, irregular	Strong, regular
Muscle tone	Limp	Some flexion	Active movement
Response to stimuli	None	Weak response	Cry
Colour	Blue or pale body	Pink body, blue extremities	Completely pink

Clinical features and treatment: resuscitation

If an infant is *not* pink and breathing well at birth, follow the algorithm in Figure 2.1.

Figure 2.1 Neonatal resuscitation algorithm. (Modified from ILCOR. Pediatrics 2006;117:e978–e988 and South African Handbook of Resuscitation of the Newborn SAPA 2004).

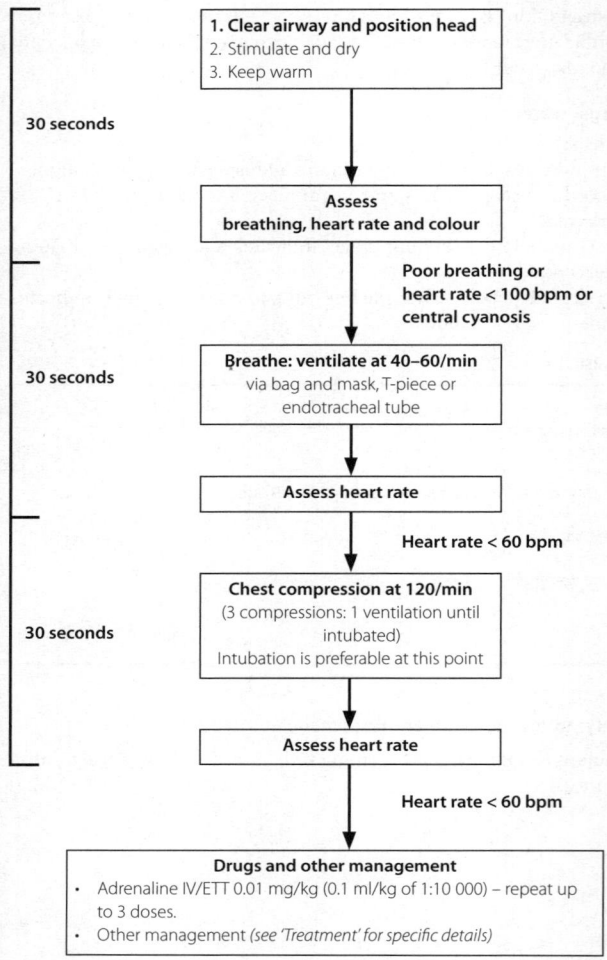

Treatment

Temperature management:
- Avoid overheating. ☆☆☆☺
- Prevent hypothermia in preterm infants < 28 weeks by placing in an open polythene bag. ☆☆☆☺

Oxygen administration:
- Avoid unnecessary exposure to 100% oxygen. ☆☆☺
- Wean as soon as possible but give 100% oxygen if central cyanosis or bradycardia persists despite adequate ventilation.

Ventilation and circulation:
- Use the lowest inflation pressure needed to achieve visible chest wall movement, increase in heart rate, and improved colour. ☆☺
- A pressure regulated T-piece (Neopuff®) with PEEP 5 cm is preferable to other devices in preterm infants. ☆☆☺
- Meconium stained liquor: tracheal suction is only indicated if the infant is *not* vigorous. ☆☆☆☆☺

Other management:
- Volume expansion: 10 ml/kg saline (not albumin) only if hypovolaemia suspected. ☆☺
- Use blood if hypovolaemic and anaemic with Hb < 10 g/dl.
- Sodium bicarbonate: no human data to suggest benefit. Animal data suggests harm. Current South African National Guidelines suggest the use of 2 ml/kg 4.25% solution in prolonged resuscitation. ☺
- Naloxone: no efficacy data. Use for reversal of maternal opiates if poor respiratory effort *after* normal heart rate and adequate ventilatory support established. Dose 0.1 mg/kg IV. ☺
- Dextrose: if ongoing resuscitation at 10 minutes and *confirmed* hypoglycaemia < 2.2 mmol/l, administer 2 ml/kg 10% dextrose IV. All infants who have required resuscitation should have their blood sugar checked as soon as possible thereafter, as hypoglycaemia is an associated morbidity. ☆☺

Hypoxic ischaemic encephalopathy (HIE)

Definitions

- HIE is an acquired syndrome of acute brain injury characterized by neonatal encephalopathy (NE) in the first 3 days of life and evidence of intrapartum hypoxia in a term infant.
- Neonatal encephalopathy is characterized by an abnormal level of consciousness, abnormal tone and primitive reflexes in the first week of life. Abnormal breathing and seizures may occur.

Clinical assessment of HIE

- Clinical signs vary with time. Moderately or severely affected infants typically develop increasingly obvious or severe signs during the first 48–72 hours.
- Cycling, posturing and myoclonus may represent seizure activity or lack of inhibition/control at a brainstem level. Seizures are often clinically silent.

The Sarnat classification

Three stages of encephalopathy are described:
- Stage 1: irritability, increased tone, poor sucking and exaggerated Moro reflex
- Stage 2: lethargy, decreased tone and primitive reflexes. Often with seizures
- Stage 3: stupor or coma, flaccid tone and seizures often clinically less apparent.

The HIE* score ☆ ☆ ☗

Table 2.2 shows the signs that are assessed by the HIE* score.
- The maximum score, based on the infant's clinical signs in the previous 24 hours, is recorded in each category and then totalled for the day.
- A peak score of 10 or less during the first 6 days with a score of 0 by day 7 predicts a normal outcome; a peak score above 15 and a score that is still abnormal on day 7 is predictive of abnormal outcome in 65%.
- The prognostic value of this score in infants treated with hypothermia may be different.

Table 2.2 The HIE* score

Grade/Score Sign	1	2	3	Score
Limb tone	Generally hypertonic	Generally hypotonic	Flaccid	
Level of consciousness	Hyper-alert, staring, *or* excessive irritability	Lethargic	Comatose *or* stuporose	
Visible fits	Infrequent < 3/day	Frequent > 2/day		
Posture	Fisting and/or cycling	Strong distal flexion	Decerebrate	
Moro	Partial	Absent		
Grasp	Poor	Absent		
Suck	Poor	Absent and/or bites		
Respiration	Hyperventilation	Transient apnoea	Apnoea needs IPPV	
Fontanelle	Full (not tense)	Tense		

*HIE score devised by CW van der Elst and evaluated by CM Thompson et al

Amplitude integrated electroencephalogram (aEEG) and cerebral function monitor (CFM)

The aEEG is a time-compressed, processed EEG that has prognostic value and is useful in diagnosing subclinical seizures. Continuous normal voltage by age 6 hours in term infants is associated with a normal outcome. A severely suppressed background persisting for 6 hours predicts a poor outcome in over 80% and if this persists beyond 24 hours, the prognosis is almost invariably poor in non-cooled infants.

Cranial ultrasound

Cranial ultrasound may show established damage at birth (oedema, infarction, ischaemia or haemorrhage) and/or evolving focal or global injury. Persistent damage is seen as densities or cystic change (leucomalacia) in the subcortex, cortex or basal ganglia. Doppler flow can provide additional prognostic information.

Magnetic resonance imaging (MRI)

MRI is the most reliable early guide to diagnosis and prognosis. This is an expensive investigation. If available it can be done at age 10–14 days to provide useful diagnostic information.

Management of HIE

Record the antenatal history, intrapartum events and management at delivery. The aim of management is to treat symptoms and minimize further organ damage. Correct standard management is more important than additional neuroprotective therapy such as hypothermia.

Central nervous system and temperature control

- Perform neurological assessment on admission and daily and apply aEEG if available.
- Obtain head ultrasound and repeat before discharge.
- Treat recurrent and persistent seizures. (*See section on Neonatal seizures*) ☆ ♦
- If moderate or severe encephalopathy is present at birth then induced hypothermia may improve the outcome if commenced as soon as possible and no later than 6 hours after birth. Core temperature should be kept at 33–34 °C for 72 hours. If head cooling is used then temperatures up to 34.5 °C may be effective. Monitor core temperature with a rectal probe or a probe insulated between the skin and mattress. Rewarming should not occur faster than 0.5 °C per hour. ☆ ☆ ☆ ♦
- If infants are not cooled, avoid *core* temperatures above 37 °C. ☆ ☆ ☆ ♦

Respiratory system

- Monitor oxygen saturation and blood gases.
- If oxygen is needed but respiratory effort is good, nasal CPAP is often adequate.
- If ventilated, ensure pCO_2, PaO_2 and SaO_2 in the normal range. ☆ ♦

Cardiovascular system

- Monitor blood pressure and keep it in the normal range.
- Treat hypovolaemia with a bolus of saline (10–20 ml/kg).
- Intrauterine hypoxia can be associated with hypervolaemia at birth, so avoid fluid boluses unless the infant is hypovolaemic. ☆ ♦
- If significant anaemia is present (PCV < 30% or Hb < 10 g%) transfuse the infant and request a Kleihauer test for fetal cells in the maternal blood.

- If there is not a sustained response to a single fluid bolus then inotropic support with dopamine and dobutamine is usually indicated.

Fluid balance and electrolytes

- Intrinsic renal failure and SIADH commonly occur.
- Initially fluid restrict to 40 ml/kg/24 hours with potassium-free 10% glucose and 0.2% to 0.45% normal saline. Adjust according to further monitoring.
- Monitor urine output, electrolytes, blood glucose and blood gases.
- If hypoglycaemia occurs, use 12% or 15% glucose as an infusion solution.
- There is no proven benefit to the use of sodium bicarbonate to treat lactic acidosis. ☹
- Treat hyponatraemia (< 130 mmol/l) with fluid restriction at 40 ml/kg but monitor urine output and sodium excretion to determine if different management is required.
- Hypocalcaemia and hypomagnesaemia should be anticipated and treated.

Multi-organ failure

- Bone marrow failure may manifest as thrombocytopaenia and hepatic failure may cause coagulopathy, hypoglycaemia and hypoalbuminaemia – monitor and treat these conditions.
- Intestinal ischaemia increases the risk of necrotising enterocolitis, hence introduce feeds slowly over the first few days – breastmilk is preferable.

Sepsis

- Chorioamnionitis is associated with intrapartum hypoxia and sepsis can be difficult to distinguish from encephalopathy.
- Screen for sepsis and treat empirically until investigations exclude sepsis.

Parental counselling

- Explain the clinical condition.
- Document the parent's version of events.
- Listen to their questions, explain the management needed and keep them informed of the prognosis based on the daily clinical assessment.

Prognosis and follow-up

- Neonatal neurological examination and aEEG are only reliable when abnormalities are severe. High doses of anticonvulsants and sedatives may obscure the clinical picture.
- Early infant neurodevelopmental assessment can be predictive of outcome. ☆☆☆☼
- Cerebral palsy and intellectual disability are common in infants who survive severe HIE and multidisciplinary follow-up is required.

Neonatal seizures

Definition

- An abnormal synchronous electrical discharge of a group of neurons in the central nervous system.
- Status epilepticus: continuous seizures lasting 30 minutes or recurrent seizures occupying 50% of the EEG recording for at least 60 minutes.

Clinical manifestations

- Clinical manifestations may be absent or subtle (eye deviation, eyelid fluttering, bucco-lingual movements or pedalling of arms and legs), focal (tonic or clonic) or generalized (multifocal rhythmic jerking, generalized posturing or myoclonic).
- Jitteriness is usually distinguished from seizures by the response to stimuli.

Causes and diagnosis

Important causes are: hypoxic ischaemic encephalopathy, intracranial haemorrhage or infarction, meningitis, hypoglycaemia, hypocalcaemia, hypomagnesaemia, hyponatraemia, hypernatraemia, and drug withdrawal.

Diagnosis:
- Measure serum glucose, magnesium, calcium and sodium.
- Do a lumbar puncture if sepsis is suspected.
- Head ultrasound may be diagnostic if intracranial bleeding, structural abnormality or ventriculitis are present.
- Consider inborn errors of metabolism if other causes are not obvious – measure serum lactate, ammonia and amino acids, and urine organic acids.
- If seizures cannot be confirmed with EEG/aEEG, treat on clinical suspicion.

Treatment

- Treat electrolyte and glucose abnormalities and sepsis.
- Ensure adequate ventilation and perfusion.
- For recurrent seizures or seizures lasting > 3 minutes treat with the following anticonvulsants, sequentially if seizures have not stopped after each dose:
  — Phenobarbitone 20 mg/kg IV infused *over 10 minutes.* ☆☆☆☙
  — Repeat phenobarbitone as above.
  — Midazolam 0.05 mg/kg IV over 5 minutes, then 0.05 mg/kg/hr. ☆☆☙ (*Double doses of midazolam can be used but EEG suppression may occur.*)
  — Intravenous lignocaine 2 mg/kg load over 10 minutes. Then infuse at 6 mg/kg/hr for 6 hours, 4 mg/kg/hr for 12 hours, 2 mg/kg/hr for 12 hours and then stop. ☆☆☙ (*Use ½ infusion doses of lignocaine if also treating with hypothermia.*) ☺

> ***Practice point:***
>
> Check that the lignocaine vial states that it is the formulation that is suitable for intravenous use.

- *Intractable seizures:*
  — Consider pyridoxine 100 mg IV/IM/PO ☺
  — Consider a third load with phenobarbitone ☆☆☙
    or clonazepam 0.1 mg/kg ☆☆☙
    or lorazepam 0.05–0.1 mg/kg. ☆☆☙
- *Preterm infants: (or term infants where lignocaine not available)*:
  — Phenobarbitone 20 mg/kg IV infused over 10 minutes
  — Phenytoin 20 mg/kg over 30 minutes as second line ☆☆☆☙
  — Midazolam 0.05 mg/kg IV over 5–10 minutes, then 0.05 mg/kg/hr.
- *If IV phenobarbitone is not available*:
  — Use midazolam, clonazepam or lorazepam as first line, and consider loading with oral phenobarbitone as crushed tablets.

The low birthweight infant

Definitions

- Low birthweight: any infant weighing less than 2 500 g at birth.
- Preterm: < 37 completed weeks intrauterine life.

- Further classification of the low birthweight baby is by weight appropriateness for scored gestational age. This assessment guides the care plan for the infant at birth. The gestational age score is based on physical and neuromuscular maturity. The weight and gestational age are plotted on a weight for gestational age chart. The baby may be:
  1. Preterm and appropriate weight for gestational age
  2. Preterm but underweight for gestational age
  3. Term but underweight for gestational age.
- Underweight babies: birthweight below the 10th centile.

Problems to anticipate

- Preterm infants: problems related to immature organ systems having to adapt to extrauterine life.
- Underweight for gestational age infants: problems related to chronic intrauterine hypoxia and undernutrition.

Table 2.3 Preterm infants compared to underweight for gestational age infants

Preterm infants' problems	Underweight for gestational age infants' problems
- Asphyxia - Hypothermia - Hypoglycaemia - Apnoea - Hyaline membrane disease - Intracranial haemorrhage - Patent ductus arteriosus - Infection - Feeding difficulties - Jaundice - Anaemia - Hyponatraemia - Metabolic bone disease of prematurity - Problems related to oxygen toxicity: eyes: retinopathy of prematurity, lungs: chronic lung disease - Poor bonding	- Asphyxia - Hypothermia - Hypoglycaemia - Meconium aspiration - Hypoxic ischaemic encephalopathy - Persistent pulmonary hypertension of the neonate - Polycythaemia - Poor bonding if long hospital stay

Care plan

- Ensure minimal handling by restricting and grouping interventions. Apply developmental care.
- Facilitate skin-to-skin ('kangaroo') care, breastfeeding if possible and rooming-in of mothers.

- Use intravenous fluids if birthweight < 1 500 g or history of intrauterine hypoxia.
- Hand hygiene (handwashing, alcohol hand rub). ☆☆☆☆☗
- Monitor: skin temperature, blood glucose, respiration, heart rate, oxygen saturation, stool and urine output, bilirubin, weight gain (15-20 g/day) and increase in head circumference (0.5-1 cm/week).
- Score infant (gestational age).
- Prescribe oral theophylline/caffeine prophylactically for apnoea of prematurity if infant scores < 35 weeks. ☆☆☆☗
- Monitor growth (weight and head circumference), check haemoglobin every 1-2 weeks and calcium, phosphate and alkaline phosphatase every 2 weeks if birthweight/gestation < 1 200 g/< 29 weeks until > 1 500 g.
- Parents: social assessment, emotional support, and regular communication about infant. Record and encourage visiting.

Fluids and feeding

- The well preterm infant over 35 weeks gestational age and 1 500 g may breastfeed if sucking is adequate at birth (see Breastfeeding p. 82).
- If sick, very growth restricted or < 1 500 g: intravenous fluids containing 10% glucose, e.g. Neolyte®, are necessary within 30 minutes of birth to prevent hypoglycaemia.
- Initial total fluid volume: 60-80 ml/kg/day. Increase daily by 20 ml/kg increments to 150 ml/kg/day (infants < 1 kg may need higher volumes).
- Start minimal enteral feeding with 12-24 ml/kg expressed breast milk (pasteurized if necessary) within 36 hours of age. ☆☆☆☗
- If well tolerated, increase milk feeds (oro/nasogastric or breast/cup) by 12-24 ml/kg/day.
- Check blood glucose every 3 hours. Maintain at 2.6-7.0 mmol/l. If it is < 2.6 mmol/l, treat as for hypoglycaemia (see p. 57). If it exceeds 7 mmol/l, for more than 3 hours, change to a solution containing 5% glucose.
- If IV fluids alone are required for more than 3 days consider parenteral nutrition.
- Feed continuously or by bolus feeds. If bolus feeds, start with hourly if < 1.2 kg birthweight, 2 hourly if 1.2-1.8 kg birthweight. Gradually increase the interval as the infant tolerates increasing volumes and establishes breastfeeding.
- Stop IV when milk accounts for 80% or more of the total.

- Stop enteral feeding if vomiting or abdominal distension occurs or if there are recurrent aspirates (> 2 ml/kg) from the stomach 1–2 hours after a feed (risk of necrotising enterocolitis).

> ***Practice point:***
>
> Give donor mother's milk or preterm formula if mother's own breast milk unavailable. Breast milk may contain insufficient nutrients for babies under 1 500 g. Suitable supplements include medium chain triglycerides, phosphate, sodium (sodium bicarbonate 4.2% or sodium chloride) and breast milk fortifiers.

Supplements
- Infants < 1 500 g on breast milk alone, add breast milk fortifier.
- If < 1 500 g and average weight gain on full enteral feeding is < 15 g/day, add medium chain triglyceride oil.
- Multivitamin drops (0.6 ml/day) once full enteral feeds. Continue until mixed feeding is well established.
- Add iron (Ferro Drops L® 0.3–0.6 ml/day) after a month. Continue until the infant has been weaned. If poor socio-economic circumstances, continue for 18 months.
- Vitamin D recommendations for infants < 1 500 g/32 weeks vary from 150–800 u/kg/day: usually supplied in multivitamin syrup.
- Check phosphate on infants < 32 weeks. If phosphate (PO_4) < 1.5 mmol/l: 0.25 mmol PO_4 8 hourly–12 hourly. Titrate to normal serum phosphate levels.

Kangaroo mother care (KMC)

This is also known as skin-to-skin care. The baby's mother becomes the baby's incubator. The technique is innovative, simple and low cost. It has improved morbidity and mortality for low birthweight babies in poorly resourced settings. It should be started at birth. ☆☆☆◊

There are 4 components:
- Position: upright, skin-to-skin between mother's breasts. Ensure airway patency.
- Nutrition: *breastmilk if possible*: breastfeeding on demand, expressed breastmilk or formula via a naso/orogastric tube or cup.
- Support: of this method of care for the mother by staff in the hospital or clinic, and family at home. This requires *education*.

- Discharge: this is possible earlier than usual. If the infant is breast-feeding well and growing, he/she may be discharged home irrespective of his/her weight. A baby should continue in KMC until his/her weight is > 2 kg. Babies need close follow-up at the infant health facility nearest to the infant's home: daily if weight < 1 600 g; frequent follow-up until weight 2 kg.

The different forms of KMC:
- Intermittent KMC: ill infants may be put into KMC for short periods, with the mother sitting next to the cot. The infants must be closely monitored.
- Continuous KMC: once an infant is clinically well, feeding well and gaining weight, he/she may be nursed in continuous KMC in a ward set aside for this purpose. The infant should wear a cap and a nappy.
- Transit KMC: KMC may be used to transfer stable infants to hospital or back home. The baby is secured between the mother's breasts over the vehicle's safety belt.

The advantages of KMC:
- Low cost
- Promotes bonding
- Promotes breastfeeding: improves lactation
- Improves immunity: breastmilk plus infants colonized with mother's organisms
- Temperature regulation better than incubator
- Infants' heart rates and respiratory rates less variable than in incubators
- Less crying
- Deep sleep enhanced
- Infants grow well. ☆☆☆☺

Hypoglycaemia

Definition
- Neonatal hypoglycaemia is a whole blood glucose < 2.6 mmol/l.
- Severe hypoglycaemia is a whole blood glucose < 1.5 mmol/l. ☆☆☆

Clinical features

- *Asymptomatic:* hypoglycaemia is detected by screening at-risk infants.
- *Symptomatic:* floppiness, jitteriness, apnoea, poor feeding and lethargy, rarely seizures and coma.

Diagnosis

Hypoglycaemia should be considered in all at risk infants:
- Underweight for gestational age (< 10th centile)
- Post mature infants (especially if wasted)
- Infants of diabetic mothers
- Prematurity
- Severe Rhesus disease
- Polycythaemia
- Septicaemia
- Hypothermia
- Hypoxic ischaemic encephalopathy.

Figure 2.2 Prevention of hypoglycaemia ☆☆☆☜ (See next page)

Treatment

Any baby who has persistent symptoms, is not tolerating enteral feeds, or is unable to maintain normoglycaemia with appropriate enteral feeds alone should be admitted to the neonatal unit and commenced on an intravenous infusion of 10% glucose.

- Start IV 10% glucose at 90 ml/kg/day (6.25 mg/kg/min) increasing by 30 ml/kg/day (2 mg/kg/min) maintaining glucose above 2.6 mmol/l.
- Beware of fluid volumes above 120 ml/kg/day.
- If normal blood glucose level is still not maintained, increase the concentration of glucose rather than the volume. If concentration exceeds 12.5% of glucose, insert a long line or umbilical venous catheter.
- If normoglycaemia is achieved, attempt to commence weaning the glucose requirement by 1–2 mg/kg/min every 6 hours.

> ***Practice point:***
>
> Babies on IV glucose should still receive breast or enteral feeds whenever possible.

Figure 2.2 Prevention of hypoglycaemia ☆☆☆◐

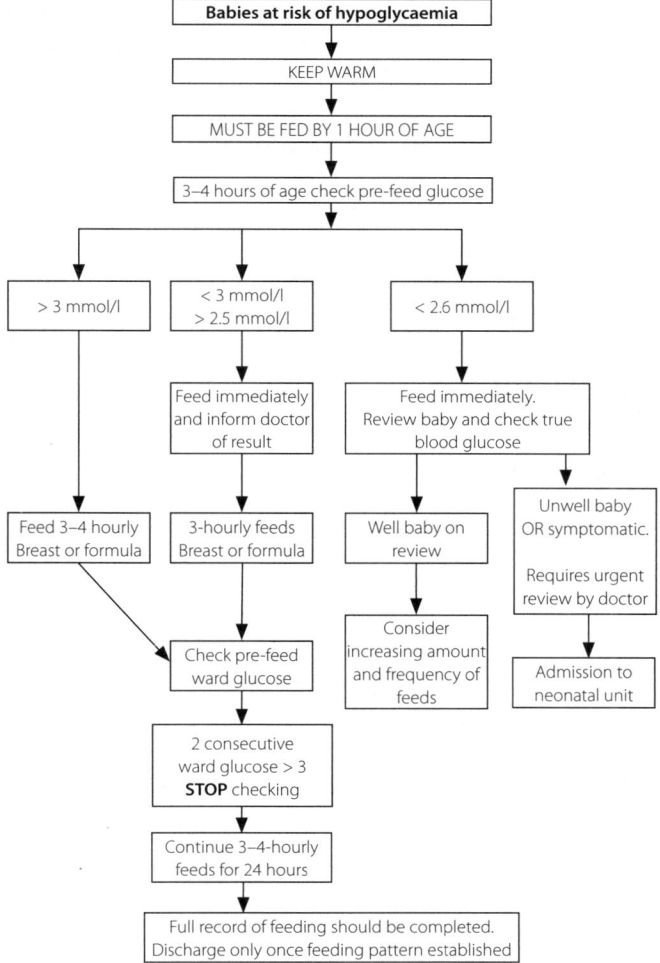

NICE Clinical Guideline 63. Diabetes in Pregnancy. March 2008.

Emergency treatment

Emergency treatment of hypoglycaemia is required if the baby is severely symptomatic or the blood glucose is persistently < 1.5 mmol/l.

- If the infant has IV access and blood glucose is low despite previous glucose infusion, give a bolus of 2 ml/kg of 10% glucose intravenously, followed by an increase in the maintenance glucose infusion. ☆☆☙
- In hypoglycaemia unresponsive to maximum glucose infusion rates, glucagon at 200 mcg/kg as an IV bolus may be useful. ☆☆☙

Complications

Symptomatic hypoglycaemia is a major risk factor for brain injury and subsequent neurodevelopmental handicap.

> ***Practice point:***
>
> Ensure that oral feeding is established before an intravenous dextrose infusion is discontinued. Sudden withdrawal can result in hypoglycaemia.

Hypothermia

Hypothermia is defined as a temperature below 36.5 °C. A newborn is more prone to develop hypothermia because of a large surface area per unit of body weight. A low birth weight baby has decreased thermal insulation because of reduced subcutaneous and brown fat.

Prevention

- Provide a warm, draught free environment (ideally 25 °C).
- Use warm towels to dry the infant at birth.
- Place the infant onto a warm resuscitation surface with radiant heater switched on.
- Dress the infant and if placed in cot, cover with two blankets.

A baby of less than 1 800 g cannot maintain body temperature without additional warmth. Incubation and kangaroo mother care provide effective control of body temperature and are used for an infant below this weight.

- Place infant in incubator.
- Dress warmly and cover head with woollen cap.
- Encourage 'skin to skin' contact (KMC) when parents visiting.

Treatment

A hypothermic baby has to be rewarmed and the method selected will depend on the severity of hypothermia and availability of staff and equipment. This would usually occur in a closed or open overhead incubator. Feeding should be continued to provide calories. If this is not possible a glucose infusion should be commenced.

Complications

Hypoglycaemia, hypoxia and *cold injury*, which is characterized by lethargy, poor feeding, bradycardia, apnoea, sclerema and pulmonary haemorrhage.

> ***Practice points:***
> - A severely cold baby can look deceptively healthy. The skin is pink because oxygen is trapped in red blood cells.
> - Every hypothermic newborn should be assessed for infection.

Infection in the newborn

All newborn, and especially preterm, babies are unable to combat infection adequately and are thus very susceptible to infection and the complications thereof.

Table 2.4 Definitions of infection in the newborn

Proven infection	Probable infection	Possible infection
- Cultured organisms from a sterile site, i.e. blood, CSF, suprapubic urine - With clinical and supporting laboratory evidence	- Clinical signs - Suggestive laboratory evidence - Negative cultures	- History of exposure and clinical suspicion

Sources of infection

Infection may be acquired from the mother before or during birth or from the environment after birth.

Antenatal: maternal infection can be transmitted to the fetus across the placenta. Vaginal bacteria may cross the membranes and enter the amniotic fluid (chorioamnionitis). Important blood-borne diseases include HIV, syphilis, rubella, cytomegalovirus (CMV) and toxoplasmosis. As a rule viral infections cause more damage to the baby when contracted earlier in the gestational period than later.

In labour: organisms may spread to the amniotic cavity through the cervix or can be acquired in the birth canal. Important agents include HIV, group B *Streptococcus* (GBS), *Gonococcus*, herpes simplex, hepatitis B, and *Chlamydia*.

Clinical signs and risk factors
- *Major*:
  - Rupture of membranes > 18 hours
  - Chorioamnionitis (infection of the intrauterine structures)
  - Maternal fever ≥ 38 °C
  - Fetal tachycardia > 160 bpm.
- *Minor:*
  - Maternal urinary tract infection
  - Rupture of membranes ≥ 12 hours
  - Low birth weight
  - Preterm labour
  - Maternal fever 37.5 °C
  - Maternal WCC > 15 000/µl
  - Multiple gestation
  - Foul-smelling lochia
  - Maternal GBS colonisation
  - Shirodkar suture.

Postnatal: cross-infection from: inadequate hand hygiene in a nursery, contaminated feeds or unsterile procedures. Important organisms: *Staphylococcus aureus, Klebsiella, Streptococcus, Enterococcus.*

Risk factors: prolonged invasive procedures, percutaneous lines, prolonged antibiotic use (especially broad spectrum) and ventilation. HIV may be transmitted in breast milk.

Clinical presentation
- Antenatal: suspect infection when:
  - Unexplained stillbirth
- Congenital abnormality, e.g. heart defect in rubella
  - Clinical signs are seen at birth, e.g. hepato-splenomegaly, rash, pallor.

- Postnatal: Hospital-acquired infections occur 72 hours or more after birth. Conjunctivitis and oral thrush are common. Cord and skin infections are less common. Group B *Streptococcus* meningitis usually occurs after 10 days of life.

Diagnosis

Clinical signs

- *Local infections*:
  - Conjunctivitis, omphalitis, skin pustules, thrush
- *Systemic infections*: the signs of invasive infections are often non-specific but the infant may present with:
  - Unstable temperature, lethargy
  - Poor sucking, failure to gain weight
  - Apnoea, respiratory distress
  - Hepato-splenomegaly, jaundice
  - Abdominal distension and vomiting

Laboratory investigations

Tests other than cultures have a 40% prediction rate. They should be used as indicators of infection in combination.

Gram staining or culture of bacteria from:
- Blood
- Cerebrospinal fluid
- Urine (catheter or suprapubic).

White cell count:
- Total count $< 5 \times 10^9/l$ or $> 20 \times 10^9/l$
- Immature neutrophils (bands) > 10% of total white blood cells
- IT ratio exceeds 0.2.

C-reactive protein (CRP) > 10: the rise may take 6 to 12 hours after clinical suspicion

Procalcitonin (PCT):
- Age and gestation dependant
- Expensive and poor marker of neonatal sepsis.

Rapid immuno-fluorescent tests

Virus identification:
- Tissue culture from blood, urine, throat swab, stool or cerebrospinal fluid. Viral particles seen, e.g. herpes simplex.
- Immunological and PCR.

Radiology

Chest X-ray: patchy infiltrates in pneumonia.

Abdominal X-ray: loops of bowel or thickened gut walls, with or without air-fluid levels and pneumatosis intestinalis in necrotising enterocolitis.

Bones: long bone abnormalities in syphilis and rubella.

Treatment

Start on immediate intravenous broad spectrum antibiotics. In a symptom free baby the CRP can be repeated in 12–24 hours. If all tests remain negative the antibiotics can then be stopped.

Important infections

Pneumonia: see p. 71

Meningitis

Organisms causing meningitis may cross the blood-brain barrier in bacteraemia. They may cross at congenital abnormalities such as a myelomeningocele. In the early stage, non-specific features of sepsis prevail.

Neurological signs are often late:
- Tense fontanelle
- Squinting
- Seizures
- Increased tone
- Coma.

Diagnosis:
- Obtain cerebrospinal fluid using a lumbar puncture.
- Microscopy: cells and organisms may be detected on a Gram stain.
- Culture, antigen screening and chemistry are of less use.

NB: Some suggest that every baby with a positive blood culture should have an LP.

Septicaemia

Bacteria can enter the blood from a colonized area or from a local infection.

Late signs are:
- Respiratory distress
- Hypothermia
- Bleeding tendency
- Sclerema/oedema.

The following complications may need to be treated:
- Hypothermia: heated crib or incubator
- Hypoxaemia: oxygen, ventilatory support
- Anaemia: packed red blood cell transfusion
- Shock: normal saline, inotropes
- Thrombocytopenia: platelet transfusion
- Bleeding tendency: Vitamin K and/or FFP
- Metabolic acidosis: volume replacement (use of sodium bicarbonate (4%) remains controversial)
- Meningitis and osteomyelitis.

Necrotizing enterocolitis (NEC)

NEC is an acute bowel disease of unknown origin usually associated with prematurity and/or events that cause bowel ischaemia.
- Early symptoms are characterized by feed intolerance, vomiting and abdominal distension. The disease may rapidly progress to gut perforation and cardiovascular shock.
- Abdominal X-rays may show evidence of thick-walled dilated bowel loops, pneumatosis intestinalis, portal venous gas, and pneumoperitoneum.
- Treatment is usually supportive and expectant. Enteral feeds are stopped and antibiotics are commenced with intensive care measures as appropriate instituted. In the case of failed medical management or bowel perforation, surgery is usually required to resect necrotic bowel.
- Despite advances in the care of premature infants, NEC remains one of the leading causes of morbidity and mortality in this population.

Urinary tract infection (see p. 224)

Organisms frequently seed out in the urinary tract in bacteraemia. An underlying abnormality such as hydronephrosis may predispose to infection. Signs are non-specific: jaundice or failure to thrive. Diagnosis depends on the growth of a single organism, with a bacterial count exceeding 100 000 organisms per mm^3 of urine. The culture must be done on a suprapubic or sterile catheter specimen of urine.

Ultrasound examination of the urinary tract is indicated.

> ***Practice point:***
>
> All babies with structural abnormalities of the urinary tract need prophylactic antibiotics and follow up.

Syphilis

Congenital syphilis may cause miscarriage, stillbirth, or severe illness in the newborn infant, or it may remain asymptomatic at birth and present only weeks or months later. All pregnant women should be screened for syphilis and treated if they test positive. An asymptomatic newborn born to a syphilis-positive untreated mother must be treated.

Clinical presentation:
- Asymptomatic
- Low birth weight
- Large/heavy pale 'greasy' placenta
- Peeling or blistering rash of hands and feet
- Hepato-splenomegaly, ascites, jaundice
- Pallor, purpura
- Respiratory distress.

Diagnosis:
An X-ray of the long bones usually shows metaphysitis (see Figure 2.3).

Serology: positive VDRL, RPR or rapid test for syphilis.

Figure 2.3 Congenital syphilis

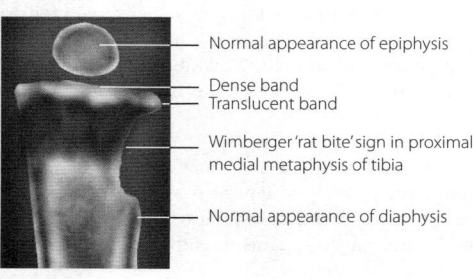

- Normal appearance of epiphysis
- Dense band
- Translucent band
- Wimberger 'rat bite' sign in proximal medial metaphysis of tibia
- Normal appearance of diaphysis

> **Practice point:**
>
> Asymptomatic infants born to women who have not been screened for syphilis often present with late signs of the disease.

Conjunctivitis (see p. 443)

Table 2.5 Treatment of important infections in the newborn ☆☆☆☆

Suspected infection	< 72 hours	Penicillin (50 000 units/kg 12 hrly) and gentamycin (5 mg/kg/day)	5–7 days
Suspected/ proven infection	> 72 hours	Penicillin as above, change gentamycin to amikacin; Amikacin (15 mg/kg/dose 24 hrly if > 32 wk gestation; 36 hrly if < 32 wk gestation)	5–7 days
Meningitis		3rd generation cephalosporins	14–21 days
Suspected listeriosis		Add ampicillin (50 mg/kg 6 hrly).	
Urinary tract prophylaxis	After acute infection has been treated	Ampicillin plus clavulanic acid 15 mg/kg/dose oral based on the ampicillin component 12 hrly/cefuroxime (10 mg/kg 12 hrly)	
Syphilis		Symptomatic infant Procaine penicillin 50 000 units/kg IMI daily OR penicillin G 50 000 units/kg IVI 12 hrly Mother incompletely treated or untreated, but infant asymptomatic Benzathine penicillin 50 000 units/kg IMI	10 days Single dose

Choices depend on culture results and varying resistance patterns.

Less serious infections

Omphalitis

Initially the skin at the base of the cord is red. A red flare may reach up towards the sternum. It later becomes oedematous and pus may ooze from the umbilicus. The risk of peritonitis or septicaemia is high. Omphalitis is caused by a variety of organisms. Obtain a swab for culture before starting treatment.

Skin pustules

Large, purulent or clear vesicles occur at any site, have a narrow red base, and contain Gram-positive cocci. *Staphylococcus aureus* is usually cultured. Skin sepsis is contagious and hand decontamination is essential.

> ***Practice point:***
>
> In a case of scattered single clear vesicles think of herpes infection. Pustular melanosis is a common benign cause of small skin pustules.

Thrush

This is caused by *Candida* species and involves the mouth or buttock area. White plaques adhere to the inner cheeks, lips, and tongue, and the underlying mucosa is red. Many napkin rashes are associated with *Candida*, especially in skin creases. The area may be red or excoriated or it may be peppered with punctate ulcers.

Treatment:
- Oral thrush: nystatin drops 1 ml PO 6 hourly
- Napkin rash: nystatin ointment to buttocks after each napkin change.

> ***Practice point:***
>
> *Candida* may contaminate the mother's nipples or vagina (treat mother as well) as well as bottles, teats, dummies, hands, or medications (educate about careful washing and hygiene).

HIV perinatal mother-to-child transmission

See Chapter 10, HIV infection.

Respiratory diseases of the newborn

Respiratory diseases usually present with acute respiratory distress. This is characterized by two or more of the following signs:
- Persistent tachypnoea
- Rib, sternal and subcostal recession
- Nasal flaring

- Expiratory grunting
- Central cyanosis.

Common causes include: hyaline membrane disease, transient tachypnoea of the newborn, meconium aspiration syndrome and pneumonia. Less common problems are pneumothorax and diaphragmatic hernia.

Hyaline membrane disease (HMD)

Definition
HMD usually occurs in premature infants due to developmental insufficiency of surfactant production and structural immaturity of the lungs.

Clinical features
Respiratory distress is apparent at birth and persists. Chest movement is impaired and the baby grunts to keep the alveoli inflated during expiration. As the disease progresses, the baby may develop ventilatory failure and apnoea. The symptoms of HMD usually peak by the third day and may resolve quickly after that.

Diagnosis
HMD is to be suspected in all preterm infants who present in the first few hours of life with respiratory distress and grunting. Chest X-ray demonstrates a diffuse granular appearance with air bronchograms, also known as 'ground glass appearance'.

Treatment
The incidence of HMD is reduced by antenatal maternal glucocorticoid administration, which should be encouraged in all potential preterm deliveries. ☆☆☆☆☾

In infants with HMD:
- Start nasal continuous positive airway pressure (NCPAP) as early as possible. ☆☆☆☾
- Keep the infant warm and ensure adequate hydration and nutrition.
- Intubate, administer surfactant, extubate (in/out) in confirmed HMD or if condition worsening. ☆☆☆☆☾
- Maintain saturations between 88 and 92%. ☆☆☆☾
- There should be minimal handling of the infant.
- If the infant deteriorates on NCPAP despite above measures, consider intermittent positive pressure ventilation (IPPV) or high frequency oscillatory ventilation (HFOV).

Transient tachypnoea of the newborn (TTN)

Definition

TTN is a self limiting disease with a higher incidence in newborns delivered by caesarean section. It has been postulated that TTN could result from delayed absorption of fetal lung fluid by the pulmonary lymphatic system. This results in reduced lung compliance and increased airways resistance.

Clinical features

Physical findings include tachypnoea with variable grunting, flaring, and recession. The infant is often described as having 'quiet' tachypnoea. Extreme cases may exhibit cyanosis.

Diagnosis

The presenting history is important. Chest X-ray demonstrates overinflation, fluid in the horizontal fissure and hilar streaking.

Treatment

The disease usually resolves within 24–48 hours. Treatment is supportive and might require supplemental oxygen via nasal prongs or NCPAP. Infants may require nasogastric tube feeding or IVI fluids in more severe cases.

Meconium aspiration syndrome (MAS)

Definition

Meconium is expelled *in utero* as a result of fetal distress. MAS occurs when infants inhale meconium into their lungs during or before delivery. This causes a pneumonitis, resulting in atelectasis and hyperinflation of alveoli.

Clinical features

Term babies, especially those who are wasted or underweight for gestation, are susceptible. Respiratory distress is present from or shortly after birth and the chest is over expanded and hyper-resonant. The umbilical cord, skin and nails may be stained with meconium.

Diagnosis

The presenting history and examination is important. Chest X-ray shows patchy shadowing throughout the lung fields with evidence of overinflation.

Treatment and prevention

The prevention of MAS remains difficult. The suctioning of meconium from the nose and throat of a vigorous baby at birth remains controversial. However, babies who are flat at birth should be suctioned below the cords if the attendant is skilled in intubation. ☆☺

The process should not delay resuscitation unnecessarily.

Treatment depends on severity. Mild cases may only require supplemental oxygen via nasal prongs while being able to feed normally. Infants may require NCPAP escalating to IPPV or HFOV.

In rare cases where ventilation fails, extracorporeal membrane oxygenation (ECMO) has been used to keep infants alive.

Pneumonia of the newborn

Definition

Bacteria may enter the lungs before, during or after birth. The group B *Streptococcus* is the most common organism. It colonizes the vagina in up to 30% of pregnant women and can be transferred to the fetus. Many infants are contaminated but few develop infection. Congenital pneumonia may complicate chorioamnionitis.

Clinical features

Preterm babies are vulnerable. Respiratory distress is present at birth or may occur later. Systemic signs of infection may predominate. These include lethargy, poor feeding, unstable temperature, cyanosis and shock.

Diagnosis

The presenting history is important. Chest X-ray demonstrates patchy shadowing and sometimes consolidation.

Treatment

Treatment is supportive and might require supplemental oxygen via nasal prongs or NCPAP in the first instance. In more severe cases the infant may require ventilation. Antibiotics should be started as soon as pneumonia is suspected and investigations performed to confirm pneumonia.

Pneumothorax and tension pneumothorax

Definition

Alveoli can rupture in any type of respiratory distress, particularly if high pressures are generated by assisted ventilation. The entrapped pleural air may compress the heart and blood vessels causing a tension pneumothorax.

Clinical features

Hyper-resonance and decreased air entry may be detected but are usually not obvious. Consider the diagnosis in an infant with deteriorating respiratory distress. Signs include cyanosis, a displaced apex beat, apnoea, pallor and poorly palpable pulses.

Diagnosis

Use a fibrescope to transilluminate the chest. A diffuse glow will be seen on the side of the pneumothorax. Chest X-ray demonstrates absence of lung markings on the affected side with collapsed lung. Tension pneumothorax is confirmed by mediastinal shift.

Treatment

Treatment is guided by the severity of signs and symptoms. Many infants who are not particularly distressed can be managed expectantly with supplemental oxygen via nasal prongs or NCPAP. If the pneumothorax is causing marked compromise or the infant is deteriorating, it requires drainage. A 10F intercostal drain should be inserted.

> ***Practice point:***
>
> CXR should not delay the insertion of an ICD in a collapsed neonate.

Persistent pulmonary hypertension

Definition

Persistent pulmonary hypertension is a cardiopulmonary disorder characterized by systemic arterial hypoxaemia secondary to elevated pulmonary vascular resistance with resultant shunting of pulmonary blood flow to the systemic circulation. Pulmonary vascular resistance remains high after birth because the vessels are inadequately dilated or are diminished or have thick musculature.

Clinical features

The infant presents with cyanosis and respiratory distress within the first day of life. A history of fetal distress, meconium stained liquor and birth asphyxia is typical.

Diagnosis

Oxygen saturation may improve after intubation, ventilation and sedation. The saturation may be significantly higher in the right radial artery than in the lower limbs, suggesting right to left shunting through the ductus arteriosus.

On chest X-ray the lung fields may be clear or show signs of meconium aspiration.

An echocardiogram demonstrates a normal heart structure with evidence of increased pulmonary pressures. The ductal shunt can be seen.

Treatment

Correct any predisposing factors, e.g. polycythaemia, metabolic acidosis. Establish adequate oxygenation (O_2 saturation above 90%). This can be difficult and may require 100% oxygen and assisted ventilation (IPPV or HFOV). Maintain normal blood pressure, with inotropes if necessary. The pulmonary vasculature can be dilated with the use of sildenafil or nitric oxide. ☆☆☆☗

Patent ductus arteriosus (PDA)

Definition

The ductus may remain patent after birth. This often occurs in preterm babies who have hyaline membrane disease.

Clinical features

A systolic heart murmur is audible in a preterm infant. Other signs include a wide pulse volume, tachycardia and cardiac failure.

Diagnosis

The clinical features are often sufficient to make a diagnosis but confirmation can be obtained by echocardiogram. Chest X-ray demonstrates cardiomegaly and pulmonary plethora. Assessment of the severity of the left to right shunt is best done by echocardiography. A large left atrium or reversed flow in the aorta may indicate a significant PDA.

Treatment

This may be required if the infant is symptomatic (tachypnoea, tachycardia, heart failure) or ventilator dependent. The decision to treat should be made by a senior clinician and is based on clinical signs and echocardiographic evidence of a large left to right shunt.

To treat:
- Restrict the intake of fluid to 120 ml/kg/day.
- Give ibuprofen intravenously (or orally but limited evidence for efficacy) in three doses of 10 mg/kg, 5 mg/kg, and 5 mg/kg at 24 hour intervals (alternative, indomethacin 0.2 mg/kg IV daily for 3 days) ☆☆◊
- Consider diuretics in refractory cardiac failure.

Neonatal jaundice

Between 50–60% of normal newborns become clinically jaundiced in the first week of life. The yellow discolouration is due to the accumulation of unconjugated bilirubin in the skin. Unbound, unconjugated bilirubin may cross the blood brain barrier, causing brain damage (bilirubin encephalopathy). Neonatal jaundice may be diagnosed as physiological or pathological. The diagnosis will indicate the management needed.

Physiological jaundice

Unconjugated bilirubin is the end product of haem metabolism. Physiological jaundice results because a newborn has:
- Increased production of bilirubin (increased erythrocyte mass and erythrocytes [containing fetal haemoglobin] with a shortened life span)
- Decreased hepatic excretion of bilirubin (low hepatocyte ligandin levels, low glucuronyl transferase activity)
- Increased entero-hepatic circulation of bilirubin (high intestinal β-glucuronidase levels, decreased intestinal motility).

Diagnosis
- Jaundice appears on day 2–3.
- It rarely lasts longer than 10 days.
- The maximum level of bilirubin is usually below 275 μmol/l.
- Only the unconjugated fraction of bilirubin is increased.
- The baby is clinically well.

Breastfeeding and breastmilk jaundice
- *Breastfeeding jaundice:* thought to be due to feeding problems, which lead to a decreased intake of milk, increased entero-hepatic circulation and sometimes dehydration.
- *Breastmilk jaundice:* diagnosed in clinically well breastfed infants who remain yellow for several weeks following physiological jaundice. The exact mechanism is unknown. A contributory factor is

thought to be breastmilk glucuronidase, which leads to increased absorption of unconjugated bilirubin via increased entero-hepatic circulation. Diagnosis is by exclusion. Breastfeeding may be continued. ☆☆☆☺

The bilirubin levels will usually stay elevated for 2 weeks, then slowly drop to normal by 4 to 12 weeks of age.

Pathological jaundice

Neonatal jaundice is considered to be pathological if it:
- Appears within 24 hours of birth, or
- Exceeds normal range for age and gestation (see phototherapy guideline charts), or
- Persists for more than 10–14 days in term infants and 21 days in preterm infants (prolonged jaundice), or
- Is mostly conjugated, or
- Is associated with systemic illness.

Pathological jaundice may result from an increase in unconjugated or conjugated bilirubin or a combination thereof (see Table 2.6). In most cases it is associated with unconjugated hyperbilirubinaemia. Conjugated hyperbilirubinaemia is rare and always pathological.

Table 2.6 Causes of neonatal hyperbilirubinaemia

Unconjugated hyperbilirubinaemia	
Excessive haemolysis	**Defective conjugation**
ABO incompatibility	Prematurity
Rhesus disease	Infection
Intracranial/other haemorrhages/haematomas	Infant of diabetic mother
Polycythaemia	Hypoglycaemia
Spherocytosis/elliptocytosis/other	Hypothyroidism
G6PD deficiency	Hypoxaemia
Conjugated hyperbilirubinaemia	
Hepatocellular injury (normal bile ducts)	Bile flow obstruction (with or without hepatocellular injury)
Congenital syphilis	Bile duct atresia
Other congenital infections	Choledochal cyst
Galactosaemia	Cystic fibrosis
Other inborn errors of metabolism	Total parenteral nutrition

Mixed unconjugated and conjugated hyperbilirubinaemia
Congenital infections
Postnatal infections
Severe haemolytic disease of the newborn

Assessment and management of neonatal jaundice

In assessing a jaundiced newborn, the aims are:
- To identify the infant who needs phototherapy or, rarely, exchange transfusion
- To make a diagnosis of the cause of jaundice, distinguishing between physiological and pathological jaundice.

Early onset jaundice: within 24 hours

This is likely to be caused by haemolytic disease of the newborn (ABO, Rh) and the following should be performed immediately:
- Check the mother's blood group.
- Check the level of total serum bilirubin (TSB) 3-hourly.
- Start phototherapy.

If mother's blood group is O, then ABO incompatibility is the most likely cause.

The following investigations are important:
- Blood groups of mother and baby – for incompatibilities
- Direct Coombs test – for antibodies on infant's red blood cells
- Haemoglobin or packed cell volume – for anaemia
- Peripheral blood smear – for abnormally shaped cells and excessive nucleated red blood cells
- Further tests are rarely required, but in unusual cases the following may be helpful: red cell enzymes (e.g. G6PD), haemoglobin electrophoresis.

Jaundice after 24 hours

A level of unconjugated bilirubin above the normal range requires careful assessment:
- Check the blood groups of mother and baby to exclude incompatibility.
- Examine the baby to exclude an obvious infection or extravasated blood/ bruising.
- Check on feeding and the baby's weight to exclude breastfeeding jaundice.
- Check the packed cell volume to exclude polycythaemia (PCV > 70).

Term baby

Often a cause will not be found. Jaundice is considered to be due to exaggeration of physiological hyperbilirubinaemia. Treatment will depend on the level of bilirubin, which should be checked daily. Phototherapy is given if indicated by the South African National Academic Hospital Guidelines: 2006 Charts (see Figure 2.5).

Preterm baby

In the absence of an obvious cause, jaundice is considered to be due to immaturity of the conjugating mechanism in the liver.

Treatment of neonatal jaundice

Prevention of Rhesus disease

- After delivery, give anti-D globulin to each Rhesus-negative mother within 72 hours of birth. It will prevent her developing anti-D antibodies if baby is Rhesus positive. Repeat the treatment after every subsequent pregnancy. ☆☆☆☆👍
- During pregnancy, any factors that can cause a significant transfer of blood from the fetus to the mother warrant the use of anti-D globulin. Includes abortion, ectopic pregnancy, antepartum haemorrhage, amniocentesis and external cephalic version. ☆☆☆☆👍

Phototherapy

Indications in term and preterm babies: see SA Neonatal Academic Hospital Guidelines: 2006 Phototherapy Chart (see Figure 2.5) www.usana-sa.co.za. ☆☆☆☆👍

- Baby birthweight < 2 kg is treated in an incubator, > 2 kg in a cot. If a transparent insulation material is necessary to maintain infant's temperature, monitor carefully as this may affect phototherapy efficacy.
- The baby is placed naked under the lights and the eyes are covered with gauze pads. Secure protective eye pads with micropore strapping or a commercial cloth harness. Remove eye pads during feeds.
- Monitor infant's temperature and ensure fluid intake is adequate (may need to supplement feeds with expressed breastmilk or formula).
- In haemolytic disease the response is unpredictable so check the serum bilirubin level several times a day.
- Position the phototherapy unit not more than 40 cm above the baby. For further details see the AAP Clinical Practice Guidelines for Management of Hyperbilirubinaemia in the Newborn Infant. ☆☆☆☆👍

Complications: rashes, loose stools, dehydration, hypo- or hyperthermia, 'spotlight' burns, separation from mother.

> ### Practice points:
>
> - Eye pads may obstruct nasal breathing.
> - Lights lose their efficacy after a certain time, depending on the type. Check and change regularly if light intensity cannot be measured.

Intravenous gamma-globulin:

In isoimmune-haemolytic disease, IV gamma-globulin is recommended if the TSB is rising rapidly, despite intensive phototherapy, or if the TSB level is within 50 mmol/l of the exchange level. Dose: 0.5 g/kg over 2 hours. This dose may be repeated. ☆☆◊

Exchange transfusion

Indications:
- Healthy full-term and preterm and ill infants of all gestations: See SA Neonatal Academic Hospital Guideline Exchange Transfusion Chart (see Figure 2.6) www.usana-sa.co.za. ☆☆☆◊
- Any infant who has clinical signs of acute bilirubin encephalopathy: immediate exchange transfusion. ☆☆☆☆◊
- Infants with severe anaemia complicated by cardiac failure who need a blood transfusion: consider exchange transfusion.

Method:
Double Volume Exchange = 160 ml/kg (term) or 180 ml/kg (preterm).
1. Umbilical venous catheter (UVC) method (push/pull): Aliquots 5 ml/kg, maximum 20 ml. Each cycle should last 1–2 minutes.
2. Peripheral method: Infuse warmed blood into peripheral IV line at 150 ml/kg/hour (12.5 ml/kg/5 minutes) and remove 5 ml/kg via arterial line every 1–2 minutes. ☆☆☆◊

> ### Practice point:
>
> Often by the time blood is available for the procedure, phototherapy has reduced the TSB to a level where exchange transfusion is no longer necessary. We do not proceed if exchange is no longer necessary.

Complications of unconjugated hyperbilirubinaemia

Bilirubin encephalopathy

Excessive levels of unconjugated bilirubin crossing the blood brain barrier can cause encephalopathy. Clinical signs vary from lethargy and poor sucking to opisthotonus, hypertonia, pyrexia, and convulsions. Late manifestations include learning disabilities, mental retardation, deafness and cerebral palsy. Kernicterus refers to the yellow-stained basal ganglia seen at autopsy.

The possibility of brain damage is increased by:
- Prematurity
- Sepsis
- Severe hypoxaemia
- Acidosis
- Drugs – especially sulphonamides.

> ***Practice points:***
> - The risk of bilirubin encephalopathy can be minimized by prompt phototherapy for unconjugated hyperbilirubinaemia, by preventing haemolytic disease caused by Rhesus sensitization, and by avoiding sulphonamides.
> - Before discharge, every newborn should be assessed for the risk of developing severe hyperbilirubunaemia (including TSB check), especially if infants are discharged before 72 hours of age. ☆☆☆☆

Severe anaemia

Severe anaemia may occur undetected in haemolytic jaundice.

Prolonged jaundice

Prolonged jaundice is defined as jaundice lasting more than 14 days in term infants and more than 21 days in preterm infants. The most common causes are breast milk jaundice, urinary tract infection, hypothyroidism, bile duct atresia (see p. 497), undiagnosed congenital syphilis and hepatitis. Less common is galactosaemia. The following steps should be taken:
- Determine whether or not the baby is breastfed.
- Collect urine to exclude infection and also test for reducing substances to exclude galactosaemia. ☆☆☆☆☆
- Measure the conjugated fraction of bilirubin and check liver enzymes.

(continued on page 82)

Figure 2.5 Phototherapy guidelines

PHOTOTHERAPY
GUIDELINES FOR ALL WEIGHTS AND GESTATIONS

In presence of risk factors use one line lower (gestation below) until 1 000 g.
If gestational age is accurate, rather use gestational age (weeks) than body weight.

Infants > 24 hours old with TSB level below threshold, repeat as follows:
1-20 μmol/l below line: repeat in 6–12 hrs, 21–50 μmol/l below line: repeat daily until levels are > 50 μmol/l below line, or jaundice is clinically resolving.

STOP phototherapy:
If TSB > 50 μmol/l below the line. Then recheck TSB in 12–24 hr.

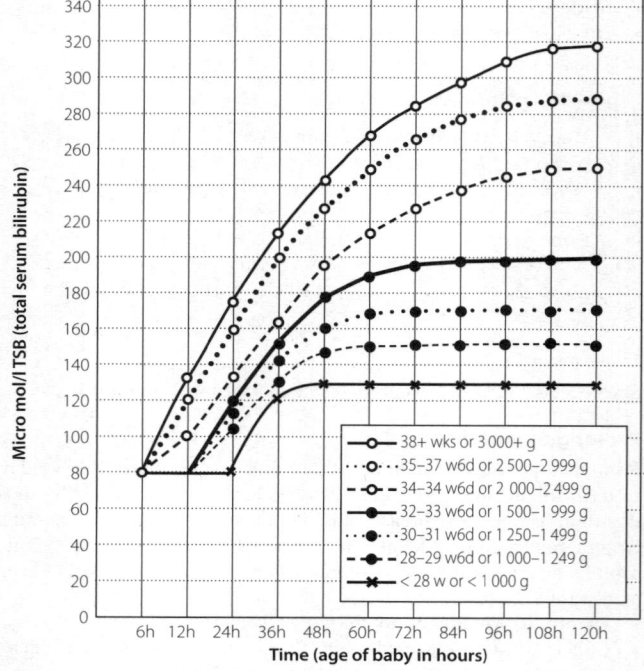

Horn AR, Kirsten GF, Kroon SM, Henning PA et al. Phototherapy and exchange transfusion for neonatal hyperbilirubinaemia. Neonatal Academic Hospitals Consensus Guidelines for South African Hospitals and Primary Care Facilities. *S Afr Med J*. 2006;96:819-824

Figure 2.6 Exchange transfusion guidelines

EXCHANGE TRANSFUSION
GUIDELINES FOR ALL WEIGHTS AND GESTATIONS

In presence of sepsis, haemolysis, acidosis, or asphyxia, use one line lower (gestation below) or levels 20 μmol lower if < 1 000 g.

If gestational age is accurate, rather use gestational age (weeks) than body weight.

> **Note:**
> 1. Infants who present with TSB above threshold should have Exchange done if the TSB is not expected to be below the threshold after 6 hours of intensive phototherapy.
> 2. Immediate Exchange is recommended if signs of billrubin encephalopathy and usually also if TSB > 85 μmol/l above threshold at presentation.
> 3. Exchange if TSB continues to rise > 17 μmol/l/hour with intensive phototherapy.

Levels for infants of 35 or more weeks based on AAP guidelines 2004 and levels for preterm infants based on guidelines by Maisels and Watchko 2003.

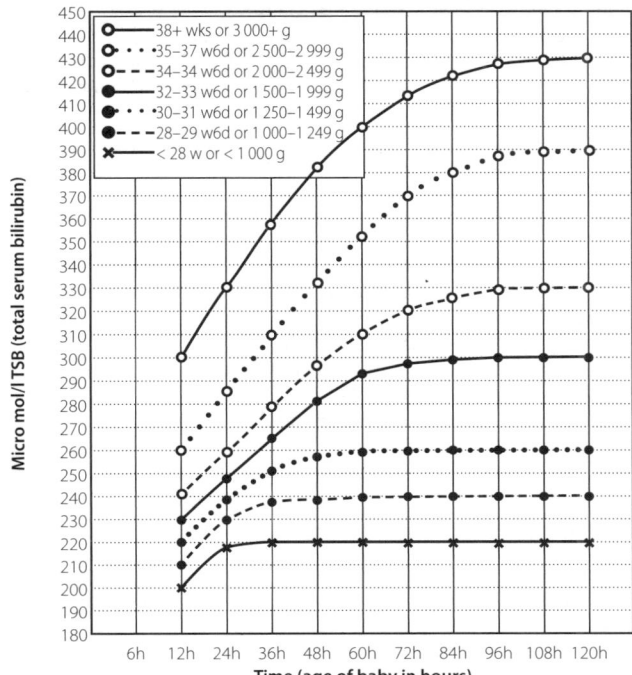

Horn AR, Kirsten GF, Kroon SM, Henning PA et al. Phototherapy and exchange transfusion for neonatal hyperbilirubinaemia. Neonatal Academic Hospitals Consensus Guidelines for South African Hospitals and Primary Care Facilities. *S Afr Med J.* 2006;96:819-824

- Test for syphilis.
- Check the infant's thyroid function (TSH and T4) to exclude hypothyroidism. ☆☆☆☆◍

Conjugated hyperbilirubinaemia

For details, see Chapter 4, Gastrointestinal problems.

Breastfeeding – getting the right start

Breastmilk is unique in that it is a living nutritional fluid. It contains cells, antibodies, enzymes and hormones. Formula has none of these. In addition, the methods of formula feeding markedly increase the risk of infection in the infant. Breastfeeding has been shown to significantly reduce infant morbidity and mortality in poorly resourced settings. ☆☆☆☆◍

It is therefore vital to encourage all mothers to breastfeed from the start to ensure the survival of their newborn infants.

WHO and Unicef launched the Baby Friendly Hospital Initiative (BFHI) in 1991 following the Innocenti Declaration of 1990. The BFHI aimed at ensuring that all maternity facilities should become centres of breastfeeding support.

The BFHI starts with 'The Ten Steps to Successful Breastfeeding'. Each maternity facility should:

1 Have a written breastfeeding policy routinely communicated to all staff.
2 Train all health care staff appropriately to implement the policy.
3 Inform all pregnant women of the benefits and management/technique of breastfeeding.
4 Help mothers to breastfeed within one half-hour of birth.**
5 Show mothers how to breastfeed and maintain lactation even if separated from their infant.
6 Give newborn infants nothing beside breastmilk to eat or drink, unless medically indicated.
7 Practise rooming in: mothers and babies to stay together 24 hours a day.
8 Encourage breastfeeding on demand.
9 Give no artificial teats or dummies.
10 Facilitate the establishment of breastfeeding support groups and refer mothers to them on discharge.

** In 2006, the Global Criteria for the BFHI were revised; Step 4 is now interpreted as 'Place babies in skin-to-skin contact with their mothers for at least an hour immediately following birth and encourage mothers to recognize when their babies are ready to breastfeed, offering help if needed.' ☆☆☆☆◍

Getting the right start

- Antenatal education of the mother is very important.
- Regarding breastfeeding, she should know the advantages, correct position and latch, how to make sufficient milk, how to prevent sore nipples, mastitis, engorgement.
- The mother's decision to breastfeed ought to be made before the birth of her infant. With adequate and factual information an *informed choice* is possible.

Breastfeeding immediately after birth

- *Early feeding* profoundly influences the establishment and maintenance of lactation. Production of prolactin and oxytocin are stimulated.
- A healthy baby should be put skin-to-skin on the mother's chest at birth. Rooting and suckling in the awake, alert baby are particularly strong for the first 40 minutes of life.
- *Caesarean section.* A baby can be placed skin-to skin in theatre if mother is fully conscious after general anaesthesia or following spinal anaesthesia.

Rooming in

- Do not separate mother and infant unless there is a medical indication.
- To initiate lactation, frequent feeding is essential and a mother needs to learn the subtle hunger cues: sucking, rooting, mouth and tongue movements, hands to mouth, wriggling and soft sounds.
- Crying is the last sign and by this time the baby is often frantic and needs a lot more time, effort and patience to get on the breast.

Positioning

- There are many ways to hold a baby for feeding and each mother and infant should be encouraged to find the most comfortable arrangement.
- Whatever the position, ensure that the baby's head faces the mothers breast. The baby must look directly at the breast. Mother and baby should be skin-to-skin, baby's tummy touching mother's tummy, nose at the same height as the nipple.

Latching

- When the infant's mouth opens in response to the rooting reflex, place the baby's mouth *over the whole areola*. This encourages the

baby to continue to suckle as the nipple is at the junction of the hard and soft palate. The more the baby suckles the more milk is produced.
- Do not permit baby to suck just on the nipple – it's hard work and frustrating for the baby. For the mother it is painful and causes sore, then cracked nipples.
- The nipples must not be washed before each feed. This disturbs natural secretions that keep the area supple.
- *Cracked nipples*: apply a few drops of colostrum before and after feeds. Important: correct the latch.

Expressing milk

This may be necessary if mother is separated from baby for any length of time, or in the case of maternal HIV. The milk can be stored until needed.
- *Hand expression.* Sit mother comfortably and instruct her to gently and rhythmically compress the areola between the thumb and forefinger. This is done vertically and horizontally while pressing the 2 fingers together. It should be painless and the breast must not be squeezed or pulled.
- *Breast pump.* This is faster but strict hygiene is necessary. Avoid devices that allow milk to flow through their suction chamber. They are difficult to clean. Rather use those that collect milk in a receptacle. *Because of infection risk, breast pumps must never be shared.*
- The more the breasts are emptied, the more milk they produce.
- Normal breastmilk may have a grey, blue or yellow tinge and the colostrum may be watery. Reassure the mother.
- *Heat-treating expressed breastmilk* (Pretoria pasteurization or flash heating) is a method of rendering breastmilk safe for the babies of HIV-positive mothers who choose to breastfeed. This is particularly applicable and the feeding method of choice for premature babies of HIV-positive mothers.

For further information, consult: www.milkmatters.org

Milk storage

- Collect milk in a clean glass, plastic or stainless steel container labelled with the mother's name and the time and date. The lid must form a tight seal. Expressed milk may be frozen.
- Donated pasteurized breastmilk is available in certain parts of the country to premature babies below 1 500 g whose mothers are unable to produce milk due to serious illness or absence. Donor milk

banks are situated in the Western Cape, Gauteng, the Free State and KwaZulu-Natal.

For further information, consult: www.milkmatters.org

Demand feeding

- Babies should feed as long and as often as they desire.
- Allow one breast to be emptied before the other is used and start successive feeds on alternate breasts. *Timing feeds, e.g. 10 minutes a side is incorrect.*
- Initially a baby may feed frequently for short periods (a few minutes each hour) as only a small amount of colostrum is available. Thereafter feeding periods are longer and less frequent. Low birth weight infants and those with certain medical conditions (e.g. infants of diabetic mothers) need to feed regularly.
- Small infants should not go longer than 3 hours without feeding.

Breast engorgement

- Uncomfortable fullness can be avoided by correct positioning, latching and by feeding frequently.
- The problem usually begins on day 3–5 and is characterized by low-grade fever and throbbing, swollen, warm, red breasts.
- Treat this promptly to prevent complications: gentle breast massage and warm compress application before a feed. Cold compresses and cabbage leaves may be used between feeds.

Mastitis

- A tender spot on the breast without fever indicates a plugged milk duct. A tender spot with fever exceeding 38 °C is most likely due to mastitis.
- Continue breastfeeding, as emptying the breast will relieve symptoms and engorgement.
- Apply warm packs to the affected area and prescribe an antibiotic (e.g. flucloxacillin) compatible with breastfeeding for 10 days.

Breast abscess

This is characterized by a red, tender fluctuating mass in the breast that requires surgical drainage, antibiotics and rest. In most cases breastfeeding may be continued as it relieves engorgement and does not prevent healing.

Exclusive breastfeeding for 6 months

- This implies no water, juice, herbal infusions, cereals or solids. It is particularly important when there is a family history of atopy or when an HIV-positive mother has opted for exclusive breastfeeding.
- Babies do not need water. Breastmilk is sufficient to quench thirst.
- Weaning foods may be introduced after 6 months.
- A mother may feed for as long as she desires. The WHO recommends breastfeeding for 2 years. In some societies 4 years is the norm.

Artificial teats and nipple shields

- Avoid teats when giving breast-fed babies expressed milk. The mechanism of sucking on a teat is quite different from suckling at the breast and can cause nipple confusion. Rather use a cup or spoon.
- Cup method. Support the baby upright on your lap and place the rim of the cup on the lower lip. Tilt the cup so that the milk surface comes in contact with the infant's mouth. Do not pour. Baby will pace the rate at which milk is lapped.
- Shields are sometimes recommended for inverted nipples. Avoid them if possible as they cover the areola and prevent stimulation during suckling thereby diminishing milk production. Correct latching will correct the inverted nipple.

Inadequate breastfeeding

Mothers sometimes stop breastfeeding because they feel their milk is insufficient.

The signs of correct feeding are:

- The infant should have at least 6 wet nappies a day, swallow regularly while breastfeeding and gain weight.
- If the infant fails to thrive and illness is excluded, check the latch, ensure one breast is being emptied before the other is used and that successive feeds are started on alternate breasts.
- Encourage the mother to hand express after each feed (preferably 2 hourly) and cup feed the baby the expressed breastmilk.
- Keep mother and baby skin-to-skin if possible.
- With increased frequency of breastfeeding the milk supply will increase.

Breastfeeding support groups

Failure to breastfeed is often attributed to a lack of time and support rather than a lack of milk. Thus breastfeeding support groups in the community play an invaluable role in successful breastfeeding.

Recommended reading

1. Hertz, GS. 2007. *Little Green Book of Breastfeeding Management* 4th ed (South African version) for further details of breastfeeding management (available from the National Department of Nutrition).
2. *South African Handbook of Resuscitation of the Newborn*. SAPA and University of the Witwatersrand. Johannesburg. 2004.
3. Horn, A. 2007. *Fluid Requirements and Supplements: Neonatal Drug Doses and Normal Values*. 2nd ed. 2007. Available from School of Child and Adolescent Health, University of Cape Town.
4. Horn, A. *et al*. Phototherapy and exchange transfusion for neonatal hyperbilirubinaemia. Neonatal Academic Hospitals Consensus Guidelines for South African Hospitals and Primary Care Facilities. *S Afr Med*. 2006; 96:819–824.

3 Respiratory problems

M. Klein, H.J. Zar

Respiratory illness is important, not only because it is a major cause of death but because it is the most common cause of acute and chronic illness in childhood. It may lead to permanent impairment of lung function and to chronic lung disease in adulthood.

An approach to cough

Cough is the most common presenting symptom of respiratory illness and the differential diagnosis includes almost all respiratory problems.

Cough is the patient's personal physiotherapist. It gets things out of the airway and prevents things from getting deep into the lung.

Only if a child has difficulty coughing will chest physiotherapy be beneficial.

Inability to cough may be an emergency.

Cough for longer than 2 weeks is a red flag for TB.

Psychogenic cough is a rare psychosocial disorder due to anxiety or stress. Patients are of school going age or older. Cough is loud, with an unnatural barking or 'honking' character. Cough is absent during sleep. Onset often follows a mild respiratory tract infection and then the cough persists. Cough itself may irritate the airway mucosa, helping to perpetuate the condition.

> *Practice point:*
>
> Because cough is beneficial it should not be suppressed. Over-the-counter cough and cold mixtures are contraindicated under 4 years of age. They should never be given under 2 months of age. Adverse effects include coma, convulsions and death.

An approach to fast breathing

Causes
- Fever from any cause
- Pneumonia
- Anxiety
- Pain
- Dehydration – metabolic acidosis
- Lung congestion – left-to-right cardiac and extracardiac shunts: VSD, ASD, PDA
- Pulmonary oedema
- Severe anaemia (Hb < 4 g/dl)
- Salicylate intoxication.

Respiratory rate limits

IMCI guidelines for primary health care workers include respiratory rates above the following limits.

Table 3.1 Respiratory rate limits for age

Age	Upper respiratory rate limit
< 2 months	60 breaths a minute
2–12 months	50 breaths a minute
1–5 years	40 breaths a minute

An approach to noisy breathing

Normal breathing is quiet. Noisy breathing implies airway obstruction.

The challenge is to identify the site of obstruction, rather than what label to 'call' the noise.

Finding the site of obstruction

The kind of noise – less helpful

Similar sounds arise from different sites (Table 3.2). So it is not helpful to decide if the noise sounds like stridor, wheezing or snoring. The sounds are not always easy to tell apart and doctors are not always in agreement as to what to call a noise.

Even if one could tell them apart with certainty it would not help to identify the site of obstruction as the same noise can arise from different sites of obstruction.

Table 3.2 Noises according to site of obstruction

	Stridor	Wheeze
Nasopharynx and throat	+	0
Larynx	+	+
Trachea and bronchi	+	+
Peripheral airways	0	+

The loudness of noise – unhelpful

Loudness of noise varies with the severity of airway obstruction (Figure 3.1). For a given level of sound (horizontal arrow) airway obstruction may be mild (*A*) or severe (*B*). Total airway obstruction is silent.

Figure 3.1 The relationship between noise and obstruction

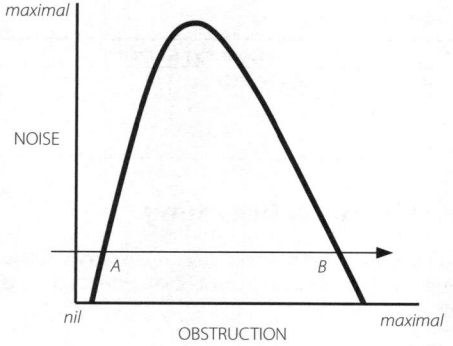

Sites of obstruction

There are 4 principal sites of obstruction: two above and 2 below the thoracic inlet.

Different conditions affect each site, thus if one knows the site of obstruction this limits the possible list of causes (Table 3.3).

Chapter 3: Respiratory problems 91

Table 3.3 Sites of airway obstruction and common causes at each site

SITE	COMMON CAUSES
Extrathoracic	
1 Nose and nasopharynx	Coryza, sleep-disordered breathing
2 Larynx	Laryngomalacia, croup
Intrathoracic	
3 Trachea and main bronchi	Vascular ring, TB nodal compression, foreign body
4 Peripheral airways	Asthma, bronchiolitis, bronchopneumonia, cystic fibrosis, aspiration syndromes: gastro-oesophageal reflux disease (GOR), chronic HIV-associated lung disease

Figure 3.2 Identifying the site of airway obstruction

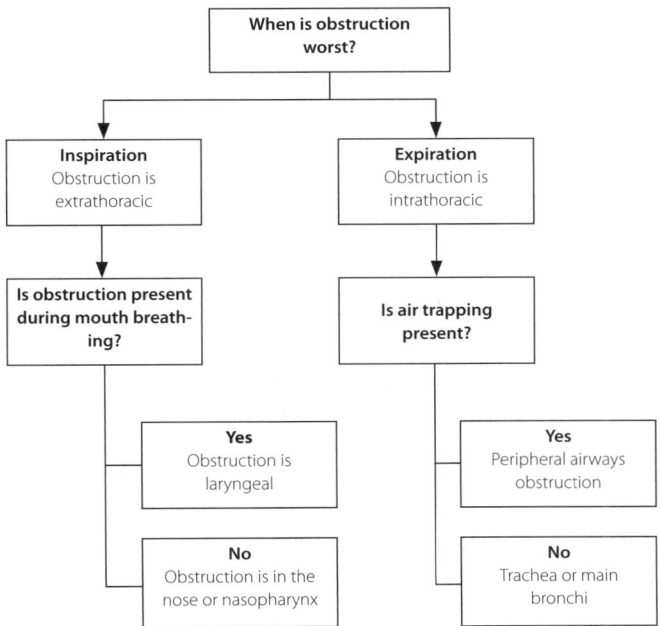

An approach to peripheral airway obstruction (PAO)

Airways divide approximately 14 times before the respiratory bronchioles and the respiratory zone of the lung are reached. Peripheral airways (beyond the fourth division) are thus the most numerous airways in the lung.

Peripheral airways are the most common site of pathology in lung disease in adults and children.

Table 3.4 Lung disorders with bilateral PAO (listed in order of probability)

Age	Acute PAO	Persistent or recurrent PAO
< 2 years old	Bronchiolitis Bronchopneumonia	Recurrent chest colds Aspiration lung disease Cystic fibrosis Asthma
> 2 years old	Asthma Bronchopneumonia	Asthma Aspiration lung disease Post-infective lung damage: HIV, adenovirus etc Cystic fibrosis

Tachypnoea, chest recession, wheezing and crackles (to a lesser extent) are all signs that can occur with PAO. However, they are often only present with severe obstruction.

There is only one physical sign that is specific for and diagnostic of PAO and which is detectable even when the other signs are absent: ***bilateral air trapping*** (BAT).

Because of the frequency and importance of peripheral airway obstruction, BAT should be screened for routinely in patients with any respiratory complaint

Clinical detection of bilateral air trapping (BAT) and PAO

Inspection: Hoover's sign: bilateral retraction of the costal margins with inspiration due to flat diaphragms in PAO. Harrison's sulcus is a fixed deformity, a groove as a result of outward flaring of the costal margins. Harrison's sulcus occurs with chronic PAO, but also with conditions such as rickets. Hoover's sign is common, Harrison's sulcus very uncommon.

Palpation: cardiac pulsation is difficult to feel. The liver and spleen are pushed down.

Percussion: resonant over areas that are normally dull: the upper border of the liver may be pushed down and cardiac dullness reduced or absent.

Auscultation: there are no auscultatory signs that are diagnostic of PAO. Wheezing is common, but it is also heard with tracheo-bronchial obstruction and occasionally even with laryngeal obstruction.

> *Practice point:*
>
> Do not miss persistent PAO. Percuss routinely for resonance over the heart and liver in all children with respiratory complaints. Missed PAO may delay the diagnosis of poorly controlled asthma, cystic fibrosis, or gastro-oesophageal reflux with micro-aspiration and severe lung disease.

Coughs and colds

All colds may go into the chest, but the chest component is usually asymptomatic or produces only a cough. It takes 6–8 weeks for post-viral airway inflammation to resolve. If the child has another cold in this time, inflammation occurs on that already present, causing a recurrence of cough or wheeze. This mechanism is responsible for most recurrent or prolonged chest infections (recurrent chest colds).

The usual causes of frequent coughs and colds are recurrent infections at day care centres, 'crèche syndrome' or parental smoking.

Smoking is a serious drug addiction. It is not easily overcome. Smokers need firm guidance, much encouragement and continuing support to help them quit. Counsel smokers to stop for the sake of their own and for their child's health.

Cigarette smoke is irritant and immunosuppressant. Passive smoking increases cough and wheeze, increases the risk of developing asthma, precipitates asthma attacks and makes asthma difficult to control. It is not sufficient for parents to avoid smoking in the presence of their child. Smokers are a source of infection. Smokers have increased carriage of respiratory pathogens and infect their own children. Thus children of smokers have more middle ear infections, croup, bronchitis, bronchiolitis, and pneumonia.

Treatment

Cough mixtures and cough suppressants are contraindicated. Pertussis is the only condition in which paroxysms of coughing are a severe problem and should be suppressed.

Use saline nose drops to liquify and promote drainage of mucus. Use oxymetazoline nose drops if nasal obstruction interferes with feeding or the child's sleep.

Pertussis: pholcodine 0.1–0.2 mg/kg/dose t.d.s. (a semi-synthetic codeine derivative) may be effective. Alternatives include salbutamol 0.15 mg/kg PO 6 hourly ☆☆☝, or chlorpromazine hydrochloride ✚ (Largactil®) 2 mg/kg orally stat. Repeat with 1 mg/kg increment every 3–4 hours until paroxysms are abolished. Then continue at that dose 6 hourly, reducing to 8 hourly and then to 12 hourly over 1 month. The objective is to abolish cough paroxysms, not the cough reflex. Control: tracheal or pharyngeal stimulation should elicit a cough but no paroxysm.

Asthma

Asthma is common. (See page 19.) With treatment, patients who are properly managed and take their preventive medicines regularly are able to live normal lives free of symptoms.

Diagnosis

The diagnosis of asthma is clinical and should be made in all children who meet the following 3 criteria:

- Recurrent wheeze, tight chest, or cough
- Wheezing precipitated by multiple triggers
- Wheeze responsive to a bronchodilator.

Asthma is one of the causes of peripheral airway obstruction. Other causes of peripheral airway obstruction (p. 92) should be considered in its differential diagnosis.

Practice point:

Do not assume that wheezing is due to broncho-constriction. It is not the only mechanism of wheeze. Do a clinical bronchodilator response test (BRT) in all children with wheezing. Only prescribe bronchodilator therapy for those who have a positive BRT: i.e. if there is an objective reduction in wheezing, respiratory rate or retractions within minutes of a therapeutic dose of an inhaled short-acting bronchodilator. Inhalation from metered dose inhaler (MDI) with small volume spacer and mask or mouthpiece is more effective than nebulization.

Laryngomalacia

This is the most common cause of noisy breathing in neonates.

Diagnosis

A confident clinical diagnosis of congenital laryngomalacia can be made if the following conditions are satisfied:
- Inspiratory noise may start at birth, but usually comes on insidiously during the first 10 days.
- The degree of obstruction and noise vary from breath to breath and often with posture. Some breaths are free and others obstructed.
- No expiratory obstruction.

Laryngomalacia may be simple or complex.

Simple laryngomalacia

This is the most common cause of noisy inspiration during infancy. The larynx is structurally normal. Malacia refers to laxity of the supraglottic soft tissues, which are sucked into the laryngeal lumen with inspiration. It is a benign condition although the noise can provoke anxiety. Obstruction and noise improve with growth and often resolve by 1 year of age.

Complex laryngomalacia

Laryngeal dysfunction is part of a more widespread neuro-developmental problem. In addition to the above symptoms there may be difficult drinking, dysphagia, laryngeal incompetence with pulmonary aspiration, or vocal cord paralysis.

Symptoms may ameliorate with growth but usually do not resolve completely.

Investigations

- Laryngoscopy. Not routinely indicated. Perform if airway obstruction severe, failure to thrive, or suspicion of complex laryngomalacia.
- Barium swallow. Gastro-oesophageal reflux (GOR) may retard resolution of laryngomalacia. A barium swallow is indicated to look for GOR if the child chokes and splutters while feeding, vomits or has frequent regurgitation, failure to thrive, or worsening obstruction, or if symptoms don't improve after 2 to 3 months.

Management

Most need reassurance only. GOR requires treatment if present (p. 151). Laser excision of excess supraglottic tissue is indicated for severe obstruction, failure to thrive, or in cases in which the parents are distressed by the noise. In complex laryngomalacia tracheostomy may be required.

Bronchiolitis

This is the most common cause of severe acute viral lower respiratory tract infection under 2 years of age.

The condition is:
- Usually caused by respiratory syncytial virus or rhinovirus and is highly infectious
- Affects the peripheral airways causing bilateral air trapping and often wheeze
- Airway obstruction is due to inflammation and oedema and not muscle constriction
- Usual source of infection: adult with common cold, but may be from another child
- Mechanism of transmission: contaminated hands. Droplet transmission is less common. Adults are generally unaware of the risk posed by their hands.

Prevention

Avoid exposure to children and adults who have colds.

Promote hand washing. No one with a cold should touch a baby without first washing their hands.

No vaccine for active immunization is available. Passive protection for RSV bronchiolitis is conferred by palivizumab (Synagis®) but it is expensive and injections must be repeated monthly during the RSV season. Palivizumab reduces RSV-related hospitalization and ICU admission in premature infants and in infants with chronic lung and congenital heart disease. It does not reduce the need for mechanical ventilation and has no effect on mortality.

Clinical features

History. Usually, the illness starts with 1 to 2 days of nasal congestion, after which breathing gradually becomes more difficult. The child may start to breathe more rapidly and may exhale more forcefully. Infants may present with apnoea.

Examination reveals:
- Tachypnoea. Bilateral air trapping from peripheral airway obstruction with positive Hoover's sign and resonance on percussion over the heart and the upper border of the liver
- Pseudo-hepatosplenomegaly due to downward displacement of liver and spleen
- Wheeze with diffuse crackles on auscultation.

The pseudo-hepatosplenomegaly, tachypnoea and crackles may result in bronchiolitis being mistaken for heart failure

Diagnosis

Viral bronchiolitis is a clinical diagnosis based on history and clinical examination. Chest X-rays and viral identification are not required

Measure the oxygen saturation on room air using pulse oximetry.

Bronchodilator response test: some infants benefit from bronchodilation therapy, however the majority do not. The only way to tell is to do a BRT.

Treatment

Admit:
- If apnoeic spells
- If not drinking
- If oxygen saturation breathing air is < 90%.

Consider admission if there are underlying risk factors for severe disease, e.g. premature baby < 6 months old.

Fewer than 5% of children with bronchiolitis require hospital admission.

Nurse alone or cohort with children > 2 years of age and no underlying risk factor for severe illness.

No medications are indicated for children with mild or moderate bronchiolitis who do not need hospital admission. The objective of hospitalization is to maintain hydration and oxygenation.

Feeding. If unable to drink, give feeds by naso-gastric tube. Use normal feed volume in frequent divided amounts to minimize abdominal distension.

Oxygen by nasal prongs. Use 100% oxygen. Unless they are very thin, prongs should be cut off so that they do not enter (and obstruct) the nostrils.

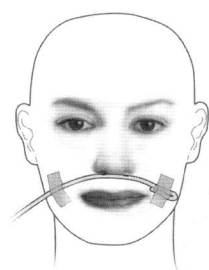

Figure 3.3 Nasal prong oxygen

Antibiotics are not routinely indicated.

Bacterial co-infection is rare in RSV bronchiolitis, except in severe cases such as those requiring ICU admission

Bronchodilator therapy is not recommended routinely and is not a reason for hospital admission. Bronchodilators can be given more effectively by MDI, with spacer and mask than by nebulizer.

Some infants with bronchiolitis respond to an inhaled bronchodilator but most do not. Assess whether wheezing children actually benefit from inhaled bronchodilators by administering a test dose of inhaled bronchodilator, i.e. do a clinical bronchodilator response test (BRT). If there is minimal improvement, inhalations should not be used. The idea that adrenaline may be more effective than ß-2 agonists has been disproved.

Intravenous fluid, if used, should not exceed 65 ml/kg/day unless diarrhoea is present.

Oral steroids are not effective or indicated

Therapy not recommended

The following interventions are *not* therapeutic and so are *not* recommended for the acute illness or during convalescence:
- Chest physiotherapy, except in children undergoing mechanical ventilation
- Induction of cough or regular suction
- Inhaled corticosteroids
- Oral corticosteroids.

Discharge and follow-up

Send the child home as soon as he or she is drinking and oxygen saturation is > 92% in air. Some tachypnoea, air trapping and crackles may persist for up to 4 weeks.

See hospitalized children 6–8 weeks after discharge, by which time air trapping has usually resolved. If air trapping is still present consider:
- Another intercurrent viral infection
- Cystic fibrosis
- GOR with micro-aspiration.

Post-bronchiolitic wheezing

Counsel parents that the child may cough or wheeze with every cold for about 2 years, that it is probably not asthma (but may be – most asthma attacks are precipitated by viral URTIs in young children) and does not respond to asthma medication, that the episodes will get progressively milder and less frequent and will finally stop, leaving no permanent lung damage.

The episodes will be more frequent, more severe, and persist for longer if the parents smoke.

Croup

Acute viral croup is the paediatric equivalent of adult acute laryngitis. Adults suffer from hoarse voice and cough and occasionally feelings of 'tight chest'. Adults rarely develop serious airway obstruction. This is common in young children because of their small airway dimensions.

Clinical features

A confident clinical diagnosis of acute viral croup can be made in children fulfilling all of the following criteria:
- Previously well
- Immunized against diphtheria
- Initial runny nose
- Cough and difficult noisy breathing (inspiratory stridor) and chest retractions developing gradually over a few hours
- Age 4 months to 4 years. Peak incidence in second year.

The following features are **not** typical of acute viral croup (Table 3.5).

Table 3.5 Features that are not typical of acute viral croup

Features	Condition
Sudden onset, very severe obstruction	Foreign body
< 4 months old	Congenital subglottic stenosis
Incomplete immunization	Diphtheria
Severe oral thrush	*Candida* laryngitis
Fever, erythema	Staphylococcal tracheitis
Fever, sore throat, dysphagia, drooling	Epiglottitis, retropharyngeal and peritonsilar abscess
Aphonia, previously hoarse	laryngeal papillomatosis

Diagnosis

Record oxygen saturation in air. Saturation < 92 % is rare in croup and should lead to a review of the diagnosis. Blood gases are unhelpful and unnecessary.

X-ray confirmation is indicated only if atypical features are present. A steeple sign on AP view is diagnostic of subglottic narrowing.

Severity. Treatment depends on the severity of airway obstruction, not on the noise (stridor).

The degree of airway obstruction is graded, not the stridulous noise, which gets softer as obstruction increases.

Criteria used in grading:
- Inspiratory obstruction: inspiratory noise (stridor), retractions, tracheal tug
- Expiratory obstruction: visible or palpable contraction of rectus abdominus muscles during expiration.
- Pulsus paradoxus: pulse becomes weak or disappears with inspiration. This can only be felt by pressing hard enough to just feel the pulse. Variation in the pulse force with breathing cannot be felt with strong pressure.

Table 3.6 Grades of obstruction

Grade	Inspiratory obstruction	Expiratory obstruction	Pulsus paradoxus
I	+		
II	+	+	
III	+	+	+
IV	Extremis: marked retractions, apathy, cyanosis		

Treatment

For all grades of obstruction give *corticosteroids*.

On diagnosis of acute viral croup give prednisone 2 mg/kg stat or dexamethasone 0.15–0.3 mg/kg. Give as a single dose. Oral and parenteral steroids are equally effective.

Benefit is seen in children with all levels of severity of croup, including mild cases.

Although there is no data to support it, a further dose may be given after 24 hours, but it should not be repeated.

If airway obstruction is worse 4 hours after receiving steroids, the diagnosis should be reviewed.

Grade 1 obstruction

Children with grade 1 obstruction can be sent home after getting steroids, with instructions to return if airway obstruction gets worse

Grade 2 obstruction

- Admit to hospital.
- Monitor oxygen saturation.

- Record vital signs and grade of obstruction 3-hourly until there is consistent improvement.
- Give adrenaline nebs as below.
- Comfort the child.
- Encourage parents to stay.
- Avoid everything that may induce crying as this will make the obstruction worse.
- Continue normal feeds.
- No blood tests.
- No IV unless child not drinking.
- Sedate with chloral hydrate if the child is not consolable.

Nebulized adrenaline

> **Practice point:**
>
> Adrenaline 'buys time' for steroids to do their work. It does not alter the course of the disease. All children who receive nebulized adrenaline must also receive steroids. All children who receive nebulized adrenaline must be observed for at least 3–6 hours to ensure no relapse occurs.

Mix 2 ml adrenaline 1:1000 (2 mg) with 2 ml saline. Nebulise the entire volume with oxygen at 5-6 l/min. Repeat half-hourly until the obstruction improves.

Tachycardia is frequent with severe croup and is not a contra-indication to adrenaline nebs. Tachycardia secondary to adrenaline occurs with systemic absorption if nebs are given to children with mild (Grade 1) obstruction. Tachycardia with grade 2 or more severe obstruction is an indication for adrenaline, not a contraindication.

Grade ≥ 3 obstruction

Grade 3 obstruction means the subglottic airway is narrowed to a slit. This is life threatening.
- Admit to ICU.
- Give continuous adrenaline nebs with oxygen.
- If 6 hours after giving steroids, obstruction remains grade ≥ 3, endotracheal intubation is advised.

Continued ICU observation beyond this time is only warranted under special circumstances.

Discharge and follow up

Stop nebs when obstruction is grade 1. Hospitalized children may be discharged 6 to 8 hours after their last required adrenaline. Routine post-discharge follow-up is not necessary. Croup may recur but recurrences seldom require hospitalization.

Febrile dysphagia syndrome

In order of frequency of occurrence, febrile sore throat and dysphagia occur with:
- Retropharyngeal abscess
- Epiglottitis
- Peritonsilar abscess
- Tonsillitis.

Epiglottitis

Epiglottitis is a cellulitis-like inflammation, spreading rapidly from its origin in the lingual tonsil to envelop the larynx and surrounding tissues from outside. The usual cause is *H. influenzae* type b. This has been rare in South Africa as it has been virtually eradicated by HiB vaccine.

Symptoms
- Fever
- Pain in the throat
- Difficulty swallowing
- No hoarseness
- Airway obstruction subtle despite risk of acute total occlusion.

Differential diagnosis

Peritonsilar and retropharyngeal abscess cannot be differentiated from epiglottitis on clinical grounds. Large retropharyngeal abscess may cause considerable airway obstruction but does not carry the risk of acute unpredictable obstruction, as with epiglottitis.

These may also compromise the airway through a mass effect. Epiglottitis is the most dangerous because it is unpredictable and fatal airway obstruction can occur suddenly without warning.

Diagnosis

Febrile dysphagia is an emergency. Call for specialist ENT and anaesthesia help. If none is available proceed with deliberate caution.

Inspect the throat if the mouth is opened willingly. *Never use a spatula* – gagging can precipitate total obstruction.

Lateral neck radiograph should only be requested if:
- Intubation equipment and someone who can use it accompany the patient.
- The child is allowed to adopt its own position of comfort and is not touched by anyone trying to position it for the X-ray.
- An experienced person is available to interpret the X-ray.

Management

Endotracheal intubation
Elective endotracheal intubation is the safest treatment for epiglottitis. Those with prior experience of the condition may elect to personally observe the child in an ICU for a few hours to assess the response to antibiotics and steroids.

Intubation technique:
- Select a tube one size smaller than predicted.
- *NEVER* attempt to see the vocal cords because it is impossible. They are hidden by the swollen epiglottis and surrounding tissues.
- Keep calm.
- Identify the epiglottis. It is markedly swollen anteriorly and curved backwards, *BUT* there is a groove along its posterior surface. Identify the posterior dimple at the tip of the epiglottis which is start of the posterior groove.
- Orientate the bevel of the endotracheal tube anteroposteriorly so that the tip makes a sharper point. Slide the point along the posterior groove of the epiglottis. This leads directly into the glottis which is usually entered without difficulty.
- Extubation can usually be attempted after 48 hours.

Figure 3.4 Intubation technique

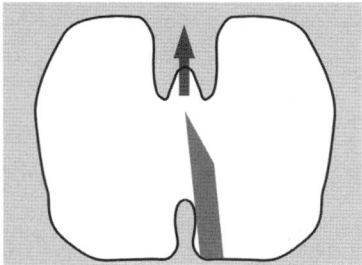

Antibiotics:
- Ceftriaxone 100 mg/kg IV stat, then 50 mg/kg after 24 hours and stop.
- Alternatives include cefotaxime or cefuroxime intravenously until extubation. Then complete a 5-day course with oral amoxycillin.

Corticosteroids:
- Methylprednisolone (2 mg/kg stat PO, maximum 60 mg) or dexamethasone (0.15–0.3 mg/kg IM/IV, maximum 12 mg). Prednisone or prednisolone (2 mg/kg) PO or by nasogastric tube 24 hours later.

Pneumonia

Community acquired pneumonia (CAP) is a common severe manifestation of lower respiratory tract infection. Prompt diagnosis and treatment reduces mortality and morbidity.

Primary health workers should follow IMCI guidelines on assessment and management of pneumonia.

Clinical features

Commonest symptoms are cough, difficulty breathing and fast breathing.

Respiratory rate and lower chest-wall indrawing are the most useful signs for diagnosis.

Pneumonia is diagnosed when a child has a cough or difficult breathing with tachypnoea (Table 3.7).

Severe/very severe pneumonia is diagnosed when a child has lower chest wall retractions or stridor or a general danger sign.

Diagnosis

Pulse oximetry should be performed on all children seen at a hospital to assess oxygenation.

Chest X-ray is indicated if:
- Clinical pneumonia is unresponsive to standard ambulatory management
- Suspected pulmonary TB
- Suspected foreign body aspiration
- Hospitalized children to detect complications.

Perform tuberculin skin testing (Mantoux method) and induced sputum or gastric lavage when TB is suspected.

Perform blood culture in hospitalized patients.

Other specimens for aetiological diagnosis may be required if clinically indicated, e.g. pleural fluid, induced sputum or respiratory secretions.

Treatment

All children with hypoxia (room air saturation of < 90–92%) should be given oxygen.

Malnourished children need nutritional rehabilitation (p. 153).

HIV-infected children should be considered for antiretroviral therapy (p. 307) and require broader antibiotic coverage, and treatment for additional pathogens such as *P. jirovecii* or CMV.

Children with pneumonia require ambulatory antibiotics, while those with severe pneumonia require hospitalization and antibiotics (Table 3.8). HIV-infected children may progress rapidly and require additional therapy (see Chapter 10, HIV infection).

Table 3.7 Clinical signs and severity of pneumonia

Clinical sign	Pneumonia category	Management
Lower chest indrawing	Severe pneumonia	First dose of IM/IV antibiotic Hospital referral Oxygen
Tachypnoea	Pneumonia	Oral antibiotic
No tachypnoea, No lower chest indrawing	No pneumonia	Supportive treatment

> ***Practice point:***
>
> Prevent unnecessary or prolonged hospitalization for pneumonia. This exposes children to life-threatening nosocomial infection.

The following is an admission and discharge guide:

Admission criteria: failure to drink or oxygen saturation < 92% in air. Need for IV antibiotics, but many cases of pneumonia can be treated with oral antibiotics from the start or can be changed from IV to oral as soon as there is definite improvement.

Discharge when the child is improving and the indications for admission have resolved, the child is drinking, saturation is > 92% in air and the child is on oral medication.

Antibiotic therapy

All children with pneumonia should receive antibiotics.

Table 3.8 Antibiotic therapy for pneumonia

	Ambulant	Hospitalized
0–2 months	Recommend hospitalization of all children less than 2 months of age	Ampicillin/Penicillin IV + aminoglycoside IV or Ceftriaxone/cefotaxime IV
> 2 months to 5 years	High dose oral amoxicillin (30 mg/kg/dose tds)	Ampicillin IV/amoxicillin PO high dose. or Cefuroxime IV/amoxicillin-clavulanic acid or Cefotaxime/ceftriaxone IV Add: cloxacillin if suspect *Staphylococcus aureus*
5 years onwards	Amoxicillin PO high dose or Macrolide PO (erythromycin/clarithromycin/azithromycin) –if suspect *Mycoplasma pneumoniae* or *Chlamydia* spp	Ampicillin IV/amoxicillin PO high dose or Cefuroxime IV/amoxicillin-clavulanic acid or Cefotaxime/ceftriaxone IV Add: cloxacillin if suspect *Staphylococcus aureus* Add: macrolide if suspect *Mycoplasma pneumoniae* or *Chlamydia* spp

The first antibiotic is the antibiotic of choice.

Add an aminoglycoside to all hospitalized children known to be HIV infected or if the child is suspected of being HIV infected or if severely malnourished.

Add a macrolide if *C. trachomatis* is suspected in children younger than 6 months.

Add cotrimoxazole (10 mg/kg IV load then 5 mg/kg IVI qid) if PCP is suspected in an HIV exposed child less than 1 year of age and in any HIV infected child not taking PCP prophylaxis and not on antiretrovirals (☆☆☆☆◉). Consider oral PCP treatment (double IV dose) if not severely ill. For children with suspected PCP and hypoxia, corticosteroids (prednisone 1 mg/kg tapered over 10–14 days) may be of benefit.

S. aureus should be suspected in children who fail to respond to therapy in 48 hours or those with suggestive CXR changes such as the presence of a pneumatocoele, empyema or abscess.

Mycoplasma pneumoniae and *Chlamydia* spp should be suspected if there is no clinical response to beta-lactam within 48 hours of starting treatment, or if there is wheezing in children older than 5 years of age. Treat with a macrolide.

> **Practice point:**
> Do not overuse intravenous antibiotics. Oral antibiotics are as effective for non-immunosuppressed children for pneumonia.

Consider high dose oral amoxicillin (30 mg/kg per dose tds) in hospitalized children who are not severely ill or immunosuppressed, older than 3 months and in whom there is no risk of aspiration. Unless there is a specific indication for a longer course, antibiotics should be given for 5–7 days.

Sleep-disordered breathing (SDB)

SDB is the preferred term for upper airway obstruction during sleep. It encompasses the spectrum from mild to very severe airway obstruction with intermittent totally obstructed episodes (TOES). Obstructive sleep apnoea syndrome (OSA or OSAS) is a sleep-laboratory diagnosis and is too restrictive to be of clinical use.

> **Practice point:**
> SDB is common but is often missed because health workers may not screen routinely for snoring. Serious adverse effects may occur, resulting in severe complications.

Severely affected children may appear normal when awake or have problems that may not immediately suggest the diagnosis. Screen for snoring during routine child care visits.

SDB is associated with increased respiratory effort, impaired ventilation, impaired oxygenation and impaired sleep quality. Complications from SDB include growth impairment, behaviour problems, neurocognitive impairment, cor pulmonale, and death. Children under 2 years of age are particularly vulnerable.

Table 3.9 Adverse effects of SDB according to presumed pathogenesis

Fragmented sleep	Asphyxia	Negative pleural pressure

· **Developmental delay**
· Failure to thrive
· Learning difficulties
   Inattention
   Blunted intellect
· Behavioural disorders
   Hyperactivity
   Aggression
· Pathological shyness
· Social withdrawal
· Morning headache
· **Restless sleep**
   Sleep walking
   Enuresis
   Nightmares
· Daytime somnolence
	· **DEATH**
	· Near-SIDS
	· **Permanent CNS damage**
	· Cardiac arrhythmia
	· Pulmonary hypertension
	· Congestive heart failure
	· Systemic hypertension
		· Aspiration pneumonia
		· 'Bronchitis'
		· Chest deformity
		· Pulmonary oedema

Fragmented sleep probably accounts for most complications. There is considerable interaction between mechanisms: adverse neuro-developmental outcomes are due to summed effects of sleep fragmentation and asphyxia.

Children with SDB are usually normally grown or thin, unlike adults with SDB who are often obese.

History

The diagnosis of SDB can usually be made on the history alone, supplemented when in doubt by cell phone video of the child sleeping. Only in rare cases is hospital admission and close observation with saturation monitoring necessary. No special investigations are necessary to prove the diagnosis or assess severity as a guide for surgical treatment.

Snoring. Snoring is common in childhood. It affects 18–20% of infants, 7–13% of 2–8 year-old children, and 3–5% of older children. Isolated snoring for < 3 months is usually benign.

The absence of daytime symptoms and a normal physical examination, normal radiology and normal endoscopy in an awake child do not rule out SDB.

Examination

Awake: usually normal, although severely affected children may have snoring sounds and mouth breathing even when awake.

Asleep: noisy breathing and increased respiratory efforts usually corroborate parental accounts.

Diagnosis

- X-ray postnasal space: to confirm that the adenoid is present.
- FBC: polycythaemia is rare and does not exclude life-threatening obstruction.
- ECG: usually normal. ECG is an extremely insensitive test for pulmonary hypertension.
- Cardiac ultrasonography: a degree of pulmonary hypertension is present in only about a third of the most severely affected children. It is therefore a very insensitive guide to the severity of SDB.

Treatment

Treat allergic rhinitis (p. 325).

Use saline or long acting decongestant oxymetazoline or xylometazoline drops at bed-time for snoring with blocked noses from colds. Ephedrine nose drops should no longer be prescribed. Oral cough and cold medicines are contraindicated under 4 years of age.

Indications for adenoidectomy:
- History of snoring every night for > 4 months with failure of medical management
- Snoring of any duration, which is associated with a history suggestive of episodes of totally obstructed breathing (TOES) or cyanosis
- Frequent snoring with any complication listed in Table 3.9
- Presence of adenoidal tissue (not enlargement) on X-ray of postnasal space or on nasal endoscopy with a classical history as above.

Tracheostomy may be required if SDB is due to anatomical abnormality of the nose or pharyngeal airway, e.g. Pierre Robin syndrome.

Emergency airway relief for SDB

Continuous insufflation of pharynx (CIP) is an effective, simple, safe alternative to endotracheal intubation or emergency tracheotomy prior to adenoidectomy for children with life-threatening obstruction. CIP should be continued for about 12 hours after adenoidectomy as operative swelling, blood clots and retained secretions may obstruct the airway at this time.

Before children are discharged after adenoidectomy they must be closely observed for a full sleep cycle to confirm that the obstruction has been relieved.

Aspiration lung disease

Aspiration lung disease results from recurrent aspiration of milk or other food. Lung damage results from hydrolysation of aspirated milk fat and gastric pepsin, not the acid. Therefore antacids have limited benefit.

Causes

The list is in descending order of incidence. All are important to recognize. GORD is the most difficult to diagnose.
- Gastro-oesophageal reflux disease (GORD)
- Laryngeal incompetence
- Oesophageal obstruction and spill-over
- Tracheo-oesophageal and broncho-oesophageal fistula.

GORD-associated PAO (GORD-PAO)

GOR is by far the most common cause of the aspiration syndrome

Diagnosis

Two criteria are required for the diagnosis of GORD-associated PAO: PAO without other cause and demonstration of GOR.

PAO. Presence of persistent peripheral airways obstruction for which there is no obvious cause such as BPD, previous severe viral pneumonia, CF, etc.

The clue to the possibility of an aspiration syndrome is persistent peripheral airway obstruction. The key is to routinely check for bilateral air trapping by percussion when examining a child's lungs. Consider the possibility of GORD in all children with persistent PAO.

GORD. Demonstration of one or more episodes of gastro-oesophageal reflux into the proximal carina during a 30 minute period by nuclear medicine 'milk scan', or if that is not available, the demonstration a similar frequency of proximal reflux by intraluminal oesophageal pH or impedence manometry.

Contrary to expectations, regurgitation and vomiting are very uncommon in children with GORD-associated persistent PAO, possibly because the large milk boluses elicit airway protective reflexes

Micro-aspirations are not seen radiologically or by isotope studies. If barium or isotope labelled feed enters the airway during swallowing then laryngeal incompetence, laryngeal cleft or tracheo-esophageal fistula are present (see below). Proximal reflux in association with laryngeal incompetence is a malignant combination.

Fat laden macrophages in BAL fluid are non-specific, are commonly found in ICU patients with acute lung injury, and should not be used for the diagnosis of milk aspiration.

Treatment

Medical treatment should include the use of thick cereal feeds, postural positioning and acid suppression.

Because GOR-induced oesophagitis is common and because oesophagitis may worsen reflux, it is reasonable to treat for oesophagitis empirically for 1 month: omeprazole is the acid suppressor of choice (preferable to H_1 antihistamines) with the addition of alginate for the first week only. The surgical treatment of GOR induced persistent PAO is fundoplication. The severity of reflux should be re-evaluated before doing fundoplication.

Gastric acid inhibitors may increase the risk of pneumonia and gastroenteritis, so their long-term use is not encouraged.

Laryngeal incompetence

Laryngeal incompetence is the aspiration of fluid while drinking.

Causes of laryngeal incompetence:
- Congenital (rare): laryngeal cleft
- Neuromuscular dysfunction: transient: following prolonged endotracheal intubation or severe croup. Chronic: cerebral palsy, familial dysautonomia, myositis, scleroderma.

Diagnosis

Contrast enters the airway on barium swallow. Identification of laryngeal cleft requires rigid bronchoscopy. The cleft may be invisible unless some pressure is put on the laryngeal inlet with the rigid scope.

Treatment

Treatment is surgical closure of the cleft.

The principle of medical management: liquid is aspirated, semisolids are not.

All nutrients should therefore be given in semisolid form, i.e. they must not run out of the spoon when it is tipped. The only liquid given is unflavoured water. Water often elicits a cough but its aspiration does the lung no harm

Tracheo-oesophageal (TOF) and broncho-oesophageal fistula

Table 3.10 Congenital and acquired tracheo-oesophageal and broncho-oesophageal fistula

Congenital TOF • With oesophageal atresia • Isolated – extremely rare	Presents at birth Presents with aspiration syndrome at any age. Specific TOF barium study and rigid bronchoscopy required for diagnosis
Acquired	TB node erosion may create fistula between oesophagus and trachea or bronchi. The fistula is usually large and demonstrated on conventional barium swallow

Bronchiectasis

Bronchiectasis is the irreversible structural dilatation of bronchi. The term is occasionally used more loosely to include reversible dilatation associated with atelectasis.

Classification of bronchiectasis

Symptoms and disability in patients with bronchiectasis are related to 2 factors: the severity of sepsis (as measured by quantity of sputum production) and the severity of peripheral airway obstruction. With this in mind, patients can be categorized into 4 groups with type A being the least, and type D being the most, disabling.

Table 3.11 Classification of bronchiectasis

		Peripheral airways obstruction	
		Absent	Present
Sputum	**Absent** (dry)	A	B
	Present (wet)	C	D

Where peripheral airway obstruction is absent (types A and C), the primary insult is localized to bronchial obstruction by a foreign body or tuberculous node. Secondary infection destroys the dependent lobe or lung but the remainder of the lungs are normal and the primary cause may have resolved by the time the patient is seen

Where peripheral airway obstruction is present (types B and D) there has been diffuse lung injury by causes such as recurrent aspiration, severe viral pneumonia (e.g. adenovirus), recurrent HIV-associated or agammaglobulinaemia-related pulmonary infections, and cystic fibrosis. These causes do not affect the lung homogeneously. The same injury produces chronic bronchiolitis in one place and bronchiectasis in another.

Clinical features

Bronchiectasis = clubbing with chronic cough and purulent sputum and halitosis.

Diagnosis

Bronchiectasis is primarily a clinical diagnosis.

CT scanning to confirm bronchiectasis is only justified if the patient's clinical condition and symptoms suggest that resection may be warranted. If bronchiectasis is not obvious clinically, it should not be sought.

In addition to being dilated, bronchiectatic airways are shortened and have fewer branches, due to the destruction of surrounding lung tissue.

Bronchography, the gold standard, is no longer available. CT gives reliable information regarding diameter and can identify mucus retention in the most severely affected airways.

Treatment

Medical:
- Promote sputum drainage with physiotherapy and bronchodilators.
- Control halitosis with metronidazole. When halitosis is recurrent use maintenance metronidazole 200 mg 12 hourly.
- Other antibiotics are used only for acute exacerbations and never for maintenance: *H. influenzae* is the most common chronic bacterial pathogen in non-CF bronchiectasis. In children with CF, *P. aeruginosa* is commonest and specific strategies to prevent colonization or reduce bacterial growth should be used (see p. 140).

Surgery:
- Surgery is the treatment of choice for type B and D patients where feasible. The aim is to reduce sputum and the symptoms associated with it. Surgery will not benefit the symptoms of PAO and may make them worse. Type A patients generally do not warrant surgery.

Cystic fibrosis (CF)

Exclude CF in all children with persistent peripheral airway obstruction (air trapping). See p. 140.

Choking and foreign body inhalation (FB)

Choking

Choking on a FB is potentially life-threatening.

If a choking patient has an effective cough (alert, loud cough, able to vocalize, and able to take a breath before coughing), all manoeuvres are unneccessary and potentially dangerous.

If the child can't breathe and is unconscious, proceed directly to CPR. Finger sweeps are contraindicated as they may push a FB further into the airways. Inspection and removal under direct vision is recommended if time allows. If the child is conscious but has an ineffective cough perform 5 back blows followed by 5 chest thrusts in infants < 1 year and 5 abdominal thrusts (the Heimlich manoeuvre) in children > 1 year.

FB inhalation

FB inhalation may be chronically asymptomatic, chronically symptomatic or acutely life threatening.

> ***Practice point:***
>
> Acute life-threatening FB aspiration is the *only* cause for the unexpected sudden onset of extreme breathing difficulty with very marked retractions – sternum virtually touching spine. Give oxygen and arrange for immediate bronchoscopy. Under no circumstances send the child for X-rays or give sedation.

Fortunately, the manifestations of FB aspiration are usually more subtle.

Diagnosis

History:
- In a child with respiratory symptoms, a history of choking makes the diagnosis of FB aspiration. But choking may not have been witnessed or the child may be too young to tell.
- The sudden onset of cough, wheeze or difficult breathing in a previously well, awake child should always be regarded as FB aspiration unless another explanation is found.
- Rarely, occult chronically retained FB may cause necrotizing pneumonia in patients with no previous history suggestive of FB aspiration.

Examination:
- Breathing may be noisy and laboured. Unilateral soft breath sounds are typical of FB in a main bronchus.

Radiology:
- Airway FBs are usually invisible. Ball-valve obstruction produces obstructive emphysema of a lower lobe or entire lung. If long-standing, there may be collapse instead. **A normal X-ray does not exclude a FB.**

FBs are not a cause of atelectasis affecting only upper lobes or right middle lobe. FBs are not a cause of the so-called right middle lobe syndrome.

Treatment

Although the threshold for bronchoscopy is low, not all children require bronchoscopy after choking.

Following a choking episode or the sudden onset of difficult breathing bronchoscopy is mandatory if any of the following are present:
- Tachypnoea, wheeze or cough
- Any abnormal finding on respiratory examination
- Any abnormality on chest X-ray
- A clear history of FB aspiration.

Pleural collections

Empyema, pleural effusion, pneumothorax and pyopneumothorax are overlapping conditions, which may be present concurrently.

Diagnosis

Clinical examination should focus on assessing for sepsis or mass effect and should guide management. All other investigations are subsidiary to this examination.

Pleural fluid chemistry in order to see if it is transudate or exudate may be misleading. Pyogenic collections are protein rich but often clot, consuming protein, trapping cells, and forming pockets (loculi). The resultant supernatant fluid may be protein and cell depleted, resembling transudate.

Table 3.12 Classification of pleural collections

Clinical Groups	Probable cause	Investigations	Management
1 SEPTIC Empyema and pyopneumothorax Febrile, acutely ill, toxic	Pyogenic infection: *S. pneumoniae, S. aureus, H. influenzae*	No needle aspiration. Send fluid from ICD for Gram stain and culture	ICD IV ampicicillin, cloxacillin or cefuroxime. Modify according to Gram and culture results Fibrinolytics for empyema
2 ASEPTIC Afebrile or low-grade fever	TB or malignancy	Needle aspiration Tuberculin skin test Serum LDH Pleural fluid for cytology and TB culture	Draw off enough liquid to render patient comfortable. TB: antimicrobials plus steroid Malignant: refer
3 MASS EFFECT	Commonly pyogenic but can occur from any cause	As for SEPTIC group	As for SEPTIC group

Empyema and pyopneumothorax

Ill, septic febrile patients with clinically detectable fluid or tension pneumothorax should be treated with immediate intercostal tube drainage (ICD) with a 12F tube inserted midway along the mid-axillary line on the affected side. In acutely ill patients drainage should not be delayed for confirmatory X-rays. There is no place for CT chest or pleural ultrasound examination in the initial management.

Do not attempt needle aspiration in acutely ill febrile patients to prove or disprove whether the child has pus in the pleural cavity. False negative taps are common with pus (dry tap obtained due to thick pus/clot blocking needle) or air may be obtained giving a false impression of pneumothorax if the lung is punctured during the tap procedure.

Treatment

Febrile septic patients

Immediate
The principles of treatment are:
- Get rid of pus.
  Pus, of itself, is extremely toxic and can lead to systemic inflammatory response syndrome and multiple organ failure. Pneumococcal empyema can cause haemolytic uraemic syndrome.

- Relieve pressure effects if present.
  Large pleural collections impair respiratory function and may produce cardiac tamponade (tension pneumothorax).
- Kill pathogens.
  Common: *S. pneumoniae, S. aureus*, and less commonly *H. influenzae*. Rare: anaerobes or Gram negative colifoms. The inclusion of an aminoglycoside or metronidazole is not empirically indicated except in HIV-infected or malnourished children.
- Breakdown and prevent loculations.
  Loculated pockets of pus or air commonly form with pyogenic infections and delay healing. Where available, instil a fibrinolytic at the time of initial ICD insertion. This reduces the need for subsequent surgical evacuation and shortens hospital stay.
  Fibrinolysis: Within an hour of ICD insertion instil 4 mg tissue plasminogen activator (TPA) in 40 mL of 0.9% saline down tube. Clamp for 1 hour. Unclamp and put on low suction. Repeat twice a day 12 hours apart for 3 days.
- Treat pain.
- ICD insertion (see p. 535) and drainage is painful and requires good analgesia to ensure comfort and promote cough. Ensure adequate analgesia while the drain is in-situ: Paracetamol (10–15 mg/kg/dose PO) and ibuprofen (6–10 mg/kg/dose PO) OR clonidine 1–5 mcg/kg/dose PO) and valoron (1 mg/kg) OR morphine infusion (20–80 mcg/kg/hour) OR morphine PO (0.2–0.4 mg/kg/dose)

Continuing management
Subsequent measures should be guided by the clinical picture (failure of fever resolution), rather than the radiological appearance.

Persisting fever with loculated collections requires surgical drainage: the choice between mini-thoracotomy or video-assisted thoracoscopic surgery depends on local expertise.

X-rays may be misleading in differentiating between (intrapulmonary) lung cysts/breakdown and pleural collections. Multiple air bubbles, pseudocysts, > 1 cm in diameter which do not conform to anatomical lobar boundaries are pleural collections and not intrapulmonary breakdown. Multiple cystic spaces within the lung take weeks, not days, to develop.

Management of aseptic collections

An aseptic collection is one in which the Gram stain is negative and conventional culture is negative.

A negative tuberculin skin test virtually rules out tuberculous pleural effusion in non-immunosuppressed, well nourished children.

Medication for TB effusion is as for tracheo-bronchial compression (p. 120). Tuberculous effusions resolve within days on steroid therapy. For anti-tuberculous therapy see p. 273.

Respiratory muscle dysfunction

Examine the respiratory muscles explicitly in all patients with signs of muscle weakness or unexplained tachypnoea. The only way in which respiratory muscle function can be assessed is by inspection.

Table 3.13 Assessment of muscle fuction

Muscles	Signs of weakness
INSPIRATORY	
Airway muscles:	
Ala nasi	Sucked inwards with inspiration. Usually no clinical effect
Pharynx dilators	Hypotonia and weakness contribute to sleep disordered breathing
Vocal cords	
Bilateral	Severe inspiratory obstruction
Unilateral	Hoarse voice, rarely aspiration of fluids
Pump muscles:	
Intercostal muscles	Paradoxical rib cage motion with inspiration
Diaphragm	Poor or paradoxical abdominal motion with inspiration
EXPIRATORY	
Airway muscles	Weak cough
Vocal cord paralysis	
Pump muscles	
Rectus abdominus	Weak cough

Notes:
- Bilateral vocal cord paralysis is rare.
- The diaphragm is the main muscle of inspiration. During quiet breathing the chest expands only slightly because the diaphragm is doing the work. When the diaphragm is working properly all one sees is the abdomen moving outwards as the diaphragm descends during inspiration. In tachypnoeic children, when the diaphragm is unable to cope with breathing on its own, excessively 'good' chest movement results. When the diaphragm is weak the rib cage expands more than usual and the abdomen expands little or is sucked in (paradoxical abdominal motion).
- Cough is the best test of integrated respiratory muscle function. A good cough recruits all the respiratory muscles. Impaired cough is life threatening and is an indication for mechanical ventilation in patients with reversible causes of weakness such as in Guillain-Barré syndrome.

Tracheo-bronchial obstruction

Causes of tracheo-bronchial obstruction can be divided into congenital and acquired.

Table 3.14 Causes of tracheo-bronchial obstruction

Congenital	Vascular ring, aberrant right subclavian artery
	Oesophageal stenosis with proximal distention
	Funnel trachea: a long segment tracheal stenosis
	Congenital lung cyst
	Tracheomalacia at site of surgically corrected congenital tracheo-oesophageal stricture
Acquired	Extrinsic compression
	Lymph nodes: tuberculous or malignant. HIV lymph nodes do not compress airways, even when very large
	Oesophageal distension above stricture or achalasia
	Intraluminal foreign body

Tuberculous adenopathy is a relatively common cause of obstruction of the bronchus intermedius, the left main bronchus and less commonly of the trachea itself.

Clinical features

Noisy breathing (see p. 89) with predominant expiratory obstruction. In severe obstruction noise and difficult breathing are present during both inspiration and expiration, which makes it difficult to tell clinically if obstruction is laryngeal or tracheo-bronchial.

There is no air trapping unless obstruction is extreme or some cause of peripheral airway obstruction such as viral bronchiolitis is also present.

Diagnosis

The site and extent of the obstruction are best defined radiologically. Endoscopy rarely yields sufficiently detailed information.

Conventional films. The trachea and main bronchi should be seen throughout their extent on well penetrated conventional AP films. Stenosis is suggested by a gap, or vanishing airway. The fact that the airway is filled with air proximally and distally does not mean that it is patent between those landmarks

LODOX (www.lodox.com), a propriety very low dose digital radiology system originally developed to screen workers on South African diamond mines provides the best images of the trachea and bronchi

Penetrated high KV films are helpful if LODOX is not available.

CT scans are subject to artefact and provide inferior delineation of the airways. While virtual bronchoscopy image reconstruction is technically feasible with CT, the radiation dose in children is unacceptably high.

Treatment of TB nodal compression

Nodal compression is virtually diagnostic of TB. The diagnosis should be confirmed by tuberculin skin test (Mantoux) and culture, but treatment should be started before the results are known.

- Antimicrobials
  RIMCURE. Number of tablets = body wt kg/4. Round off upwards to nearest half tablet. e.g. wt 3 kg = ¾ rounded up to 1 tablet. Weight-based category charts for dosing may result in too low a dose, near category boundaries.
- Corticosteroids
  Prednisone 2 mg/kg/day in single morning dose for 7 days, then the same dose Monday, Wednesday and Friday mornings (modified alternate day regimen) for a month. Stop. Tapering not required.
- Surgery
  Bilateral main bronchial obstruction is life threatening. Some clinical response to steroids is usually obvious within 2 days. If breathing remains difficult after 5 days of steroids, surgical drainage of the subcarinal nodes is indicated.

Recommended reading

1. Rudan I, Boschi-Pinto C, Biloglav Z, Mulholland K, Campbell H. Epidemiology and etiology of childhood pneumonia. *Bull World Health Organ*. 2008. 86:408–416.
2. Gray D, Zar HJ. Community acquired pneumonia in HIV-infected children: a global perspective. *Curr Opin Pulm Med*. 2010;16:208–216.
3. Green RJ, Zar HJ, Jeena PM, Madhi SA, Lewis H. South African guideline for the diagnosis, management and prevention of acute viral bronchiolitis in children. *S Afr Med J*. 2010;100:320–5.
4. Green RJ, Feldman C, Schoub B, Richards GA, Madhi SA, Zar HJ, Lalloo U; Guideline Committee of 1999, Klugman K, Phillips D, Cameron NA, Eggers RR. Influenza guideline for South Africa – update 2008. *S Afr Med J*. 2008;98:224-30.
5. Zar HJ. Chronic lung disease in human immunodeficiency virus-infected children. *Pediatr Pulmonol*. 2008;43:1–10.
6. Zar HJ, Jeena P, Argent A, Gie R, Maathi S. Diagnosis and management of community acquired pneumonia in childhood – South African Thoracic Society Guidelines. *S Afr Med J*. 2005;95: 977–990.

4 Gastrointestinal problems

M.L. Cooke, R. De Lacy, L. Goddard, E. Nel

Gastroenteritis

This is also called acute diarrhoea. Diarrhoea is the passage of loose or watery stools, usually more than 3 daily or any number of loose stools containing blood (dysentery). Acute diarrhoea results in increased loss of water and electrolytes in the stool. Most cases are due to intestinal infections. Extra-intestinal infections may cause mild diarrhoea (parenteral diarrhoea).

General
- Vomiting is common in the first days. It usually resolves with rehydration. Bile stained or persistent vomiting may indicate a surgical condition
- Fever (> 40 °C higher probability of bacterial infection, e.g. *Shigella*)
- Loss of appetite
- Mild respiratory symptoms occur in viral infections
- Stools may be blood stained. This usually indicates infection with an invasive organism such as *Shigella*.

Dehydration and shock

Loss of weight is the most accurate measure of dehydration. The clinical estimation of dehydration is imprecise and does not rely on a single sign.

> ***Practice point:***
> Shock may occur even in the absence of other signs of dehydration.

Assessment of shock

The following signs occur in shock.
- Cold peripheries
- Prolonged capillary refill time > 3 seconds

- Tachycardia
- Thready pulses
- Decreased blood pressure
- Decreased level of consciousness.

Decreased blood pressure is a late sign of shock in children.

Treatment of shock is urgent.

Attend to the airway and breathing. Provide facemask oxygen. Boluses of 20 mls/kg (10 ml/kg in severe malnutrition) of resuscitation fluid (Ringers lactate or normal saline) should be given by rapid infusion. Reassessment for resolution of shock and presence of any complications should take place immediately after boluses, and repeat boluses may be required. See flowchart 'the management of hypovolaemic shock' on p. 464.

Assessment of hydration

Signs of (extravascular) dehydration include (see 'Signs of dehydration' on p. 466).
- Loss of weight ☆☆☆
- Loss of skin turgor ☆☆☆
- Acidotic breathing ☆☆☆
- Thirst
- Decreased (and concentrated) urine output
- Dry eyes (crying without tears)
- Dry mouth
- Sunken eyes
- Sunken fontanelle.

Diagnosis

No routine investigations are indicated as most children will recover within a few days regardless of the causative organism. Urine dipstick and fingerprick blood glucose should be performed in all hospitalized children.

Laboratory tests
- Electrolytes and serum acid base determination:
  - All severely dehydrated children
  - Moderately dehydrated children with an atypical clinical presentation
  - Malnourished children
  - Children requiring intravenous rehydration

- In the presence of complications such as seizures, severe irritability, ileus.
- Blood glucose:
  - Seizures
  - Hypernatraemia.

Microbiological investigations

Stool cultures are only indicated in the following scenarios:
- Dysentery
- Children for whom antimicrobial therapy is considered, e.g. immunocompromised, neonates
- Persistent diarrhoea
- To exclude an infectious aetiology when conditions such as inflammatory bowel disease or allergic proctocolitis are considered
- Monitoring of an outbreak.

Other microbiological investigations such as blood cultures and urine cultures are indicated if the patient is at high risk of an extra-intestinal bacterial infection (e.g. immunocompromised, severe malnutrition, premature babies).

Treatment

The loss of water and electrolytes is the principal cause of death and morbidity in acute diarrhoeal disease. Treatment therefore focuses on preventing and treating these complications. Antibiotics are not routinely used and are restricted to situations where there are definite indications.

> *Practice point:*
>
> Antidiarrhoeals and antiemetics should never be used.

Mild to moderate dehydration

Oral rehydration is the first line treatment of these children. Children who refuse to take oral fluids or vomit can be given the solution in smaller regular increments or can be given oral rehydration solution (ORS) by the nasogastric route. Home-made sugar salt solution (p. 466) may be used.

The volume of ORS varies according to the degree of dehydration. If the child's weight before the onset of the diarrhoea is known, the weight deficit can be used to estimate the fluid requirement. See p. 465 for rehydration volumes for degrees of dehydration. After 4 hours the child should be reassessed. If the child's signs of dehydration are improving, continue with oral rehydration. If the child has become severely dehydrated initiate intravenous rehydration.

Shock and severe dehydration

Identify these children promptly (effective triage in outpatients) and treat aggressively. *Reassess children regularly!*

The rehydration route of choice is intravenous (intra-osseus (IO) if IV access is not available immediately). Oral rehydration should only be used if intravenous fluids or IO access are not available. Treat shock first and then severe dehydration according to the guidelines on p. 463.

Prevention of dehydration

Once dehydration has been corrected, or in children with no signs of dehydration, stool losses are corrected with ORS. If they are thirsty, allow them to drink as much as they want. A useful guide for correction of losses per loose stool is:
- Under 2 years: 50–100 ml
- Two up to 10 years: 100–200 ml

Feeds

As far as possible the normal diet should be continued during an episode of diarrhoea.
- Only interrupt feeds to correct shock and initial dehydration (do not interrupt longer than 4–6 hours in children with mild to moderate dehydration).
- Continue and encourage additional breastfeeding.
- Do not dilute formula.
- Gradual reintroduction of feeds is not necessary.
- Lactose free and hydrolysed formula are not routinely required for acute diarrhoea.
- Avoid fluids with a high sugar content (fruit juices, carbonated beverages).
- Encourage additional feeds as soon as the child's appetite allows.

Supplements

Zinc
Zinc supplementation reduces the duration of acute and chronic diarrhoea in developing countries. Supplementation is continued for 2 weeks.

Dose (zinc acetate or zinc gluconate):
- 10 mg daily below 6 months of age
- 20 mg daily in older infants and children.

Vitamin A
Vitamin A supplementation reduces the severity of diarrhoea in populations with a high prevalence of vitamin A deficiency. Refer to Vitamin A supplementation guidelines on p. 161.

Potassium
If hypokalaemia, correct according to guidelines on p. 480.

Drugs
There is no indication for the routine use of antidiarrhoeal or antiemetic drugs.

Antibiotics
Indications for antibiotics:
- Dysentery (*Shigella*, *Campylobacter*)
- Cholera with severe dehydration
- Immune compromised and other children at high risk for possible bacteraemia and extra-intestinal infections
- Severe malnutrition
- Neonates and young infants with suspected systemic infection.

Probiotics
Probiotics may reduce the duration of acute infectious diarrhoea.

Complications
Electrolyte and metabolic disturbances (for management see Chapter 20, Fluids, electrolytes and acid-base).
- Hypoglycaemia
- Hypokalaemia (particularly in malnourished children and with recurrent episodes of diarrhoea). This causes hypotonia, paralytic ileus, cardiac arrhythmias, and impaired renal function
- Hypernatraemia. This may cause severe central nervous system complications. Rehydration is slow
- Hyponatraemia. Often occurs in secretory diarrhoea (e.g. *Shigella*) and malnourished children. Correction of dehydration leads to normalisation of sodium. If very low or symptomatic, give hypertonic sodium slowly
- Hypocalcaemia

- Hypomagnesaemia
- Metabolic acidosis. Children may have acidotic breathing. This usually indicates significant dehydration
- Hyperglycaemia (often with hypernatraemia).

Other complications:
- Seizures. These are common in infants with diarrhoea. Consider:
  - Febrile seizures
  - Hypoglycaemia
  - *Shigella* dysentery
  - CNS infections (meningitis, encephalitis)
  - Electrolyte disturbances (hyper- and hyponatraemia)
  - Tetany (not true seizures) due to hypocalcaemia and hypomagnesaemia
  - Vascular complications (venous sinus thrombosis)
- Renal failure:
  - Usually prerenal – resolves with rehydration
  - Occasionally due to acute tubular necrosis after severe dehydration, shock, or rhabdomyolysis
  - Consider renal vein thrombosis if frank haematuria.
- Ileus. Consider hypokalaemia.

Persistent diarrhoea

Definitions

Persistent diarrhoea (PD) starts acutely and lasts longer than 14 days. Specific chronic diarrhoeal disorders and malabsorption syndromes such as coeliac disease are excluded. Children who are thriving despite a history of chronic diarrhoea may have non-specific chronic diarrhoea of childhood. PD has a higher morbidity and mortality than acute diarrhoea and accounts for a disproportionately high percentage of diarrhoeal disease deaths.

Risk factors for persistent diarrhoea:
- Age < 6 months
- Immunocompromised (including HIV infection)
- Malnutrition
- Recurrent episodes of acute diarrhoea
- Early cessation of breast feeding
- Certain enteropathogens, e.g. Enteroaggregative *E. coli*, *Shigella*, *Cryptosporidium parvum*.

Complications:
- Dehydration
- Electrolyte abnormalities (potassium, sodium, magnesium, calcium, phosphate)
- Malnutrition
- Micronutrient deficiency
- Protein losing enteropathy (PLE)
- Malabsorption
- Extra-intestinal infections:
  - Bacteraemia
  - Pneumonia
  - Urinary tract infections.

Diagnosis

History:
- HIV status
- Previous medical history, e.g. intestinal surgery, previous episodes of diarrhoea
- Family history: allergy, lactose intolerance
- Diet: association of diarrhoea with specific feeds (e.g. dairy products for children with lactose intolerance), fruit juice (may cause an osmotic diarrhoea)
- Systemic symptoms: fever, arthritis or rash (possibly inflammatory bowel disease)
- Stool: watery (secretory or osmotic), pale, foul smelling, greasy stools (steatorrhoea), blood and mucus (colitis), undigested vegetable matter (non-specific chronic diarrhoea).

Special investigations

For persistant diarrhoea consider:
- Stool culture and microscopy (alert the laboratory if pathogens such as *Cryptosporidium* or *Clostridium difficile* are suspected)
- Tests for malabsorption (send watery component of stool for investigations):
  - Stool reducing substances
  - Faecal osmolar gap: $290-2([Na]+[K])$. If FOG is < 50 diarrhoea is secretory. If it is > 100 then there are additional osmotically active substances in the faeces and the diarrhea is osmotic. Between 50 and 100 is not specific
  - Stool α-1-antitrypsin clearance (for suspected PLE)
  - Osmotic diarrhoea will resolve after 12–24 hours interruption of feeds; secretory diarrhoea persists.

- Biochemistry
- Haematology
- Urine culture
- Blood culture
- HIV status
- Immunology evaluation (think of primary immune deficiency)
- Evaluation for food allergy.

For other causes of chronic diarrhoea consider in addition:
- Stool analysis
  - Steatocrit and histology for free fat
  - 72 hour stool fat determination
  - Elastase.
- Breath hydrogen test
- Sweat test
- Coeliac serology
  - Anti-tissue transglutaminase antibody
  - Anti-gliadin antibody.
- Radiological assessment
  - Ultrasound (TB lymph nodes, intra-abdominal tumours)
  - Contrast imaging (malrotation, other anatomic abnormalities)
  - CT abdomen (TB abdomen, intra-abdominal tumours).
- Endoscopy with biopsy of the small (e.g. coeliac disease) and large intestine (IBD).

Treatment

Treatment focuses on providing nutritional support, correcting dehydration and electrolyte abnormalities and preventing and treating complications. Diets should provide adequate energy and protein for age and provide additional energy and protein for catch-up growth (approximately 1 kcal/ml; 2–3 g/kg /day protein).

Figure 4.1 Treatment of diarrhoea (see next page)

Oral treatment of small bowel overgrowth: ✚
- Cholestyramine 1 g 6 hourly for 5 days
- Gentamycin 50 mg/kg/day for 3 days (q 6 hourly, maximum dose 360 mg/d) OR neomycin 100 /kg/day for 3 days (q 6 hourly, maximum dose 200 mg)
- Metronidazole 7.5 mg/kg/8 hourly for 5 days.

Figure 4.1 Treatment of diarrhoea

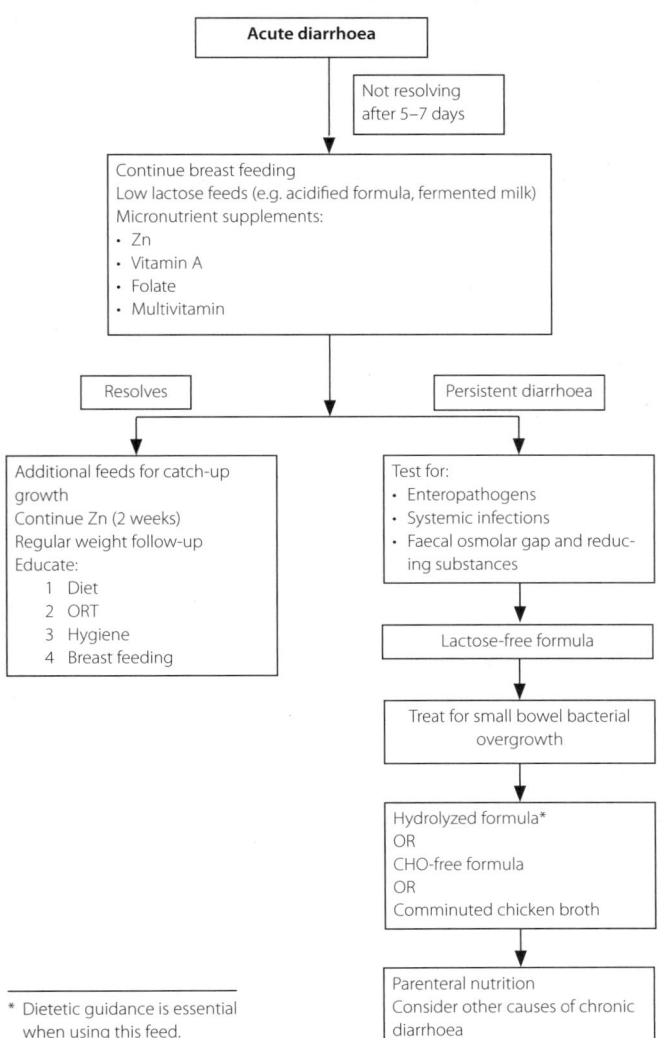

* Dietetic guidance is essential when using this feed.

Approach to blood in stool

Blood in the stool usually indicates bleeding from the gastrointestinal tract. Non-gastrointestinal causes include swallowed blood (epistaxis and haemoptysis) and rarely, food colourants.

Diagnosis

Assess severity. If haemodynamically unstable:
- Immediate resuscitation
- Treat the presumptive diagnosis (e.g. oesophageal varices) based on history and physical examination. A definitive diagnostic evaluation is delayed until the patient is stabilized.

Less significant rectal bleeding is managed with a step-wise diagnostic and therapeutic approach.

Identify the source of bleeding. The description of the stool and associated symptoms and signs provide valuable clues as to the source of bleeding. In addition the age at presentation gives clues as to possible likely aetiologies.

Sources of bleeding:
- Non-GIT sources of bleeding:
  — Epistaxis
  — Haemoptysis.
- Streaks of blood on the stool:
  — Anal fissure (associated painful defaecation, fissure visible on inspection)
  — Distal polyps.
- Frank red blood:
  — Colonic bleeding
  — Large proximal gastrointestinal haemorrhage (e.g. oesophageal varices) with rapid intestinal transit.
- Loose, mucoid stools with associated abdominal pain:
  — Infections (e.g. *Shigella*)
  — Allergic proctocolitis (usually in infants that appear healthy, most often before 6 months, may be exclusively breastfed)
  — Ulcerative colitis
  — Crohn's disease.
- Diarrhoea:
  — Infectious causes
  — Protein sensitization.
- Constipation:
  — Anal fissure.

- Signs of chronic liver disease and portal hypertension:
  - Oesophageal and gastric varices
  - Portal hypertensive gastropathy.
- Skin and mucous membranes:
  - Spider naevi:
    - Chronic liver disease with portal hypertension.
  - Rash:
    - Henoch-Schönlein purpura (often also abdominal pain)
    - Inflammatory bowel syndrome.
  - Cutaneous haemangiomas:
    - Haemangiomas of intestine.
  - Peutz-Jeghers syndrome (lips, oral mucosa),
    - Intestinal polyps.
- Soft tissue and bony tumours:
  - Intestinal polyps (Gardner's syndrome).
- Peritonitis:
  - NEC
  - Peptic ulcer
  - Crohn's disease with perforation:
- Abdominal distention, pain, mass
  - Intussusception
  - NEC (predominantly premature neonates)
  - Other surgical conditions of the upper gastrointestinal tract, e.g. peptic ulcer or variceal haemorrhage, haemangioma, duplication cyst
  - Meckel's diverticulum.

Special investigations

Special investigations are used to assess the severity of the blood loss (e.g. anaemia), confirm the cause of bleeding, and search for comorbid conditions.

> ***Practice point:***
>
> Exclude local causes, e.g. anal fissure before embarking on any special investigations.

The following investigations are often indicated:
- Confirmation of blood in the stool:
  - Haemocult
  - Stool microscopy

- Full blood count – pay special attention to the Hb and platelet count
- Clotting profile (liver disease, septicaemia)
- Liver biochemistry (in children with suspected liver disease)
- Upper and lower intestinal endoscopy (after stabilization)
- Radiological assessment if indicated by the differential diagnosis, e.g. ultrasound for suspected intussusception, contrast studies for suspected polyps, plain abdominal radiograph for suspected NEC
- Confirm or exclude a Meckel's diverticulum by technetium scan and enterocolitis by stool microsopy and culture. A colonic cause is confirmed by barium enema and colonoscopy
- A laparotomy is necessary if investigations are negative and bleeding is severe and persistent.

Treatment

Supportive:
- Treatment for hypovolaemic shock
- Blood transfusion
- Clotting factors (fresh frozen plasma, cryoprecipitate)
- Iron supplement.

Specific:
- Specific treatment is determined by the diagnosis.
- In some instances a trial of therapy is warranted, e.g. for allergic proctocolitis.
- Octreotide for variceal bleeding. May be of value for other causes of massive GIT bleeding.
- Emergency sclerotherapy/banding.

An approach to jaundice

Jaundice is a yellow discolouration of the skin and mucous membranes due to raised levels of bilirubin. Bilirubin is formed mainly from haem catabolism, and jaundice occurs when there is an over-production of bilirubin (including haemolysis), defective bilirubin metabolism or defective excretion of bilirubin from the body. Jaundice is classified into unconjugated and conjugated hyperbilirubinaemia. An important surgical cause of conjugated hyperbilirubinaemia with acholic stools is biliary atresia (see p. 497).

> **Practice point:**
> Acholic stools indicate total obstruction and require urgent referral if the patient is less than 3 months of age.

Jaundice that lasts longer than 14 days in a neonate needs investigation.

Unconjugated hyperbilirubinaemia

For neonatal unconjugated hyperbilirubinaemia see p. 75. Causes of unconjugated hyperbilirubinaemia in older children include haemolysis (see p. 497) and hereditary enzyme deficiencies such as Gilbert's and Crigler-Najjar syndromes.

Conjugated hyperbilirubinaemia

Conjugated hyperbilirubinaemia is a direct bilirubin level > 34 mmol/l or > 15% of the total bilirubin.

Diagnostic approach

- History and examination
- Liver function tests. Determine conjugated and unconjugated bilirubin levels, LFTs and cholesterol
- Determine if complete obstruction by the stool observation test. Examine stool daily. Do not rely on carer description of stool colour. Stools must be visualized by examining doctor. If acholic (white) it indicates complete obstruction and the patient must be referred urgently to exclude biliary atresia (see surgical section on p. 497). Complete obstruction can also be assessed with a hepatobiliary scan
- Exclude treatable infective causes. Perform urine dipsticks ± culture and blood cultures and treat accordingly
- Exclude treatable metabolic conditions
- Determine genetic conditions.

Causes of conjugated hyperbilirubinaemia

Table 4.1 Causes of conjugated hyperbilirubinaemia

Infective	Viral	Hepatitis A, B, CMV, HIV, rubella, herpes simplex
	Bacterial	Syphilis, septicaemia, UTI
	Protozoal	*Toxoplasmosis gondii*

Biliary	Extrahepatic biliary atresia
	Choledochal cyst
	Alagille's syndrome
	Bile plugs
	Congenital hepatic fibrosis
Metabolic/genetic	α-1-antitrypsin deficiency
	Tyrosinaemia Type 1
	Galactosaemia
	Wilson's disease
	Hypothyroidism/hypopituitarism
	Cystic fibrosis
	Familial intrahepatic cholestasis
	Enzyme deficiencies: rotor and Dubin-Johnson sydrome
Drugs/toxins	Total parenteral nutrition
Autoimmune	Autoimmune hepatitis
	Sclerosing cholangitis

Figure 4.2 Evaluation of infants with conjugated hyperbilirubinaemia (see next page)

Hepatitis

Hepatitis A (HAV)

Hepatitis A is spread via the faecal-oral spread. Incubation is 15–50 days.

Clinical features
- Often asymptomatic in the preschool child.
- During the prodromal phase nausea, anorexia and malaise are common. Thereafter jaundice, dark urine and a tender palpable liver may be noted.
- Fulminant hepatitis is rare (0.1%),
- Chronic infection does not occur.

Diagnosis
Hepatitis A IgM antibody indicates recent infection. These antibodies can persist for 4–6 months after infection. Raised IgG antibodies indicate previous infection or successful immunization.

Figure 4.2 Evaluation of infants with conjugated hyperbilirubinaemia

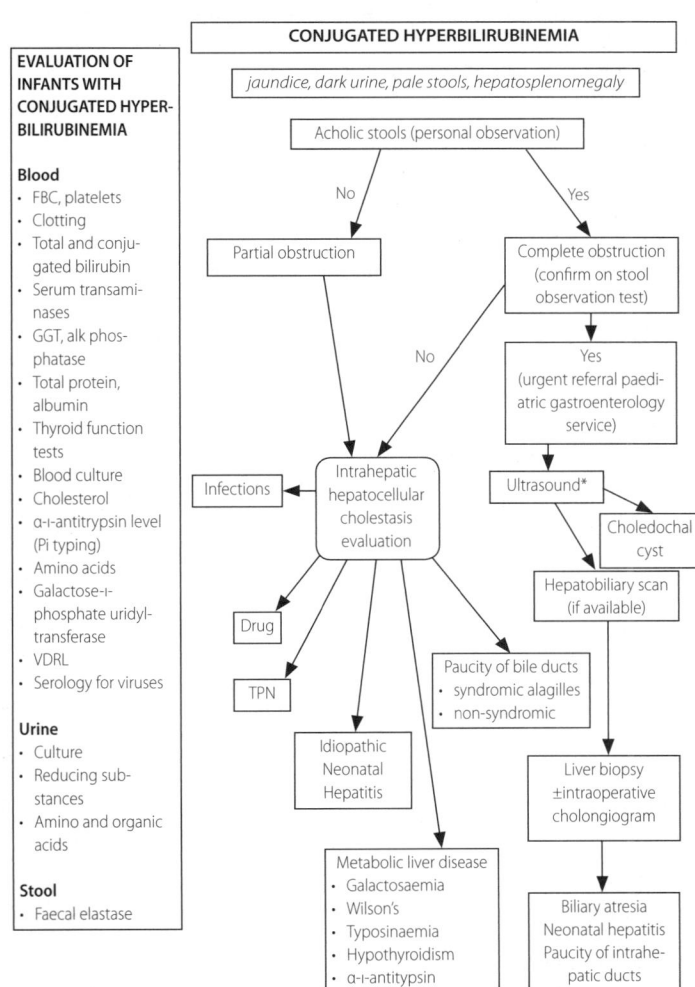

Management ☆☆

- Supportive treatment, hydration and avoidance of hepatotoxic medication
- Hand washing to decrease spread
- High-energy/low protein diet
- Investigate if jaundiced and symptomatic: Hepatitis A IgM, blood glucose, liver function tests and prothrombin ratio (INR). These results will determine the follow up or admission of the patient
- Admit with the following danger signals: protracted vomiting, dehydration, continuing fever, hypoglycaemia, confusion, intercurrent infections and increased INR
- Infected patients are most contagious for 1–2 weeks prior to onset of illness. Isolate if in hospital for 1 week after the onset of jaundice.

Prevention

- *Active immunization.* Hepatitis A vaccine (HAV) is inactive and is licensed for children over 1 year of age (dose is 0.5 ml IMI with a second dose given 6–12 months later). HAV can be given concurrently with passive immunization. It is recommended for children with chronic liver disease, haemophilia and for children in crèches.
- *Passive immunization.* Post-exposure (< 14 days) or pre-exposure prophylaxis: hepatitis A vaccine (preferable) or a single dose of pooled human immunoglobulin (0.04 ml/kg IM (minimum 1 ml) ☆☆☆◊

NB: Hepatitis A is a notifiable condition.

Hepatitis B (HBV)

Transmission of hepatitis B is via the horizontal, vertical or parenteral route (infected blood or blood products). The incubation period is 2–6 months.

Diagnosis

- HBV may be indistinguishable from hepatitis A, but can be more insidious with a longer prodrome of non-specific ill health.
- *Acute infection*: the diagnostic characteristics of all viral hepatitis are similar except that HBV presents with serological markers, i.e. HBsAg, HBeAg.
- *Chronic infection*: about 90% of neonates and 30–40% of children with acute HBV infection become chronic carriers. Initially they have asymptomatic disease. Some develop chronic hepatitis, cirrhosis and hepatocellular carcinoma.

Table 4.2 Markers of Hepatitis B infection

	HBsAg	HBsAb	HBeAg	HBeAb	HBcAb	HBN DNA	Liver enzymes
Acute infection	+	−	+	−	IgM	+	Raised
Chronic hepatitis * eAg positive (high risk)	+	−	+	−	IgG	++	Raised
eAg negative (low risk)	+	−	−	+	IgG	+	Raised
Inactive 'carrier'	+	−	−	−	−	−	Normal
Resolved infection	−	+	−	+	IgG	−	Normal
Successful vaccination	−	+	−	−	−	−	−

Key: HBV – hepatitis B virus
HBsAg – surface antigen
HBsAb – surface antibody
HBeAg – e antigen
HBeAb – e antibody
HBcAb – core antibody

* Chronic hepatitis: persistence of HBsAg for ≥ 6 months or HBeAg ≥ 3 months

Treatment

- *Prevention*: hepatitis B immunoglobulin in non-immune individuals exposed to HBV. A dose of 2 ml IMI (3 ml in adults) is recommended and should be given as soon as possible between 1–7 days after exposure. In proven high-risk exposure, give a second injection 1 month later. Hepatitis B immunoglobulin should be given to infants born to HBsAg-positive mothers (0.5 ml IMI within 12 hours of birth). Hepatitis B vaccine is part of routine immunization and is given to all infants at 6 weeks, 10 weeks and 14 weeks of age.
- *Infection*: Treatment options for chronic hepatitis B (eAg + or eAg −) include standard α-interferon, pegylated interferon and nucleotide/sides entecavir, tenofovir and lamivudine.

Acute liver failure (ALF)

ALF in children is uncommon but is a medical emergency. It refers to fulminant hepatic failure without pre-existing liver disease. It appears within a few weeks of the onset of the illness. Causes include viral hepatitis (particularly A and B), Reye's syndrome, drugs (paracetamol, anti-TB drugs), and toxins (including traditional medicines).

Diagnosis and investigations

- Protracted vomiting, jaundice (not in Reye's syndrome), disturbed mental function, coma, bleeding diathesis, various metabolic and renal disturbances, and infection
- Liver function tests, plasma proteins and prothrombin ratio, blood ammonia and glucose, serum electrolytes, and acid-base studies. FBC, crossmatch and blood culture
- Liver ultrasound, viral serology, urine and serum toxicology and tests for other specific causes may be indicated.

Prognosis

The overall mortality rate is 70%. Liver transplantation can be life-saving but is only available at specific hospitals.

Treatment

Withdraw any hepatotoxic drugs and avoid sedatives.

Encephalopathy

- Early encephalopathy may manifest as subtle signs such as irritability, changes in sleep pattern, lethargy and mild degrees of disorientation.
- Monitor grade of coma.
- Restrict dietary protein to 1.0 g/kg/day until the level of coma improves.
- Give sufficient lactulose to produce loose stools. Initially use a Fleet® or Microlax® enema.
- Give oral kanamycin/neomycin.

Cerebral oedema

- Give IV fluids at two-thirds of normal maintenance requirement.
- Nurse child with head elevated at 20 degrees.
- Give mannitol 0.5–2 g/kg over 1 hour (7 mls/kg of 20% mannitol). Repeat every 6–8 hours for a maximum of 48 hours. Do not repeat if there is no clinical response. Beware of causing hypovolaemia and oliguria (urine volume < 1 ml/kg/hour).

NB: Signs of fluid overload may occur in oliguric patients. Treat by dialysis.

Bleeding diathesis

- Inject vitamin K 5–10 mg IV and repeat daily. (Avoid intramuscular injections if there is a bleeding tendency.)
- Give fresh frozen plasma daily if bleeding or awaiting transplantation..
- Cryoprecipitate, platelets and NovoSeven® (very expensive) can be used to cover invasive procedures.
- NovoSeven® can be considered for resistant bleeding not responding to the above measures or when limited by fluid volume.

Gastrointestinal bleeding

> ***Practice points:***
>
> - Nasogastric tube – monitor contents
> - Prevent GIT bleeds – sucralfate and omeprazole or cimetidine.

Metabolic disturbances

Hypoglycaemia is common. Hyponatraemia and hypernatraemia, hypokalaemia, hypocalcaemia, and hypomagnesaemia may occur.

- Monitor glucose regularly. Maintain blood glucose above 4 mmol/l.
- Give high carbohydrate feeds or an IV dextrose infusion (10% at least).
- Correct acid-base status if necessary. Respiratory alkalosis and metabolic acidosis may occur.

Renal failure

- Pre-renal uraemia secondary to hypovolaemia
- Acute tubular necrosis secondary to hypotension, septicaemia, or drugs
- Hepatorenal syndrome.

Infections

- Provide broad-spectrum antibiotic cover. Prescribe amoxycillin or third-generation cephalosporins.
- Provide anti-fungal cover (mycostatin).

Amelioration of liver injury

Use N-acetylcysteine 5–10 mg/kg/hour for 48–72 hours

Chronic hepatic disease

Chronic liver disease does occur in children. Any abnormal liver profile needs to be investigated. The management of chronic liver disease is to treat the complications, with special attention to nutrition.

Complications and management of chronic liver failure

Table 4.3 The complications and management of chronic liver failure

Complication	Management	
Malnutrition and growth failure	Nutritional support	
	Energy	120–150% RDA
	Carbohydrate	15–20 g/kg/day
	Protein	3–4 g/kg/day
	Fat	8 g/kg/day (50% MCT)
	Fat soluble vitamins	(A, D, E, K)
Coagulopathy	Vitamin K (2.5 – 10 mg/day)	
	Fresh frozen plasma	
	Cryoprecipitate, platelets	
Portal hypertension	Resuscitate	
Hypersplenism	Intravenous octreotide (3–5 mcg/kg/hr)	
Varices – acute bleed	(50 mcg/kg in 50 ml 5% dextrose at 5 ml/hr)	
	Injection sclerotherapy/banding	
Prophylactic	Propranolol	
	Injection sclerotherapy/banding	
Ascites	Avoid excess sodium	
	Spironolactone (3 mg/kg)/furosemide	
	Albumin infusion with furosemide	
	Paracentesis if respiratory compromise	
Encephalopathy	Low protein diet (2 g/kg)	
	Lactulose	
	Neomycin/gentamicin	
Infection	Cefotaxime, ampicillin, metronidazole	
Pruritus	Cholestyramine (1–2 g/day)	
	Ursodeoxycholic acid (20 mg/kg/d)	
	Phenobarbitone (5–15 mg/kg/d)	
	Rifampicin (50 mg/kg/d)	

Cystic fibrosis

Cystic fibrosis is an autosomal recessive condition with multi-system features due to obstruction of tubular structures with abnormally viscous mucus. It is one of the most common genetic defects in Caucasian children, occurring in 1:2 000 live births.

Clinical features

- Usually presents in the first year of life.
- Usually a combination of failure to thrive with chronic diarrhoea/steatorrhoea due to pancreatic insufficiency and recurrent chest infections (typically *Staphylococcus aureus* and *Pseudomonas aeruginosa*); can present with severe malnutrition with oedema.

> ***Practice point:***
>
> Cystic fibrosis can present as severe malnutrition with oedema in patients younger than 6 months

- Electrolyte derangements include hyponatraemia with hypochloraemic metabolic alkalosis.
- 10-15% present with features of neonatal bowel obstruction due to meconium ileus.
- Other complications include: rectal prolapse, neonatal hepatitis (obstructive jaundice), cirrhosis with portal hypertension, pancreatitis, GOR, IDDM, bronchiectasis, allergic bronchopulmonary aspergillosis, progressive loss of lung function and respiratory failure.

Diagnosis

- Positive sweat test (> 60 mmol/l chloride)
- Alternatively demonstration of the 2 deletions for CFTR on chromosome 7 (commonest in South Africa being delta F508 and 3120 + 1G→A)
- Screen with sweat conductivity (> 80 mmol/l sodium)
- Low faecal elastase (< 100 mg/g) strongly supports pancreatic insufficiency and the diagnosis of CF.

Treatment ☆☆☆☆☼

- This is specialized and is best carried out in a multidisciplinary CF unit – refer for workup and/or treatment.
- The course of cystic fibrosis varies substantially depending on nutritional status. Almost all the manifestations of the disease – including the pulmonary effects – can be mimicked or made worse by specific nutritional deficiencies.
- Nutritional support and rehabilitation includes pancreatic enzyme replacement therapy and aggressive caloric, fat soluble vitamin and calcium supplementation.

- Regular daily physiotherapy for lung disease and regular surveillance of colonizing bacteria through sputum specimens.
- Chronic *P. aeruginosa* (> 6 months) colonisation of respiratory tract – macrolide antibiotic (azithromycin) 3 times a week and alternate month aminoglycoside nebulisations twice daily.
- Use recombinant DNAse (Pulmozyme®) nebulizations or hypertonic saline nebulizations twice daily for children with moderate to severe lung disease.
- Prompt treatment of respiratory exacerbations with antibiotics effective against colonizing bacteria.
- Annual influenza immunisation.

The approach to a child with hepatosplenomegaly

The signs of hepatomegaly and splenomegaly are shared by many common diseases, but may also exist in isolation. Associated features with the organ enlargement may help narrow down the differential diagnosis (e.g. jaundice, anaemia, signs of chronic liver disease, cardiac or neurological signs and dysmorphology).

Summary of pathophysiological mechanisms
- Inflammation
- Reticulo-endothelial cell hyperplasia
- Venous congestion
- Storage products
- Space occupying lesions
- Fat infiltration – typical of kwashiorkor and malnutrition
- Metabolic disorders.

The causes of hepatomegaly, splenomegaly and hepatosplenomegaly

'Apparent' hepatosplenomegaly is caused by air trapping, pushing the liver and spleen inferiorly, leading to a false impression of organ enlargement. Causes of massive splenomegaly include chronic myeloid leukaemia (CML), Gauchers disease, splenic sequestration in sickle cell anaemia and Langerhans cell histiocytosis (LCH). Causes of a spleen much bigger than a liver include portal hypertension (most common), infections such as malaria, kala azar and leishmaniasis, CML, LCH, lipid storage diseases and congenital haemolytic anaemias.

Table 4.4 The causes of hepatosplenomegaly

ENLARGED	LIVER AND SPLEEN	LIVER ONLY	SPLEEN ONLY
INFLAMMATION			
Infection			
Congenital infections: CMV, Herpes simplex, toxoplasmosis, rubella, syphilis	✓	✓	✓ (CMV)
Viral hepatitis: EBV, HIV, Hep B	✓	✓	✓ (EBV)
Parasites: hydatid, amoebiasis, bilharzia		✓	
Fungal: histoplasmosis, coccidomycosis	✓	✓	
Recurrent malaria			✓
Typhoid			✓
Endocarditis			✓
Autoimmune hepatitis	✓ (PHT)	✓	
Toxins and drugs	✓	✓	
Biliary tract obstruction	✓	✓	✓
SLE, Stills disease (RA)		✓	✓
RETICULOENDOTHELIAL HYPERPLASIA			
Septicaemia	✓	✓	✓
Malignancy			
Lymphoma	✓	✓	
Leukaemia	✓	✓	✓ (CML)
Neuroblastoma		✓	
Granulomatous response TB	✓	✓	
Haemolytic anaemia	✓		✓
Haemoglobinopathy	✓		✓
VENOUS CONGESTION			
Congestive heart failure		✓	
Pericardial effusion, constrictive pericarditis		✓	
Budd Chiari	✓ (PHT)	✓	
Veno-occlusive disease	✓ (PHT)	✓	
Portal / splenic vein thrombosis			✓

ENLARGED	LIVER AND SPLEEN	LIVER ONLY	SPLEEN ONLY
STORAGE DISORDERS			
Carbohydrate storage disease: Glycogen storage disease, galactosaemia	✓	✓	
Mucopolysaccharidosis	✓	✓	✓
Lipidosis: Gauchers, Niemann Pick, Tay Sachs	✓		✓ (Gauchers)
Tyrosinaemia	✓ (PHT)	✓	
Langerhans cell histiocytosis	✓		✓
SPACE OCCUPYING LESIONS			
Abscess	✓	✓	
Primary and secondary neoplasms		✓	
Cysts	✓	✓	✓
FAT INFILTRATION			
Malnutrition		✓	
Hyperalimentation		✓	
Uncontrolled diabetes mellitus: Mauriac syndrome		✓	
Hepatotoxic drugs: TB treatment		✓	
Reye's syndrome		✓	
METABOLIC DISORDERS			
Wilson's disease	✓ (PHT)	✓	
Cystic fibrosis	✓ (PHT)	✓	
Galactossaemia	✓ (PHT)	✓	

PHT = pulmonary hypotension

Infantile colic

An otherwise healthy infant who is distressed or cries for more than 3 hours per day, for more than 3 days per week and for at least 3 weeks.

Clinical features

History:
- Feeding – breast/bottle
- Change in weight
- Stool consistency/colour/blood
- Vomiting or reflux
- Timing and duration of crying.

Symptoms:
- Inconsolable cry
- Drawing up of knees
- Flatus.

Examination:
- Normal.

Diagnosis

Clinical, no investigations if history is suggestive and examination and growth pattern are normal.

Differential diagnosis:
- Reflux oesophagitis
- Lactose intolerance
- Cow milk protein allergy (CMPA)
- Intussusception
- Volvulus
- Strangulated hernia
- Torsion of testis
- Non-accidental injury
- Maternal depression/anxiety.

Treatment

- Reassure as most infants improve after 3–4 months
- Parental support
- Reduce overstimulation

- One week trial of lactose-free formula. If no improvement a trial of a hypoallergenic formula may be considered if CMPA is being considered
- Anticholinergic drugs are contraindicated, as serious side effects may occur.

Functional gastrointestinal disorders

Definition
Abdominal pain is a common complaint in childhood and adolescence. There are many organic causes of recurrent abdominal pain, but a benign common cause is recurrent abdominal pain syndrome (RAPS) or irritable bowel syndrome of childhood.

Causes
- Recurrent abdominal pain syndrome
- Constipation
- Parasites / TB
- UTI
- Lactose intolerance
- Gastritis/peptic ulcer/oesophagitis
- Abdominal migraine.

Features suggesting an organic cause of abdominal pain
- Age of onset: < 5 years or > 14 years of age
- Pain localization: away from umbilicus
- Nocturnal pain
- Food intake: aggravates or relieves pain
- Associated features: fever, arthralgia, rash, jaundice
- Loss of appetite, weight loss
- Alteration in bowel habit
- Positive family history: peptic ulcer, inflammatory bowel disease
- Abdominal distension, mass or visceromegaly
- Faecal soiling
- Anal skin tags
- Occult blood positive stools.

Clinical features of RAPS
Gradual onset of vague, constant peri-umbilical pain with minimal radiation unrelated to meals or activity and without night waking. It

predominantly affects children aged 5-14 and may occur in clusters lasting days to weeks with intervening pain-free periods. Pain may occur only at school and not be present on weekends or holidays. Occasional associated features include headache, pallor, nausea, dizziness, fatigue and low grade fever.

Diagnosis

If RAPS is suspected do only:
- FBC and ESR
- Urine dipstix
- Stool analysis for parasites and occult blood.

For suspected organic pathology also consider:
- Abdominal X-ray
- Ultrasound abdomen
- Stool reducing substances
- Gastroscopy.

Treatment of RAPS

- Reassure the patient and parents.
- Medications have very little place.
- Modify the diet to increase fibre.
- With firm reassurance, complete resolution can occur in 30-50% of children within 6 weeks of presentation.

Constipation and faecal impaction

Definitions

Chronic constipation is characterized by infrequent passage of hard stools, often with associated pain and retentive posturing.

Faecal impaction/loading occurs when there is retention of stools in the colon and rectum from repeated incomplete evacuation of faeces. The cause is often multi-factorial, including low-fibre diet, poor fluid intake, little exercise and a fear of defecation, either due to an episode of painful defaecation (e.g. fissure-in-ano) or unpleasant school facilities/rigorous toilet-training.

Soiling/faecal incontinence is the involuntary passage of liquid stool usually due to rectal dysfunction caused by faecal impaction.

Encopresis is the purposeful passing of normal stools in inappropriate areas. This behaviour should be referred to child psychiatry.

Clinical features

Symptoms include constipation, loose stools, faecal incontinence, mild abdominal distension, and abdominal pain. The condition can be misdiagnosed as chronic diarrhoea or recurrent non-specific abdominal pain of childhood (RAP). Recent onset of constipation and/or blood in the stool with painful defecation are commonly caused by an acute anal fissure.

Examination must include assessment of growth, abdominal examination for faecal masses, inspection of the rectum and perianal area and rectal examination, and thorough neurological examination.

Although uncommon, *organic causes* of constipation such as Hirschsprung's disease, metabolic conditions such as hypothyroidism or hypercalcaemia, anatomic malformations, neuropathic conditions (e.g. tethered cord) or drug ingestion should be considered.

Diagnosis

Faeces may be palpable on both abdominal and rectal examination. Investigations, including abdominal X-rays (AXRs) are unnecessary for diagnosis. Blood tests (calcium, thyroid function) should not be routine and only done in resistant cases. If there is suspicion of Hirschsprung's disease the child should be referred for a rectal biopsy.

Treatment

This consists of counselling and education of parents and child, along with behaviour and dietary modification. Maintenance oral therapy is always necessary even after clearing impaction if present. ☆ ☆ ☆ ◈

The colon can be cleared rectally with repeated phosphate-containing enemas, (1 paediatric or ½ adult daily times 3 days in children older than 2 years), or with a balanced electrolyte polyethylene glycol (PEG) solution.

Golytely®, or Kleen Prep® is given at a rate 15–25 ml/kg/hour. Encourage older children to drink these large volumes with artificial sweeteners or diabetic drinks (do not add any sugar-containing mixture) but smaller children will usually require NGT infusion. An enema should be given within the first hour of starting the preparation. Observe closely as there is a risk of aspiration. The solution should be continued until the rectal effluent is clear (usually after 6–8 hours). The efficacy of clearance can be determined clinically (soft, mass-free abdomen) and an AXR is not necessary. Movicol®/Pegicol® also contains PEG and can be used for clearout and subsequent maintenance therapy.

Maintenance therapy may include osmotic laxatives (lactulose or sorbitol), Movicol®/Pegicol® and stool lubricants (liquid paraffin). Stimulant laxatives are not recommended in children but can be used for short periods in the child who is difficult to treat. Continue maintenance for several months/years as premature withdrawal invariably results in a relapse. For the child under 1 year, glycerine suppositories can be used as well as small doses of stool softeners, and prune/other fruit juice.

Treat an associated anal fissure and painful defecation with a local anaesthetic cream applied regularly to the anal verge, together with stool softeners.

Encourage more fibre in the diet and supplement with bulk laxatives (ispaghula husk) and encourage increased fluid intake (water or fruit juice). ☆☆◊ This will not be adequate as the only form of treatment.

Adherence and success of treatment is dependent on parental and child education and understanding of the condition and treatment aims. Behaviour modification includes a regular daily bowel routine for the toilet trained child and increased exercise. A star/reward chart can be very useful. Children should not be blamed for faecal incontinence.

An approach to vomiting

Definitions

Regurgitation is the passage of refluxed gastric contents into the oropharynx, which is often effortless.

Vomiting is the passage of refluxed gastric contents into and out of the mouth, usually with effort.

Vomiting is a symptom, not a diagnosis. The diagnosis depends on the age of the child and the presence or absence of associated features (fever, diarrhoea, headache). The differential diagnosis varies with the character of the vomitus.

> ***Practice point:***
>
> Bile stained vomiting is surgical until proven otherwise.

Figure 4.3 The differential diagnosis of vomiting

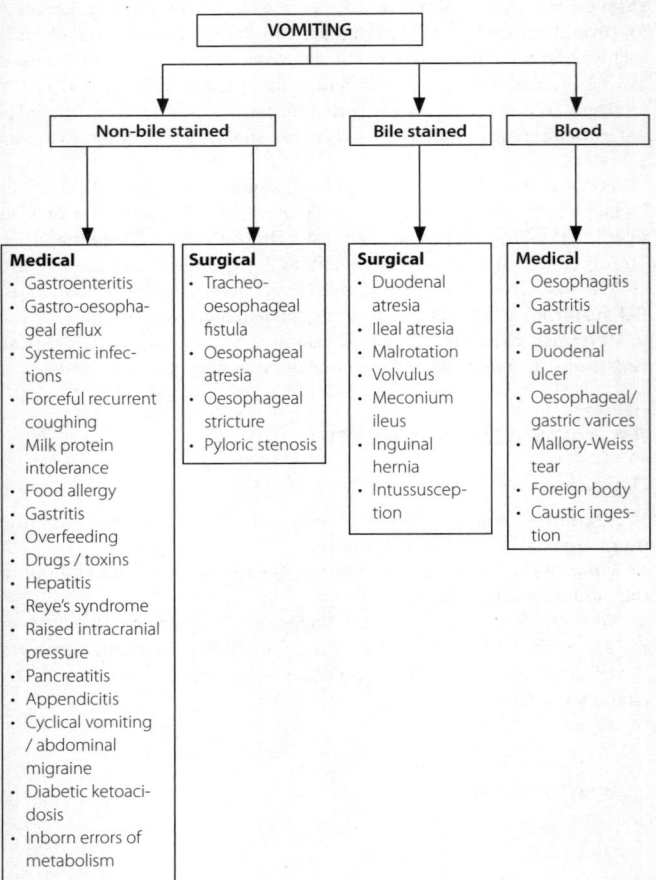

Gastro-oesophageal reflux

Gastro-oesophageal reflux (GOR) is the involuntary passage of gastric contents into the oesophagus. It is a normal physiological process that occurs throughout the day in healthy infants, children and adults. Episodes are into the distal oesophagus and are brief (< 3 minutes) and asymptomatic. Content comprises food, drink, saliva, gastric, pancreatic and biliary secretions.

Gastro-oesophageal reflux disease (GORD) is a spectrum of *disease*, defined as such when the reflux of gastric contents causes troublesome symptoms and/or complications, such as:
- Poor weight gain
- Oesophagitis: irritable, poor feeding, haematemesis, anaemia, dysphagia
- Respiratory: laryngitis/stridor, aspiration pneumonia, reactive airway disease
- Apparent life threatening events.

GORD is likely when reflux episodes to the upper oesophagus or into the carina are demonstrated by any method.

Diagnosis

History and examination: In infants and toddlers there are no symptoms that are diagnostic of GORD.

Investigations of GORD:
- Barium swallow. Useful for defining the presence of anatomical abnormalities (malrotation, hiatal hernia, oesophageal stricture) that may cause symptoms similar to those of GORD.
- Nuclear scintigraphy (nuclear medicine 'milk scan'). This is a non-invasive test, which quantifies the volume, frequency and height of the reflux. It is useful in detecting disorders of swallowing, oesophageal motility, pulmonary aspiration and oesophagitis.
- Oesophageal pH monitoring. This gives a quantitative measure of oesophageal acid reflux. It is useful in monitoring the effect of therapy.
- Combined multiple intraluminal impedence monitoring (MII) and pH monitoring. These detect acid and non-acid reflux episodes. However the role of these investigations in the evaluation of children with GORD has yet to be determined.
- Endoscopy and biopsy. This combination is used to identify and grade oesophagitis. Histology may demonstrate oesophagitis even

if the oesophagus looks macroscopically normal. It is also useful to exclude other conditions such as eosinophilic oesophagitis.

Treatment

A stepwise approach is warranted according to the severity of the symptoms. No treatment is necessary for GOR, whereas therapy is needed for GORD.

Dietary changes

For suspected milk protein sensitivity a trial of extensively hydrolyzed feed may be used. Thickening may decrease vomiting but does not decrease frequency of oesophageal reflux episodes.

The mode of feed delivery may be changed to either smaller volume feeds, continuous, nasogastric feeds or nasojejunal feeds.

Positioning

The prone position best is best, but sudden infant death syndrome (SIDS) risk is increased, so supine positioning is recommended from birth to 12 months.

Pharmacological treatment

Acid suppression with proton pump inhibitors (omeprazole 0.7–1.4 mg/kg in the morning 20 minutes before breakfast) or histamine receptor antagonists.

Surgical management

See Chapter 21, Surgical problems. Antireflux surgery may be warranted in certain children with GORD who have failed optimal medical treatment.

Recommended reading

1 *Functional gastrointestinal disorders.* Rome 3 Criteria: www.romecriteria.org
2 Kelly, DA. Managing liver failure. *Postgrad Med Journal.* 2002;78:660–667
3 Guidance for the evaluation of cholestatic jaundice in infants: Recommendations of the North American Society for Pediatric Gastroenterology, Hepatology and Nutrition. *J Pediatr Gastroenterol Nutr.* 2004;349:115–128
4 Pediatric gastroesophageal reflux clinical practice guidelines: Joint recommendations of the North American Society for Pediatric Gastroenterology, Hepatology and Nutrition (NASPGHAN) and the European Society for Pediatric Gastroenterology, Hepatology and Nutrition (ESPGHAN). *J Pediatr Gastroenterol Nutr.* 2009;49:498–647

5 Growth and nutrition

M. Hendricks

Malnutrition

Malnourished children, irrespective of severity, are at great risk of dying. The Food Fortification Baseline-1 Survey (2005) showed that among South African children aged 1–9 years 9.3% were underweight, 18% were stunted, 10% were overweight and 4% were obese.

Nutritional assessment

The nutritional status of each child attending a health facility should be assessed:
- Take a dietary history from the caregiver. Ask about the type of feeding, appetite and symptoms of underlying illness e.g. HIV and TB.
- Enquire about the family size, income and social support.
- Check the immunization status.
- Assess weight, length/height and weight-for-height: recumbent length (< 2 years), standing height (> 2 years). Plot measurements on growth charts and on the RTHC; assess the growth curve.
- Examine for severe wasting, symmetrical oedema and signs of nutrient deficiency (Table 5.1). In a child with severe malnutrition look for complicating factors such as fever, hypothermia, hypoglycaemia and underlying infection.

Table 5.1 Clinical features of nutrient deficiency

Parameter	Clinical features
Skin	• Palmar pallor (e.g. anaemia) • Hypo- or hyperpigmentation, desquamation and ulceration (zinc or protein deficiency)
Eye	• Night blindness, xerosis conjunctivae, xerosis corneae, Bitot's spots, keratomalacia, corneal scars (vitamin A deficiency) • Conjunctival pallor (e.g. anaemia)
Hair	• Depigmentation, sparsity (severe malnutrition)

Parameter	Clinical features
Mouth	• Cheilosis, glossitis, magenta tongue (B vitamin deficiency) • Bleeding gums (vitamin C deficiency)
Subcutaneous tissue	• Reduced (deficient energy) • Oedema (severe malnutrition)
Muscle bulk	• Wasting, weakness (severe malnutrition)
Bones	• Craniotabes, rickety rosary, wide metaphyses, frontal bossing, wide anterior fontanelle, delayed dentition, bow legs (vitamin D deficiency) • Bony tenderness, pseudoparalysis (vitamin C deficiency)
Abdomen	• Hepatomegaly (fatty liver)
CNS	• Apathy (severe malnutrition, iron deficiency anaemia)
Cardiac	• Cardiac failure (thiamine deficiency)
Thyroid	• Goitre (iodine deficiency)

Classification of malnutrition

Anthropometric indices are reported using percentiles or Z-scores:
- Z score:
  - Z scores express the anthropometric value as a number of standard deviations (SD) above or below the reference mean or median value.
  - The Z-score is calculated by subtracting the observed value from the median or mean of the reference population and dividing by the standard deviation (SD) of the population.
  - Curves are normally distributed with a fixed Z-score interval corresponding to a fixed weight- or height-for-age difference.
  - Z-score charts are included (see Appendix).
  - Cut-off values are a Z-score <–2SD (< 3rd centile) or > +2SD (> 97th centile)
- Percentiles:
  - Rank individuals according to a reference distribution.
  - Useful clinically but the curves are not normally distributed and cannot be used for population studies.

Based on the clinical examination a child can have:
- *Good growth*. Growth curve follows the percentiles.
- *Growth faltering or failure*. Growth curve is flat or drops off for 2 consecutive months.

- *Underweight.* Z-score of < –2 SD (< 3rd percentile) may indicate acute or chronic malnutrition. However, it may be normal for a few children to grow below, but parallel to, the –2 SD cut-off.
- *Stunting.* Z-score < –2 SD (< 3rd percentile) indicating long-term changes in nutritional status.
- *Wasting.* Weight-for-height Z-score of < –2 SD indicating recent loss of weight.

Malnourished children should be classified using the World Health Organization classification (Table 5.2).

Table 5.2 Classification of malnutrition (WHO)

	Moderate malnutrition	**Severe malnutrition**
Symmetrical oedema	No	Yes. Oedematous malnutrition[1]
Weight-for-height	–3 ≤ SD Score <–2 (70–79%) Moderate wasting	SD Score < –3 (< 70%) Severe wasting[2]
Height-for-age	–3 ≤ SD Score <–2 (85–89%) Moderate stunting	SD Score < –3 (< 85%) Severe stunting

1 In terms of the Wellcome Classification, includes the child classified with kwashiorkor and marasmic-kwashiorkor;.
2 May include the child previously classified with marasmus.

Moderate malnutrition

This includes children with wasting and stunting. The child with growth faltering and underweight should be similarly managed based on the Integrated Management of Childhood Illness (IMCI) guidelines.

Management
- Assess feeding and counsel mother/caregiver to:
  - Exclusively breast or formula feed
  - Following the introduction of complementary feeding, increase the energy density of feeds by adding a teaspoon of margarine, vegetable oil or peanut butter to feeds
  - Increase frequency of feeds (5 meals per day)

- Provide a varied and affordable diet using staples, e.g. maize meal, pulses, vegetables, fruit, meat and milk.
- Screen for and treat associated infections, e.g. TB, HIV and anaemia
- De-worm with mebendazole or albendazole
- Give high-dose vitamin A (Table 5.3), multivitamin syrup and iron as required
- Refer to the Nutrition Supplementation Programme for supplementation
- Follow up feeding problem in 5 days; if no feeding problem, follow up in 14 days.

Severe malnutrition

Definition

Children with severe malnutrition who require hospitalization usually have severe wasting and/or oedema. To reduce mortality, physiologic and metabolic changes in the severely malnourished child need to be recognized and strict attention given to appropriate management.

Clinical presentation

- *Oedematous malnutrition*. Weight may be above the 3rd centile. There may be pallor, apathy, and changes in skin, mucous membranes and hair (Table 5.1). The abdomen is protuberant with an enlarged, firm liver.
- *Severe wasting*. The child is emaciated, does not have hair, skin, mucous membrane or mental changes and the serum protein concentrations are relatively normal.
- All children with severe malnutrition have atrophic lymphoid tissue with poorly palpable lymph nodes and small tonsils. However, severely malnourished children with HIV or TB may have generalized lymphadenopathy and splenomegaly.

Investigations

Useful investigations include blood glucose, urine dipsticks (and culture if UTI suspected); electrolytes and urea, total protein, albumin; FBC; blood culture; chest X-ray, Mantoux and gastric washings and HIV test (if HIV not excluded by prior investigation).

Treatment

Admit the child who has severe wasting, or oedematous malnutrition. Children with severe stunting will require admission if they have severe

illness. Involve the mother in treatment, counselling and rehabilitation from the start. WHO recommends 10 steps to manage the severely malnourished child. The case fatality rate has been significantly reduced in settings where these guidelines have been implemented. ☆☆☆☆☜
These may be applied in two phases:
- Stabilization (1–7 days): management of acute problems
- Rehabilitation (2–6 weeks): ongoing management.

1 Treat/ prevent hypoglycaemia (blood glucose < 3 mmol/l):

> *Practice point:*
>
> Prevent hypoglycaemia by early feeding or giving oral 10% dextrose on admission.

- Monitor the blood glucose 4 hourly for first 48 hours.
- Feed every 2 hours for 48 hours then 3 hourly. Where this is not feasible consider using continuous nasogastric feeds, especially in the first 48 hours.
- *If hypoglycaemia develops:*
  - Feed or give 50 ml 10% dextrose orally or by NGT
  - Feed every 30 min for 2 hours for 24 hours, then 2 hourly
  - Give 5 ml/kg IV 10% dextrose if child unconscious, lethargic or convulsing.

2 Treat/prevent hypothermia (axillary temperature < 35 °C):
- Prevent this by frequent feeding, maintaining a warm and draught-free environment, avoiding exposure, and clothing the child and letting him/her sleep with the mother.
- *If hypothermia develops:*
  - Clothe (including head) and keep dry.
  - Use heater, lamp, warming blanket.
  - Feed 2 hourly.
  - Monitor the temperature 2-hourly until 36.5 °C.
- Hypothermia and hypoglycaemia often occur together and may indicate underlying infection.
- Hypothermia causes slow capillary filling; do not mistake this for *hypovolaemia* and overcorrect with excess fluids.

3 Treat/prevent dehydration:

> *Practice point:*
>
> IV fluids only for shock; otherwise rehydrate orally or by NGT. ☆☆☆☆☆

- Difficult to estimate dehydration in a severely malnourished child so assume that children with watery diarrhoea are dehydrated.
- Guideline for rehydration:
  - 10 ml/ kg/ hour for first 2 hours;
  - 5–10 ml/kg/ hour next 4–10 hours.
  - Offer breast or formula feeds no later than 4 hours following the start of oral rehydration.
  - Assess the progress of rehydration by checking respiratory rate, pulse rate, urine and stool frequency hourly.
  - If signs of overhydration, stop fluids and reassess after 1 hour.

4 Correct electrolyte imbalance:
- K^+: 3–4 mmol/kg/day: < 5 kg KCl 250 mg PO 8 hrly; 5–10 kg KCl 500 mg PO 8 hourly; > 10 kg 1 g 8 hourly orally until the oedema has resolved. In renal failure carefully monitor serum K^+ concentrations and the ECG tracing, and withhold potassium or use smaller doses
- Mg^{++}: 0.4–0.6 mmol/kg/day: Give either magnesium chloride 50 mg/kg/day (solution with 440 mg elemental magnesium per 5 ml) orally or magnesium sulphate (50%) 0.2 ml/kg/day IMI
- Give potassium and magnesium until oedema subsides
- Phosphate 2–3 mmol/kg/day if low.

5 Treat/prevent infection:

> *Practice point:*
>
> Assume that all children have underlying infection and *treat every child with broad spectrum antibiotics.* ☆☆☆☆

- If the child is severely ill (apathetic or lethargic) or has complications (hypoglycaemia, hypothermia, broken skin, and lower respiratory tract or urinary tract infection) give:
  - Ampicillin 50 mg/kg/dose IV 6 hourly and gentamicin 7.5 mg/kg/day IV for 7 days
  - Metronidazole 7.5 mg/kg 8 hourly orally for 7 days

- Where specific infections are identified treat according to the antibiotic sensitivity.
- If the child appears to have no complications give:
  - Co-amoxicillin/clavulanate (Augmentin®) 15 mg/kg/dose 8 hourly (if no diarrhoea) or cefuroxime 10–15 mg/kg/dose 12 hourly for 5 days. In situations where these antibiotics are not available follow the WHO recommendation of giving amoxicillin 15 mg/kg/dose 8 hourly for 5 days.

For all children:
- Give measles vaccine if child not immunized and > 6 months.
- Give mebendazole or albendazole orally.
- Treat TB when suspected.

6 Correct micronutrient deficiencies:

> *Practice point:*
>
> Do not give iron until oedema has resolved (usually 7–10 days) and the child is gaining weight.

Give daily for 2 weeks:
- *Multivitamin syrup* 5 ml/day for 3 months
- *Vitamin A* on day 1 (Table 5.3)
- *Folate* 2.5 mg/day
- *Zinc* 2 mg/kg per day orally, 2–6 months 10 mg daily, > 6 months 20 mg daily
- Do not give iron until oedema has resolved (usually 7–10 days) and the child is gaining weight. Thereafter give *ferrous gluconate* 3 mg/kg/day for 12 weeks if there is anaemia.
- *Vitamin K* is given when there is a bleeding tendency or an international normalized ratio (INR) greater than 2.

7 Start cautious feeding:
- Start feeding as soon as possible after admission and provide sufficient energy and protein to maintain the physiologic processes.
- If the child is breastfed, encourage the mother to continue.
- If replacement fed, use:
  - Low osmolarity and low lactose feeds. A slow cautious approach is essential; give oral or nasogastric tube feeds
  - 100 kcal/kg/day
  - 1–1.5 g protein/kg/day
  - 130 ml/kg/day (100 ml/kg/day if oedematous).

- Day 1–2: 2 hourly feeds; day 3–5: 3 hourly feeds; from day 6 onwards: 4 hourly feeds
- Keep a record of intake and output; check daily weights.

8 Achieve catch-up growth:
This occurs during rehabilitation and is associated with a return of appetite. During this phase:
- Give the child 150–200 kcal/kg/day and protein 4 g/kg/day but there should be a gradual transition to high-energy feeds.
- Ready to use therapeutic food (RUTF), a lipid-rich, energy dense food that is not water-based, is recommended.
- Increase feed volumes.
- If the child is breastfed, encourage the mother to continue.
- Monitor the pulse and respiratory rate to avoid precipitating cardiac failure.
- Weigh the child and record the intake daily:
  - Weight gain should exceed 10 g/kg/day.
  - Failure to maintain catch-up growth indicates an undiagnosed infection or inadequate intake.

9 Provide sensory stimulation and emotional support:
- Involve the mother in feeding, bathing, comforting and play
- Provide:
  - A stimulating environment
  - 15–30 minutes of structured play daily
  - Physical activity when the child is well.

10 Prepare for follow-up after recovery:
- Child considered to have recovered if weight-for-length is −1 SD.
- Consider discharge when gaining weight, infection is treated, oedema has resolved and biochemical indices are normal.
- Advise/counsel mother caregiver to:
  - Feed with energy dense foods (see IMCI recommendations).
  - Provide structured play.
  - Apply for a child support grant (consult with social worker).
  - Attend local clinic and community projects (provide letter).

Treatment of associated conditions
Anaemia:
- Transfuse (10 ml/kg) of whole blood if Hb < 4 g/dl or if there is respiratory distress and Hb is between 4–6 g/dl. Transfuse over

4-6 hours ✢ and give 1 mg/kg of furosemide at the **start** of the transfusion. Monitor for signs of cardiac failure.
- Dermatosis. Apply zinc and castor oil to raw areas and omit nappies so that the perineum can stay dry. Treat associated fungal infection with topical clotrimazole and oral nystatin. If bacterial skin infection is suspected treat with topical antibacterial creams and oral antibiotics.
- Eye problems. If there are eye signs of vitamin A deficiency, give vitamin A on days 1, 2 and 14. To prevent corneal rupture instil chloramphenicol or tetracycline eye drops 3 hourly for 7–10 days; use atropine eye drops 3 times daily for 3–5 days; cover the eyes with saline-soaked pads and bandage them.

Nutrient deficiencies

Vitamin A

The vitamin A (VA) status is marginal in 1 out of 3 children < 6 years of age. The main signs of vitamin A deficiency (VAD) are outlined in Table 5.1. VA supplementation can reduce the all-cause mortality rate in children aged 6 months to 5 years by 23% ☆☆☆☆◐ especially from diarrhoea, measles and HIV infection.

All children < 5 yr should be supplemented routinely every 6 months with VA (Table 5.3). Check to see if the child requires VA and record the dose given on the RTHC. Give an additional dose of vitamin A for severe malnutrition, persistent diarrhoea, measles and xerophthalmia. Do not give vitamin A if a dose was given in the previous month. If there is measles or xerophthalmia the dose must be repeated after 24 hours, and again on day 14 for xerophthalmia.

Table 5.3 National vitamin A supplementation programme

Target group	Dosage	Duration
Non-breastfed infants 0–5 months	50 000 IU	single dose at 6 weeks
6–11 months	100 000 IU	single dose at 6 months, or up to 11 months
12–60 months	200 000 IU	single dose at 12 months, and then every 6 months until 60 months
All post-partum women	200 000 IU	single dose at delivery (no later than 6–8 weeks after)

Vitamin D

Figure 5.1 provides an approach to rickets.

Vitamin D-deficiency rickets results from failure of bone matrix mineralization at the growth plate. Deficiency results from inadequate exposure to sunlight or a poor dietary intake. The main signs are outlined in Table 5.1. Recurrent chest infections may occur. Radiologically there is osteopenia, cupping, fraying and flaring of the metaphyses, and delay in epiphyseal development. Biochemical changes include hypophosphataemia and elevation of alkaline phosphatase. Hypocalcaemia is variable. A generalized aminoaciduria may result from the secondary hyperparathyroidism. Treat with oral vitamin D 5 000 IU per day for four weeks and thereafter ensure an intake of 400 IU per day.

Zinc

According to a recent national survey, 45% of South African children aged 1-9 years are deficient in zinc. Zinc deficiency in children is associated with an increased risk of diarrhoea, respiratory infection and growth failure. There is also an increased risk of mortality from diarrhoea, respiratory infection and malaria. Zinc supplementation reduces the frequency of: diarrhoea (14%); severe diarrhoea (15%); persistent diarrhoea (25%); respiratory illness (8%) and LRTI (20%). It also reduces stunting and mortality in SGA infants.

WHO currently recommends supplementation of all children with diarrhoea and severe malnutrition. The recommended dosage: < 6 months 10 mg daily; > 6 months 20 mg daily for 10–14 days. ☆ ☆ ☆ ☆ ☆

An approach to failure to thrive

Definition

Failure to thrive (FTT) broadly includes children whose weight is below the norm for gestation corrected age, gender, genetic potential and medical condition. It is a process that may lead to malnutrition. There is no consensus regarding the definition of FTT but it includes any of the following in the child where growth is observed over time:
- Weight < 3rd percentile for gestation corrected age on more than 1 occasion (note that there are special growth charts for children with Down's syndrome, Turner's syndrome and cerebral palsy).
- Weight for length/ height < 10th percentile.
- Weight gain decrease in two or more major percentile lines.
- A daily weight gain less than expected for age (Table 5.4).

Figure 5.1 An approach to rickets

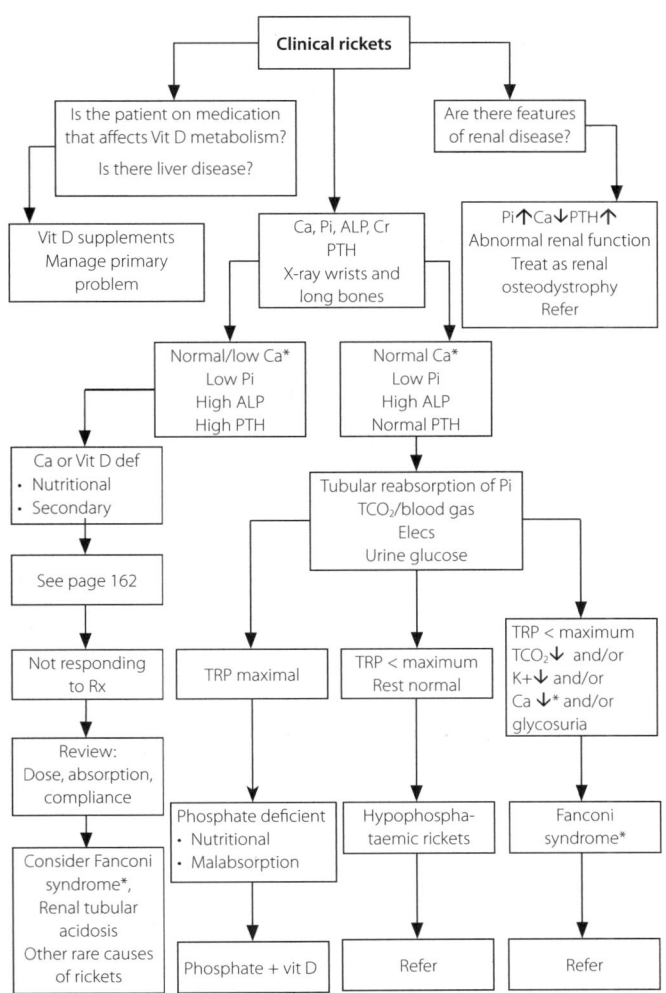

*Fanconi syndrome may start with only one abnormality and develop several over time

Children with genetic short stature, prematurity and intrauterine growth restriction with an appropriate weight for length and normal growth velocity are not included in the definition of FTT.

Table 5.4 Rate of daily weight gain expected for age

Age (months)	Daily weight gain (g/day)
0–3	26–31
3–6	17–18
6–9	12–13
9–12	9–13
12–36	7–9

Aetiology

The causes of FTT are inadequate energy intake, inadequate nutrient absorption or increased energy requirements. The majority of cases are due to inadequate energy intake as a result of poor feeding or psychosocial problems.

Table 5.5 Causes of failure to thrive

Inadequate nutrient intake	Inadequate nutrient absorption	Increased nutrient requirements/ ineffective utilization
Feeding problems: • Poor feeding technique • Insufficient lactation • Inadequate preparation • Inadequate quantity • Inappropriate type • Food fads Poverty Disturbed child/caregiver relationship Mechanical: • Cleft palate • Nasal obstruction • Dental lesion Dysfunctional sucking/ swallowing: • Hypoxic ischaemic encephalopathy • Cerebral palsy Gastro-oesophageal reflux	Malabsorption: • Infection/parasites • Lactose intolerance • Milk allergy • Cystic fibrosis • Inflammatory bowel disease • Coeliac disease Intestinal obstruction: • Pyloric stenosis • Hernia • Malrotation Biliary atresia/cirrhosis Short bowel syndrome	Chronic/recurrent infection: • Tuberculosis • HIV • Urinary tract infection Chronic disease: • Juvenile idiopathic arthritis • Bronchopulmonary dysplasia • Anaemia • Cardiopulmonary/renal disease Genetic syndromes Metabolic problems: • Galactosaemia • Storage disease • Hypercalcaemia Endocrine: • Hyperthyroidism • Diabetes mellitus

History

Include details of the following:
- Medical:
  - Perinatal: prenatal exposure to toxins, e.g. alcohol, anticonvulsants; birth weight and gestation; any neonatal problems
  - Previous chronic or recurrent illnesses
  - Family illnesses, weight/height of family members and developmental delay
  - Review systems for underlying symptoms.
- Diet and feeding:
  - Nutritional intake and feeding (quantity, type of foods, frequency, enrichment, duration of meals)
  - Food preferences
  - Inappropriate nutrient intake, e.g. low calorie juices or teas
  - Dietary restrictions.

Family and psychosocial:
- Determine the following:
  - Primary caregiver
  - Family composition
  - Family income, food security and support systems
  - Psychosocial stressors (involve social worker).

Development:
- Enquire about the child's developmental milestones and behaviour.

Examination

Examine for the following signs:
- *General:* observe interaction of caregiver with child; nutritional status as outlined; dysmorphism (e.g. FAS); microcephaly; cataracts (galactosaemia, congenital infection), clubbing (e.g. chronic lung disease, cystic fibrosis); lymphadenopathy (HIV, TB); bruising of skin (child abuse) and hyperthyroidism
- *ENT:* cleft palate, drooling, oropharyngeal lesions (e.g. candidiasis)
- *Cardiovascular system:* congenital or acquired heart disease
- *Respiratory system:* chest deformities, hyperinflation, wheezing and crackles (chronic lung disease)
- *Abdomen:* distension (malabsorption); hepatosplenomegaly (liver disease; storage disease; malignancy)
- *Central nervous system:* spasticity and increased reflexes (cerebral palsy); hypotonia and weakness. Also assess the child's *development*.

Investigations

These depend on the underlying symptoms and signs. Recommended baseline tests include urinalysis and culture (if UTI suspected), urinary reducing substances, full blood count, ESR, electrolytes, urea and creatinine, TB and HIV screen, stool pH, reducing substances, fat stain and parasites, sweat chloride test, barium swallow or milk scan (if GOR suspected).

Management

A multidisciplinary approach is recommended that includes a dietician, gastroenterologist, speech therapist, psychologist/psychiatrist and social worker.

Indications for hospitalization include significant medical problems, severe malnutrition, child abuse, neglect and psychosocial problems not responding to outpatient care. Parenteral feeding is indicated if there is impaired intake or increased requirements cannot be met by oral feeds. The diagnosis should guide further management of FTT.

Recommended reading

1. Ashworth A, Khanum S, Jackson A, Schofield C. *Guidelines for the inpatient treatment of severely malnourished children*. Geneva. World Health Organization. 2003.
2. World Health Organization (WHO). *Management of severe malnutrition: a manual for physicians and other senior health workers*. Geneva. WHO. 1999.
3. Ahmed T, Ali M, Ullah MM, Choudury IA, Haque ME, Salam MA, Rabbani GH, Suskind RM, Fuchs GJ. Mortality in severely malnourished children with diarrhoea and use of a standardised management protocol. *Lancet* 1999; 353: 1919-1922.
4. Kirkland R. *Etiology and evaluation of failure to thrive (undernutrition) in children younger than two years*. In: UpToDate, Drutz JE, Augustyn M, Motil KJ (Eds), Waltham. MA. 2008.

6   Cardiovascular problems

R. De Decker, J. Lawrenson, H. Pribut, L. Zühlke

Cardiovascular disease in infants and children manifests in various ways: cyanosis, respiratory distress, shock, irregular heart rhythm, murmurs, and cardiac failure. This chapter provides an approach to these categories, with discussion of specific congenital and acquired conditions. Cardiac examination in general will not be discussed, although the importance of a thorough clinical examination of the patient cannot be over-emphasized. In particular, do not disregard parental concerns regarding cyanosis.

An initial approach to the diagnosis of congenital heart disease

It is often not possible (nor useful) for the general practitioner to make a precise diagnosis. However, it is possible for patients to be categorized into broad groups and managed appropriately. A good starting point is the presence or absence of cyanosis.

The clinical impression of cyanosis can be confirmed by pulse oximetry. In the neonate especially, a normal saturation does not rule out a heart lesion as the duct may still be patent. Discharge saturations should be higher than 95%.

Figure 6.1 Approach to the child with cardiac disease

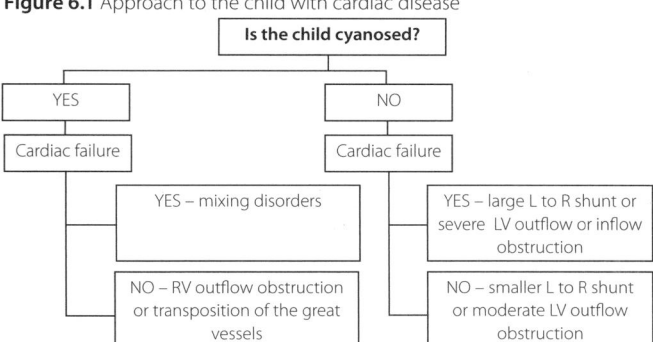

Cyanosis absent

- *Left to right shunt*: ventricular septal defect, patent arterial duct, atrial septal defect or combinations thereof.
- *Inflow or outflow obstruction*: mitral stenosis, coarctation, aortic stenosis or combinations thereof or pulmonary stenosis.

Cyanosis present

- *Mixing disorders – increased pulmonary blood flow/heart failure.*
  Oxygenated and deoxygenated blood mix within the heart or vessels or in both and there is increased flow to the lungs and signs of congestive heart failure. Pulmonary flow depends on pulmonary vascular resistance, which is high at birth. As the child gets older, the pulmonary flow increases and results in congestive failure. The child will develop symptomatic heart failure around 6 weeks of age, e.g. common arterial trunk.
- *Right ventricular outflow tract obstruction – reduced pulmonary blood flow.*
  An admixture of oxygenated and deoxygenated blood within the heart, as well as a markedly reduced pulmonary blood flow, occurs in these abnormalities. The admixture (and hence the degree of cyanosis) is determined by the severity of RV outflow narrowing, e.g. Tetralogy of Fallot.

Table 6.1 Common heart conditions in babies

Lesions	Cardiac failure	Cyanosis	Chest X-ray	Clinical group
The first month				
Hypoplastic left heart syndrome	+++ Shock	+	Cardiomegaly Plethora	LVOTO
Coarctation of the aorta	+++	–	Cardiomegaly	LVOTO
Transposition of the great arteries	+	+++	Cardiomegaly Plethora	'Mixer'
Obstruction to the right heart, e.g. pulmonary atresia	–	+++	Oligaemia	RVOTO
Arrhythmias	++	±	Normal	Arrhythmia
1–3 months				
Complex VSD (+ PDA or ASD)	++	–	Cardiomegaly Plethora	L to R shunt
Intracardiac mixing, e.g. TAPVD	++	+	Cardiomegaly Plethora	'Mixer'

Lesions	Cardiac failure	Cyanosis	Chest X-ray	Clinical group
Atrioventricular canal (AVSD)	+++	±	Cardiomegaly Plethora	L to R shunt
Functionally single ventricle/ TGA+VSD	++	++	Cardiomegaly Plethora	mixer
Common arterial trunk	++	++	Cardiomegaly Plethora	mixer
3–12 months				
Left to right shunts	+	–	Cardiomegaly Plethora	L to R shunt
Myocarditis/cardiomyopathy	++	–	Cardiomegaly Congestion	Acquired heart disease
Tetralogy of Fallot	–	++	Oligaemia Normal sized heart	RVOTO

Key:
- PDA = patent ductus arteriosus
- ASD = atrial septal defect
- VSD = ventricular septal defect
- TAPVD = total anomalous pulmonary venous drainage
- TGA = transposition of great vessels
- AVSD = atrioventricular septal defect
- Plethora = increased pulmonary flow
- Oligaemia = decreased pulmonary flow
- Congestion = decreased pulmonary venous drainage
- LVOTO = left ventricular outflow tract obstruction
- RVOTO = right ventricular outflow tract obstruction

Common symptom complexes

The neonate with central cyanosis

- Does the baby have cyanotic congenital heart disease or respiratory disease?
  - The neonate with respiratory disease is often premature and has significant respiratory distress. In addition the X-ray shows obvious parenchymal changes. Blood gas analysis reveals hypoxia with normo- or hypercarbia. Blood gases or saturation measurements return to normal with the administration of the highest concentration of oxygen possible.
  - The neonate with congenital heart disease is more likely to be full term with mild tachypnoea at most. Blood gas analysis reveals

hypoxia with normo- or hypocarbia. The infant fails to improve after the administration of oxygen.

> **Practice point:**
>
> The analysis of the effect of oxygen administration on transcutaneous saturation measurements to differentiate between respiratory and cardiac disease has not been formally compared to the hyperoxia test that uses blood gas analysis.

Management of the neonate with cyanosis

- Treat all suspected cyanotic heart disease as though there is a lesion with a duct-dependent circulation. In infants less than 6 weeks old give prostaglandin E_2 by nasogastric tube to open the arterial duct. Prostaglandin E_2 (dinoprostone (Prostin-E_2®)): ¼ tablet (125 µg) half hourly, crushed and dissolved in 2–5 mls water. Increase to ½ a tablet every 15 minutes if necessary. ☆☆☆☆☆
- Potential side effects include apnoea, profuse watery dehydrating diarrhoea, hypothermia, acidosis (even in the absence of diarrhoea) and hypoglycaemia.
- Ensure that the airway, breathing and circulation are adequate. Administer oxygen (highest concentration possible) and establish intravenous access. Provide warmth (in an incubator) and maintain a normal blood glucose level.
- If cyanosis does not improve, commence assisted ventilation prior to the use of intravenous prostaglandin. Prostaglandin E_1 (alprostadil (Prostin VR®)) causes significantly more apnoea than oral prostaglandin, particularly at high infusion rates. In South Africa, intravenous prostaglandin use is limited to regional or tertiary hospitals. Recommended infusion rate is 0.005 µg/kg/minute up to 0.1 µg/kg/minute (60 µg/kg alprostadil in 50 ml saline run at 0.5 ml/hr will provide 0.01 µg/kg/minute). Do not use IV prostaglandin if equipment and personnel to intubate and ventilate the patient are not readily available.
- Transfer the patient when stable. Consider the use of air transportation if the child is more than an hour from a major referral centre.

The older child with cyanosis

Cyanotic heart disease presents mostly in early infancy. Over 3 months of age less severe right ventricular outflow tract lesions predominate. The most common is Tetralogy of Fallot. Consider cyanotic heart disease in the older child who has cyanosis with clubbing and an abnormal cardiovascular examination without obvious respiratory pathology or CO_2 retention.

Problem: hypercyanotic spells

These occur in congenital heart defects with right ventricular outflow tract, e.g. Tetralogy of Fallot or in any complex defect with severe pulmonary stenosis. Such spells – thought to be the result of infundibular muscle spasm – can be precipitated by diarrhoea, mild upper respiratory infections, anaemia or emotional upset.

Clinical presentation

Cyanosis, tachypnoea and acidosis intensify during a spell and murmurs diminish in intensity or disappear.

Prevention

- Correct or avoid precipitating factors such as crying. Avoid hot baths that cause systemic vasodilatation. Treat mild gastroenteritis aggressively to avoid dehydration and acidosis. Correct iron-deficiency anaemia.
- Explain the precipitating factors to the parents and ensure that they remain with their child throughout hospitalizations to avoid emotional upset.
- Oral β-blockers (propanolol 3–5 mg/kg per day in 3 divided doses) can be used to prevent spells.

Management

- A hyper-cyanotic spell is an emergency and a single episode warrants referral to a specialist centre for prompt evaluation.
- Encourage the caregiver to console the child.
- Give oxygen 100% by facemask; allow the child to remain in the arms of the parent if possible.
- Bend the legs at the hips and knees ('squatting' while supine). This increases the systemic vascular resistance and decreases the right to left shunt.
- Morphine: 0.1 mg/kg IV or subcutaneously if IV access is not available. Chloral hydrate (50 mg/kg orally) or midazolam (IV preparation – 0.5 mg/kg rectally) may be given during the early stages of a mild spell to sedate the child and hopefully terminate the event.
- Insert an intravenous cannula and infuse normal saline or Ringer's lactate (10 ml/kg) rapidly; repeat the 10 ml/kg boluses if there is no improvement. Liberal use of intravenous fluids is encouraged.

- Sodium bicarbonate 8.4 %: 2 ml/kg IV.
- Monitor the response to therapy with transcutaneous oxygen saturations. As the muscle in the infundibulum relaxes and blood is ejected into the pulmonary artery the ejection murmur returns.
- If these measures fail, administer ketamine (0.5–1 mg/kg IV). Intubate and ventilate the patient if the patient remains cyanosed and acidotic. A transfusion of blood is needed if the haemoglobin concentration is less than 10 g/dl.
- If the emergency management fails, an urgent Blalock-Taussig shunt (surgical connection of a subclavian artery to a pulmonary artery) is required and the patient must be transferred to the appropriate centre as quickly as possible.

> *Practice point:*
>
> The intravenous ß-blocker esmolol is no longer available in South Africa. This drug (if available) is typically administered prior to the administration of ketamine.

Problem: the neonate with cardiovascular collapse

A neonate with an obstructive left heart lesion (such as coarctation, critical aortic stenosis, hypoplastic left heart syndrome, and interrupted aortic arch) is often incorrectly assessed as having septic shock or a metabolic abnormality.

Consider a cardiac lesion:
- If there is no response to fluid boluses in a shocked neonate.
- If a neonate presents with poor feeding, lethargy, tachypnoea, poor peripheral perfusion, an enlarged liver and has an enlarged heart and pulmonary oedema on chest X-ray.

Management
- Resuscitation includes maintenance of an airway, control of body temperature and placement of an intravenous cannula.
- If the diagnosis can be confirmed at the referral centre, do not administer oxygen at all to avoid pulmonary flooding. If the diagnosis is not known, do not administer more than 40% oxygen.
- Start prostaglandin (see above) to ensure duct patency and transfer the patient to a specialist centre.

Problem: congestive cardiac failure

Clinical features result from the inability of the cardiovascular system to meet the demands placed on the heart:

- Pulmonary venous congestion results in dyspnoea, difficulty with feeding, tachypnoea, subcostal recession and wheezing. Repeated attacks of wheezing/bronchiolitis may be caused by congestive heart failure. Basal crackles are generally not heard in the chest of a small child with heart failure.
- Systemic venous congestion results in hepatomegaly and rarely in oedema.
- Pallor, sweating (particularly with feeding), cold extremities and poor pulses are a feature of increased sympathetic nervous system activity.
- Fluid retention is manifested by abnormal weight gain or a decrease in urinary output.
- Failure to thrive may be the only manifestation of heart failure.

Treatment of acute severe heart failure

- Oxygen 40%
- Intravenous diuretic: furosemide 1–2 mg/kg/dose
- If the response is poor, use an intravenous inotropic agent such as dopamine but obtain a specialist opinion beforehand.
- The patient may require intubation and ventilation for transfer to a tertiary centre.

Treatment of less severe heart failure

- Restrict fluid intake: give 60% of the total daily requirements initially. (Fluid restriction may cause unhappiness in the older child.)
- Reduce preload with diuretics:
  - Furosemide: 1–2 mg/kg/day in 2–4 divided doses (intravenously or orally).
  - Spironolactone: 1 mg/kg PO 2 or 3 times a day. In combination with furosemide it enhances diuresis and prevents furosemide-related hypokalaemia. The effects of the drug are due to its function at a tissue level rather than to its diuretic action.
- Reduce afterload with angiotensin converting enzyme (ACE) inhibitors:
  - Captopril: commence: 0.5 mg/kg/day PO divided into 8 hourly dosage (neonates 0.1 mg/kg/day). Increase by 0.5 mg/kg/day. Maintenance: 3–5 mg/kg/day. Stop potassium supplements. Monitor urea and creatinine values twice weekly in neonates and infants. In neonates, ACE inhibitors should be used only after consultation with a paediatric cardiologist.

- Caloric supplementation: this may be necessary as the basal metabolic rate is often greatly increased; poor feeding due to dyspnoea and/or anorexia as a result of gut oedema may decrease caloric intake.

> ***Practice point:***
>
> The use of angiotensin converting enzyme inhibitors and spironolactone in children with heart failure has not been studied. The use of these drugs is extended from randomized controlled trials in adults with heart failure. Digoxin has fallen out of favour as a result of a narrow therapeutic window; in addition, patients with large left to right shunts are nowadays offered surgery early in infancy. Digoxin may be used in patients with severe heart failure due to a cardiomyopathy after consultation with a cardiologist.

Problem: the well child with a cardiac murmur

- An innocent or functional murmur occurs in 60% of normal children. The detection of a cardiac murmur in a healthy child often creates a disproportionate amount of anxiety in doctors and parents.
- Auscultation of the heart reveals normal sounds and a soft vibratory murmur that is heard only in systole.
- The murmur is loudest at the left sternal edge and does not radiate. It varies with posture and does not disappear when the head is turned. Its intensity increases with fever and anxiety.
- The general practitioner should seek the opinion of a paediatrician if there is any evidence of a constitutional abnormality such as failure to thrive or if the patient has symptoms directly referable to the cardiovascular system such as tiredness, impaired effort tolerance or syncope.

Problem: the child with prior cardiac surgery

Increasing numbers of children with complex congenital heart disease are surviving into adolescence and adulthood. The pathophysiology of these lesions and their treatment is not covered in most undergraduate or many postgraduate curricula. Many patients and their parents have a limited understanding of their own disease.

When such patients are encountered – even for trivial medical problems – practitioners should contact the tertiary referral centre where the surgery was performed. Extensive patient databases are maintained at such centres to facilitate advice and treatment.

Acquired heart disease

Rheumatic fever

This is a common systemic disease affecting several systems including the heart. Rheumatic fever occurs typically between the ages of 5 and 15 years and is the commonest cause of acquired heart disease in South African children. The exact pathophysiology of the disease is unclear. Group A β-haemolytic streptococcal infection, poor socio-economic conditions and a genetic predisposition result in a disease with potentially devastating consequences. Recurrence is more likely during the first year after the initial attack and in the younger patient.

> ***Practice point:***
> Acute rheumatic fever is a notifiable condition in South Africa.

Diagnosis

The modified Duckett-Jones criteria (listed below) are helpful. The criteria are used to diagnose a first attack of rheumatic fever. A previous streptococcal infection (raised antistreptolysin O titre) and/or culture of β-haemolytic group A streptococcus plus one major and two minor criteria or two major criteria are needed to make the diagnosis. Failure to meet the criteria (which apply to the epidemiological definition of the disease rather than to the diagnosis in an individual patient) does not exclude rheumatic fever.

Major criteria:
- Carditis
- Migrating polyarthritis
- Chorea
- Subcutaneous nodules
- Erythema marginatum.

Minor criteria:
- Fever > 38 °C
- Arthralgia
- Raised erythrocyte sedimentation rate (ESR) or raised C-reactive protein
- Leucocytosis
- Prolonged PR interval on ECG.

Acute rheumatic fever and infective bacterial endocarditis may be difficult to differentiate at initial presentation. If so, it is essential to obtain blood cultures (and if possible two-dimensional echocardiography) before commencing specific treatment for acute rheumatic carditis.

In areas of high prevalence of rheumatic heart disease, it is more appropriate to use the 2002–2003 World Health Organization diagnostic criteria to allow for the diagnosis of recurrent disease and to ensure that patients receive appropriate prophylaxis against further acute episodes and ensuing valve damage.

Mitral regurgitation or aortic regurgitation detected with Doppler echocardiography alone (i.e. without clinically detectable regurgitation) is currently considered insufficient evidence to diagnose carditis.

Table 6.2 WHO criteria for the diagnosis of rheumatic fever

Diagnostic categories	Criteria
Primary episode of RF	Two major or one major and two minor manifestations **plus** evidence of a preceding group A streptococcal infection
Recurrent attack of RF in a patient **without** established rheumatic heart disease	Two major or one minor and two minor manifestations **plus** evidence of a preceding group A streptococcal infection
Recurrent attack of RF in a patient **with** established rheumatic heart disease	Two minor manifestations **plus** evidence of a preceding group A streptococcal infection
Rheumatic chorea Insidious onset rheumatic carditis	Other major manifestations or evidence of group A streptococcal infection not required
Chronic valve lesions of RHD (patients presenting for the first time with mitral stenosis or mixed mitral valve disease and/or aortic valve disease)	Do not require any other criteria to be diagnosed as having rheumatic heart disease

2002-2003 WHO criteria for the diagnosis of rheumatic fever disease (based on the revised Jones criteria).

Source: Rheumatic fever and rheumatic heart disease – report of a WHO Expert Consultation, Geneva 29 October–1 November 2001.WHO technical report series 923.p.23, Table 4.1 © World Health Organization 2004. http://www.who.int/cardiovascular_diseases/resources/trs923/en/

Treatment

- Bed rest (preferably as a hospital inpatient) until the sleeping pulse is normal and signs of rheumatic activity have resolved (evidence dated).
- Single dose of Benzathine penicillin 1.2 million units IMI or Penicillin V 250 mg PO 6 hourly for 10 days (in order to eradicate carriage of streptococci).

- Non-steroidal anti-inflammatory agents such as ibuprofen: for symptomatic relief of fever and joint pain. Non-steroidal anti-inflammatory drugs may be more effective and better tolerated than aspirin. Acetyl salicylic acid (Aspirin soluble®) 75 mg/kg/day PO may be used if ibuprofen is not available.
- Steroids: these are still used in some centres but a Cochrane review did not find good evidence for their use. ☆☆☆☆😐
- Patients with the following complications need immediate referral to a tertiary centre:
  - Low cardiac output with severe cardiac failure due to mitral or aortic regurgitation.
  - Critical mitral stenosis with low cardiac output or pulmonary oedema.
  - Carditis (persistent resting tachycardia) that recurs or fails to settle within 2 weeks.

Prevention

- *Primary:* early treatment of suspected streptococcal sore throat with Penicillin V 250 mg PO 6 hourly for 10 days. Emerging evidence suggests that 1.2 million units Benzathine penicillin is superior.
- *Secondary:* (in children who have had rheumatic fever) early treatment with 1.2 million units Benzathine penicillin. ☆☆👍

Table 6.3 Duration of secondary prophylaxis (modified from WHO guidelines)

Category	Duration of monthly penicillin prophylaxis
Patient with history of ARF but without proven carditis	5 years after last attack or until 18 years of age – whichever is longer
Patient with healed carditis or mild mitral regurgitation	10 years after last attack or until 25 years of age – whichever is longer
More severe valve disease or after surgery	Lifelong prophylaxis

Infective endocarditis

Clinical presentation

Consider the diagnosis in a patient with a pyrexial illness without an obvious cause. A history of fatigue and vague joint pain is common and clinical findings include new murmurs, anaemia, splenomegaly and haematuria. Splinter haemorrhages, Osler nodes and Roth spots are rare.

Investigations

- *Blood culture*: take at least 3 before commencing treatment. This can be done within an hour if the child is very ill. The cultures need not be obtained during fever spikes. Ensure strict asepsis when taking these specimens, as contamination with skin flora may lead to confusion. The specimens may need to be incubated for more than a week before an organism is grown.

> ***Practice point:***
>
> Ask the microbiology laboratory for a prolonged culture (2 weeks) on all specimens from patients with suspected endocarditis.

- *Echocardiography*: vegetations can usually be seen if an echocardiographic examination is performed by an experienced practitioner. Failure to detect vegetations does not 'rule out' the diagnosis. (Small vegetations may not be detected at the onset of the disease.)

Treatment

Antibiotics: the duration and choice of treatment should ideally be discussed with a bacteriologist. Refer all patients with endocarditis (especially those with prosthetic valve endocarditis) to a specialist centre early in the disease. Bacterial endocarditis is not a 'medical' condition and prompt surgical treatment is often required.

Use the following guidelines: ☆ ☆ ☆ ☆ ☼
- Unknown organism: give penicillin, cloxacillin and gentamicin IV for 4 weeks. (Use cloxacillin plus penicillin as enterococci are not always sensitive to the former.)
- *Streptococcus viridans*: give Penicillin IV (200 000 U/kg daily in divided doses 4–6 hourly) for 4 weeks and gentamicin IV (1 mg/kg every 8 hours) for 2 weeks. (Daily use of gentamicin in children with endocarditis has not been studied.)
- *Enterococcus* spp: give Penicillin IV and gentamicin IV for 4–6 weeks.
- *Staphylococcus aureus*: give cloxacillin IV (200 mg/kg/day) for 4–6 weeks. Use gentamicin IV for 3–5 days for aminoglycoside-sensitive organisms.
- HACEK organisms (fastidious gram negative organisms originating from the mouth) i.e. *Haemophilus* spp, *Actinobacillus* (recently

renamed *Aggregatibacter actinomycetemcomitans*), *Cardiobacterium hominis*, *Eikenella corrodens*, *Kingella* spp): give ceftriaxone IV for 4 weeks or ampicillin plus gentamicin IV for 4 weeks.

Prophylaxis against endocarditis

- Advise children with cardiac lesions to brush their teeth twice daily with fluoride toothpaste. Regular attendance at a dentist is recommended.
- Major revisions of endocarditis prophylaxis guidelines occurred in the USA and UK in 2007 and 2008. There is no evidence to substantiate many current practices and routine endocarditis prophylaxis is not recommended. However in developing countries, given poor dental health and standards of hygiene in general as well as the high incidence of acquired valvular heart disease, it is not unreasonable to consider endocarditis prophylaxis in selected patients. ☆☆☆
- For dental extractions use the schedule below. For similar procedures with anaesthesia, use the same scheme (ampicillin 50 mg/kg IV if the patient is nil by mouth).

Table 6.4 Antibiotic prophylaxis for dental extractions or upper respiratory tract surgery without an anaesthetic

1 hour pre-op	< 5 years	5–10 years	> 10 years
Amoxycillin*	750 mg	1 500 mg	2 000 mg
Clindamycin°	150 mg	300 mg	600 mg

* for underweight children and those less than 15 kg use 50 mg/kg
° recommended if allergic to penicillin

Previous heart valve replacement

- Children and adolescents who need valve replacement surgery usually have a mechanical bi-leaflet device inserted.
- The St Jude valve is most commonly used and the current model is visible on chest X-ray. A clinician should be become familiar with the clicking of the prosthesis. Any change in sound, even without symptoms, necessitates referral to a cardiologist.
- Important complications are thromboembolism from the valve and thrombotic obstruction of the valve.
- Prescribe prophylactic penicillin 250 mg PO twice daily in patients with rheumatic heart disease and a prosthesis in situ.
- Anticoagulant therapy: warfarin is used for life and the dosage can be supervised and adjusted aiming at an INR of 2–3.

Pericardial disease

Clinical presentation

The classical presentation of pericarditis (as in viral pericarditis) with chest pain relieved by sitting, tachycardia, and a loud pericardial rub is unusual in South Africa. Most children have a long history of being unwell and present with signs of pericardial tamponade. As there is a high prevalence of *M. tuberculosis* it is wise to treat all pericardial disease as being caused by tuberculosis.

In children with AIDS, significant pericardial effusions can occur without symptoms and are only diagnosed after a chest X-ray is taken for assessment of respiratory disease. Purulent pericarditis (due to bacteria such as *H. influenzae*) is rare.

Investigation and management

- Chest X-Ray
- Ultrasound examination of the heart
- Mantoux
- Drainage: an experienced practitioner is best qualified to perform percutaneous drainage of pericardial fluid. In an emergency, aspiration can be attempted using a large bore intravenous cannula inserted just to the left of the xiphoid process preferably with ultrasound guidance. Pericardial fluid must be sent for prolonged culture for *M. tuberculosis*.
- In the child who is not haemodynamically compromised, treatment with anti-tuberculous therapy without drainage of fluid is warranted, especially if there is a long history of being unwell.
- Tuberculous pericarditis is best treated with a 6 month course of anti-tuberculous drugs.
- Prednisolone 2 mg/kg PO for 1 month is used to decrease the possibility of constrictive pericarditis. Wean therapy slowly after 4 weeks. Start this once cultures are negative for organisms that cause purulent pericarditis. Steroids are not recommended in HIV positive children with possible TB pericarditis.

Disorders of cardiac rhythm

Complete heart block

Congenital atrio-ventricular dissociation typically presents in the neonate. The clinical consequences of the abnormal rhythm depend on the rate and nature of the ventricular escape rhythm. The patient may be asymptomatic or in severe heart failure.

Urgent referral to a paediatric cardiologist or cardiac service is appropriate in the presence of heart failure or if a coexisting congenital heart defect is suspected. In a stable patient, a review of the ECG (sent by fax to a paediatric cardiology centre) may suffice. The serum of the mother must be tested for antibodies associated with systemic lupus erythematosus. Nearly all children with congenital heart block in the absence of congenital heart lesions are born to mothers with anti-Ro and anti-La antibodies.

Indications for a pacemaker

- *Urgent:* heart failure, syncope or ventricular tachycardia during monitoring.
- *For consideration:* a neonate or infant with a heart rate less than 50/min, an older child with a heart rate less than 60/min, cardiomegaly and no increase in heart rate during exercise.

Narrow complex tachycardia

This is relatively common in infancy. The term 'supraventricular tachycardia' or SVT includes most patients who have narrow complex tachycardia but is not a specific diagnosis. Several types of tachyarrhythmias may result in a similar clinical presentation and an exact diagnosis allows the cardiologist to tailor therapy appropriately.

Clinical presentation

Sustained narrow complex tachycardias may occasionally cause heart failure and cardiogenic shock. The majority of patients are only mildly distressed at the time of presentation. The ECG shows a rapid narrow complex rhythm and P waves may be difficult to identify. Obtain an ECG recording of the arrhythmia (even from a strip recorder) as this may allow an expert to diagnose and treat the underlying disorder. Re-entrant tachycardias (atrioventricular and atrioventriculonodal tachyarrhythmias) are the most common conditions presenting as a sustained narrow complex tachycardia in children. Recurrence is common.

Medical management

- Use the diving reflex. This is safe and easy, but successful only in about 50% of cases. Hold the patient prone and submerge the face in a basin of ice-cold water for 1 or 2 seconds (the baby will not drown!).

- Adenosine (Adenocor®). Give this intravenously (start at 0.1 mg/kg in children; 0.15 mg/kg in infants, use of higher doses suggested in neonates and infants to max. 0.3 mg/kg) followed by a rapid saline flush (10 ml). After the initial dose give incremental doses of 0.05 mg/kg until a maximum dose of 0.5 mg/kg is reached. The precautions for electrical cardioversion (see below) apply to adenosine. The half-life of the drug is extremely short and side effects such as bradycardia and nausea are transient. Do not give the drug to those patients known to have atrial flutter; fortunately this is an extremely rare cause of a narrow complex tachycardia in children.

Electrical cardioversion

This is the treatment of choice if the patient is shocked and adenosine is not available.

It is safe to use electrical cardioversion to treat narrow complex tachycardia provided the following steps are taken:
- Empty the stomach beforehand, if time permits.
- Ensure that appropriate facilities are available for resuscitation and intubation.
- In 'elective' cardioversion (as opposed to cardioversion in shock) the patient should be anaesthetized with an inhalational or intravenous agent.
- Use synchronized DC electrical cardioversion at 0.5–2 J/kg. Start with the smallest level of electrical cardioversion and increase the dose if necessary. Too much electrical energy can result in myocardial damage.

Maintenance treatment

To prevent a recurrence use propranolol 1 mg/kg/dose PO 8 hourly for at least a year. All patients should be referred to a paediatric cardiology service.

Broad complex tachycardia

This is relatively rare and is seen most commonly in poisoning (typically with agents that prolong the QT interval) and in severely ill patients with fulminant myocarditis. Non-synchronized DC cardioversion (2–4 J/kg) is indicated for the patient who is severely ill. Magnesium sulphate 50% (0.05–0.1 ml/kg) can be given as a slow bolus intravenous injection to correct QT prolongation in patients with poisoning.

Recommended reading

Park, MK. *Pediatric Cardiology for Practitioners.* 5th Ed. Mosby. Elsevier. 2008.

7 Nervous system and neuromuscular problems

K. Donald, G. Fieggen, J. Wilmshurst

Every child should have a basic neurological examination to ensure adequate development for age and to detect deviations from the norm. In addition to a brief clinical assessment, this chapter includes approaches to raised intracranial pressure, headache, altered consciousness, seizures and epilepsy, paroxysms, movement disorders, hemiplegia, floppy and weak infants, neuro-regression, and CNS infections.

Clinical diagnosis
Be sure to include the following in a physical examination.

Neonate
Primitive reflexes
- Head circumference and fontanelles
- Dysmorphology.

Infant
- Conduct a brief developmental assessment including:
  - Gross motor abilities
  - Fine motor and visual abilities
  - Language and auditory skills
  - Social skills
  - Head circumference.
- Use the Glasgow Coma Scale (GCS) (or paediatric version) to comment on the level of consciousness. However, this is more difficult to apply consistently to children so fuller neurological examination is more useful.

Child
- Assess gross development, hearing and vision.
- Determine the GCS.
- Evaluate school performance.
- Score a 'draw a man' test.

Problems with the head

Microcephaly (too small)

A head circumference below the 3rd centile or significantly below the length and weight centiles is always relevant, especially if it has crossed centiles. This suggests that the brain has stopped growing (common) or cannot expand further (rare).

Refer for paediatric review.

Macrocephaly (too big)

A circumference above the 97th centile or disproportionately large compared to weight and height; this is particularly significant if crossing centiles. Manage according to the underlying condition, which may be:

- Hydrocephalus – overwhelmingly most common
- Familial macrocrania or 'external' hydrocephalus
- Other causes of chronic raised ICP (tumour, rarely chronic subdural haematoma or subdural effusion)
- Other medical conditions (e.g. neurofibromatosis 1, neuro-degenerative conditions, ricketts).

Investigate with ultrasound or CT scan (preferable) if:
- Size increases rapidly.
- Fontanelle is bulging or sutures are splayed.
- Any neurological sign is present (e.g. squint – VI nerve palsy).
- Irritability, vomiting or poor feeding are present.

Management

- Always look for the cause of hydrocephalus.
- Ventriculo-peritoneal (VP) shunt or endoscopic third ventriculostomy (ETV) for hydrocephalus.
- Exclude non-accidental injury if there is a chronic subdural haematoma.

Abnormal shape

- Posterior flattening: this is usually positional
- Anterior flattening: this may indicate coronal suture synostosis
- Elongated head: this may be caused by sagittal suture synostosis
- Look for syndromic features
- Refer to a paediatric neurosurgeon.

Brain tumours

- Are almost always primary tumours
- Are second only to leukaemia in frequency of childhood cancer; commonest solid malignancy in children
- Often present with hydrocephalus (especially posterior fossa tumours); headache and ataxia are common
- Duration of symptoms is usually short
- Surgery is the primary treatment modality usually, but paediatric oncology/radiation therapy may need to be involved
- Best treated at a centre with paediatric neurosurgical expertise
- Consider other mass lesions in the brain, e.g. brain abscess, congenital cysts, hydatid cysts, tuberculoma, haematoma (post spontaneous bleed).

Problems with the neck

Neck stiffness

This is an important sign of meningitis but also consider the following causes:
- Raised intracranial pressure with tonsillar herniation
- Subarachnoid haemorrhage
- Injury.

Torticollis ('wry neck')

Table 7.1 gives the differential diagnosis of torticollis.

Table 7.1 The differential diagnosis of torticollis

Category	Causes	Management
Congenital	Sternomastoid 'tumour'	Refer for physiotherapy
Inflammatory	Retropharyngeal abscess Post URTI	Urgent ENT referral. Symptomatic treatment
Trauma	Rotatory subluxation	Refer (orthopaedics/neurosurgery)
Neurological	Cerebellar herniation Squint (4th cranial nerve palsy) Dystonia	Urgent neurosurgery referral. Refer paediatric neurology

Problems with the back

Back pain
This is *always* significant in childhood and requires referral for investigation.

Spina bifida (spinal dysraphism)
This is usually lumbo-sacral and may be either:
- *Open* (myelomeningocele) or
- *Closed* (occult dysraphism).

Myelomeningocele
- Obvious open lesion on the back, usually leaking CSF
- Lower limb weakness related to level of the lesion
- Sphincter involvement invariably present.
- May occur with other congenital anomalies involving the vertebra and ribs, heart and urinary tract.

Management
- ABCs: (may have bulbar dysfunction due to Chiari II)
- Cover area with a sterile, saline-soaked gauze dressing.
- Optimal management entails surgical closure *within* 36 hours, so refer immediately. The purpose of surgery is to prevent infection, not reverse the neurological deficit.

Long term issues
- 90% develop hydrocephalus and need a VP shunt
- Despite this, 70% have normal IQ
- Teach parents bladder management (clean intermittent catheterization)
- Orthopaedic correction of clubfeet
- Recurrence risk for mother is greatly increased, so folate supplementation is essential commencing prior to conception
- Exclude shunt dysfunction and tethered spinal cord if there is subsequent neurological deterioration.

Occult spinal dysraphism
There is variable motor and sphincter involvement, often with a delayed onset.

Cutaneous manifestations include:
- Subcutaneous mass (usually lipoma)

- Dermal sinus (significant if eccentric, irregular, above the natal cleft, or if buttock crease is deviated)
- Other stigmata (haemangioma, hairy patch).

> *Practice point:*
>
> It is important to distinguish a sacrococcygeal sinus (very common) from a dermal sinus (rare).

Refer to a paediatric neurosurgeon.

Raised intracranial pressure

This is a medical emergency! Reduced cerebral blood flow and brain shifts (herniation) rapidly injure the brain. ☆☆☆☆ The presentation and management depend on the cause and on the age of the child (i.e. are the sutures fused or not?).

Causes

Acute:
- Haematoma (usually traumatic)
- Infection: meningitis and infective mass (abscess or empyema)
- Hydrocephalus
- Blocked VP shunt.

Chronic:
- Hydrocephalus
- Brain tumours.

Clinical features

Infant:
- If sutures are open, macrocrania as above
- Bulging fontanelle.

Older child:
- Headache and vomiting (especially if in morning)
- Ataxia, spastic legs
- Visual changes: declining acuity and squint (VI nerve palsy)
- Papilloedema (may be a late sign).

Critical signs:
- Dilated pupil (III nerve palsy)
- Depressed or deteriorating level of consciousness
- Agitation or confusion
- Cushing response (raised blood pressure, slow pulse rate).

Investigations
- Urgent CT scan
- *Do not lumbar puncture.*

Management

In general, this is aimed at treating the cause. The child should be treated at a specialist centre. Much of the literature is focused on raised ICP in head injuries. ✦☆☆

While waiting for transfer, the following apply:
- Maintain adequate cerebral perfusion. Cerebral perfusion pressure (CPP) = mean arterial pressure − intracranial pressure.
- Try to keep CPP > 50 mm Hg.
- Adequate IV fluid volume, avoid hypotonic fluids.

Positioning
- Raise the head of bed 15 degrees.
- Keep head in a neutral position.
- Avoid any constriction of the neck (dressings, collar).

Optimise sedation and analgesia.

Prevent seizures:
- Phenytoin is best.

Temperature:
- Treat pyrexia aggressively.

If suspected meningitis:
- Give a dose of ceftriaxone or cefotaxime IVI.
- Do not do a lumbar puncture before doing a CT brain scan and clinically assessing safety for the intervention.

Further steps:
- Mannitol: IV bolus 0.5 g/kg (hypertonic saline has also been used in some centres, but only under strict control). Only as emergency management while waiting for definitive treatment. ✦☆

- Use a urinary catheter.
- Dexamethasone: 1 mg/kg IV 6 hourly in divided doses. This is effective for meningitis, abscess or brain tumour. ♦☆
- Intubation:
  - Critical to oxygenate well
  - Important to control PO_2 and PCO_2 but done badly this may cause coning
  - Best done through nose after cords have been sprayed with a local anaesthetic
  - Rapid sequence induction is ideal
  - Avoid ketamine
  - Maintain a 'low normal' pCO_2 (4 to 4.5 kPa). Avoid hyperventilation
  - If unable to intubate, keep on high flow oxygen

Special considerations in the child with a VP shunt

- The long-term cognitive outcome depends on the original cause of hydrocephalus and may be excellent. 50% of shunts malfunction within 5 years of implantation. ♦☆☆☆
- A blocked shunt is an emergency as these patients can deteriorate very rapidly. Always exclude shunt dysfunction if there are any symptoms of raised ICP, abdominal symptoms or a febrile illness.
- Endoscopic third ventriculostomy (ETV) is being used increasingly for non-communicating hydrocephalus. ♦☆☆ It avoids dependence on a shunt but may also block and need urgent revision.

Headache

Obtain a detailed description of the headache, its timing, frequency, duration, triggers, location, nature, and relief factors. Check how the home and school schedule is going. Most parents are concerned that their child has a brain tumour and until this is excluded, progress in management is very difficult.

Features of pathological headache

These are:
- Headache on waking or which interrupts sleep
- Vomiting
- Squint or visual deterioration
- Altered level of consciousness
- Focal neurological signs
- Hypertension.

Management 🩸☆☆☆

If pathological features are present:
- Exclude meningitis/encephalitis: consider lumbar puncture only if safe
- CT scan (before lumbar puncture if considered necessary)
- Refer to paediatrician/paediatric neurology.

Migraine headache

Features of migraine headache:
- The child is pale and older children may describe a typical 'aura' of visual scotomata, flashing lights and a feeling of light-headedness.
- After 30 minutes or so an intense throbbing unilateral (often retro-orbital) headache will start and is associated with vomiting and photophobia.
- Headache usually resolves following sleep.
- There is a family history in 50% of cases.

Management 🩸☆☆☆

- Acute treatment includes anti-emetics, analgesia and avoiding dehydration (if vomiting).
- If available, nasal sumatriptan is the optimal acute intervention
- 'Headache hygiene': avoid trigger factors (stress, lack of sleep, dietary triggers).
- Second-line medications include propranolol (exclude asthma first) (start 1 mg/kg/day; max 2 mg/kg/day, give as 3 divided doses), pizotifen (1–3 mg/day) and low dose sodium valproate (10–20 mg/kg/day slowly incremented)
- Failure to control events:
- Referral to a paediatric neurologist.
- Topiramate (🩸☆☆☆) or levetiracetam (🩸☆) may be initiated.

Important differentials of headache

- Raised intracranial pressure (p. 187)
- Sinusitis: ask about allergies
- Sleep apnoea or hypoventilation: ask if snores at night, day time drowsiness
- Benign intracranial hypertension (BIH): check for papilloedema
- Infection: especially encephalitis or meningitis (particularly tuberculous).

Altered states of consciousness

Agitation and confusion

Possible causes: *raised* ICP, systemic illnesses, toxic conditions, seizures, infections, metabolic derangements, vascular conditions, migraine, psychological factors.

Lethargy and coma

Possible causes: *raised* ICP, trauma, epilepsy, hypoxic-ischaemic insults, vascular abnormalities, infectious disorders, metabolic disorders, systemic illnesses, migraine coma, toxic conditions.

Management

Immediate: resuscitation (See Chapter 1, Emergencies and trauma)
- Assess GCS, breathing pattern, blood pressure and pulse, pupils, fundi, deep tendon reflexes
- Bed-side tests: *blood glucose* level and *blood gas* analysis. Collect urine for future tests (toxicology, amino acids and organic acids).
- Full history and examination – pinpoint the cause anatomically.
- CT scan of the brain.
- Lumbar puncture if no contra-indications (Table 7.1).

Table 7.1 Contraindications for a lumbar puncture before neuro-imaging

Absolute contraindications
Decreased or decreasing GCS
Focal neurological signs
Evidence of raised intracranial pressure
Coagulopathy
Relative contraindications
Skin sepsis in LP area
Shock
Seizures
Neonate whose respiration may be compromised by position
Meningococcaemia

> *Practice point:*
>
> Once neuro-imaging has been performed for the above, LP is occasionally recommended but only after specialist advice. If there is a delay and meningitis is likely, commence antibiotic treatment immediately.

Seizures and epilepsy

Status epilepticus

This is a generalized convulsion lasting 30 minutes or more. Seizure activity can be continuous or the child may go in and out of ictus. There is a risk of brain damage.

The management is summarized in Figure 7.1. 🌢☆☆

Figure 7.1 Management of status epilepticus 🌢☆☆ ✚

ABC (oxygen, monitor saturation, pulse & BP)
Rectal diazepam (0.5 mg/kg)

IV diazepam (0.3 mg/kg) / lorazepam : (0.1 mg/kg)
(take blood for glucose, gas, electrolytes, FBC and culture)

IV access failure / delay – intra osseus access or
intranasal midazolam 200 µg/kg

IV phenobarbitone (20 mg/kg)

10 minutes ↓

Repeat phenobarbitone (10 mg/kg)

10 minutes ↓

Repeat phenobarbitone (10 mg/kg)

10 minutes ↓

Refer to PICU for intubation and sodium pentothal infusion

Notes:

Lorazepam: (0.1 mg/kg) is a faster-acting alternative to diazepam for bolus IV (must be stored in a locked fridge).

Midazolam: intranasally (200 µg/kg) or sublingually (500 µg/kg) if no venous access.

Midazolam: infusion loading 200 µg/kg by slow IV injection, then titrating an infusion between 30–300 µg/kg/hr.

Phenytoin: slow intravenous injection (20 mg/kg over 20 minutes) if known adverse reaction to phenobarbitone (monitor for cardiac arrhythmias).

Watch carefully for drug related respiratory depression.

Intubation, ventilation and sodium pentothal infusion should only be done in a centre with trained anaesthetic and paediatric intensive care staff.

Acute convulsion

Figure 7.2 gives a brief flow diagram approach to the child who presents with new onset seizures.

Chapter 7: Nervous system and neuromuscular problems | 193

Figure 7.2 Epilepsy flow chart 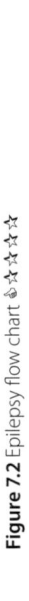☆☆☆☆

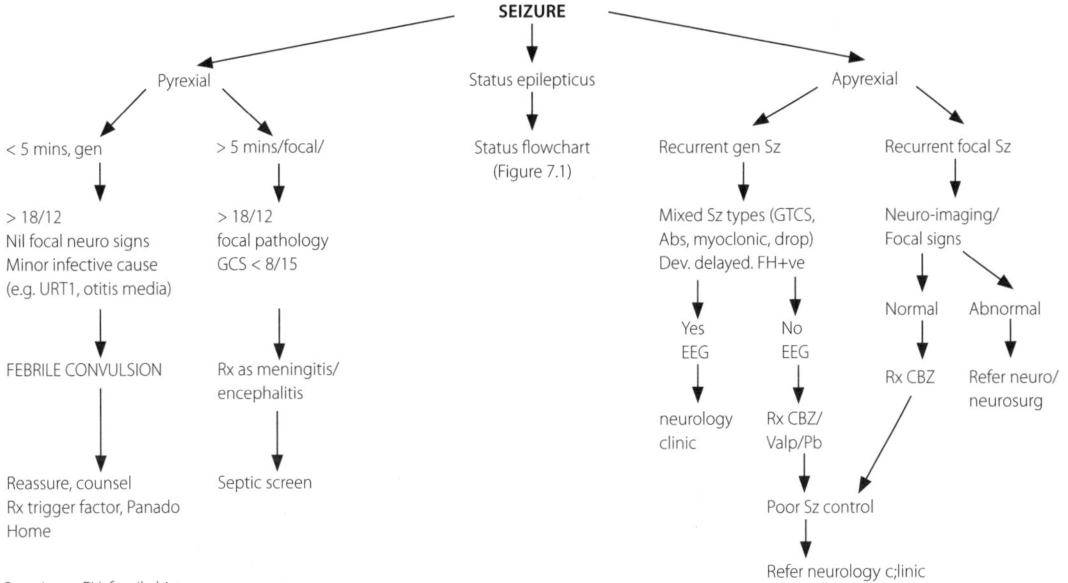

```
                                SEIZURE
           ┌───────────────────────┼───────────────────────┐
        Pyrexial              Status epilepticus        Apyrexial
                                    │
                              Status flowchart
                               (Figure 7.1)
```

Pyrexial branch:
- < 5 mins, gen
  - > 18/12
  - Nil focal neuro signs
  - Minor infective cause (e.g. URTI, otitis media)
  → FEBRILE CONVULSION
  → Reassure, counsel
     Rx trigger factor, Panado
     Home

- > 5 mins/focal/
  - > 18/12
  - focal pathology
  - GCS < 8/15
  → Rx as meningitis/encephalitis
  → Septic screen

Apyrexial branch:
- Recurrent gen Sz
  - Mixed Sz types (GTCS, Abs, myoclonic, drop)
  - Dev. delayed. FH+ve
    - Yes EEG → neurology clinic
    - No EEG → Rx CBZ/Valp/Pb → Poor Sz control → Refer neurology clinic

- Recurrent focal Sz
  - Neuro-imaging/Focal signs
    - Abnormal → Refer neuro/neurosurg
    - Normal → Rx CBZ → Refer neurology clinic

Sz: seizure, FH: family history

Febrile convulsion

Definition
- The child has a pyrexial illness and a clear focus of infection with no evidence of intracranial infection
- Generalized convulsion: duration < 5 minutes (up to 15 minutes is possible but rare).
- Convulsions do not recur
- The child is stable, more than 18 months old, and has no abnormal focal neurology.

Management
- Reassurance
- Advise that the child has a 1 in 3 risk of more events until 6 years of age
- Recommend methods to control temperature
- Lumbar puncture if below 18 months of age
- CT scan if neurological focal features
- Recurrent febrile convulsions and/or atypical features warrant referral to a paediatrician or paediatric neurologist.

Epilepsy

The child who has an initial short generalized seizure and is otherwise well does not automatically require an EEG or treatment. Always take a detailed history from an eye witness of the exact nature of the event. If there is any possibility of a focal onset, neuro-imaging is recommended.

> **Practice point:**
>
> Rather than labelling the child 'epileptic' explain to the parents that *more than one event* must occur before intervention is necessary.

Focal epilepsy

Simple partial seizures: consciousness is preserved, motor automatisms.
Complex partial seizures: loss of consciousness.

Investigations
- A sleep EEG is best.
- Neuro-imaging is necessary if there are focal features either on history, clinical examination or EEG.

Benign focal epilepsy of childhood
- Typically presents between 8 and 12 years.
- Seizures usually occur during sleep and on awakening.
- Does not necessarily require therapy.

Generalized epilepsy

Generalized tonic clonic seizures (GTCS)
- Rarely present below 1 year of age.
- Refer to neurology if there is any evidence of neuro-regression.
- Treatment – sodium valproate or carbamazepine. (Table 7.2)

Absence epilepsy
In an otherwise well child, complex partial seizures must be distinguished from absence epilepsy.

Childhood absence epilepsy (CAE)
- Commonest form, onset 4 to 6 years
- Brief episodes (10-30 seconds) of unresponsiveness and gross motor arrest, may be simple automatisms.
- Can be induced by hyperventilation
- Usually resolves by adolescence.

Juvenile myoclonic epilepsy (JME)
- This is the commonest adolescent form of epilepsy; onset 8 to 14 years
- Features include infrequent GTCS and frequent myoclonus on awakening (exacerbated by sleep deprivation)
- Also absence seizures (18-38%)
- Photoparoxysmal response on EEG (30-48%).

Atypical absences
- Usually more prolonged with atypical EEG features
- Associated with various epilepsy syndromes; poor cognitive outcome
- Medication: sodium valproate. (Table 7.2)

Tonic seizures
- May be isolated or part of epilepsy syndromes.
- Difficult to control and may be associated with serious autonomic dysfunction.
- Treatment: carbamazepine. (Table 7.2).

Myoclonic seizures
- Myoclonus, especially with neuro-regression and or ataxia, warrants referral to a neurology unit.
- There are often other seizure types associated (GTCS, tonic, drop, atypical absence events).

Drop attacks
- Usually associated with epilepsy syndromes; tonic or atonic
- Refer to neurology.

Epilepsy syndromes
- The following require prompt referral to a neurology centre.

Infantile spasms
- Neurological emergency
- Onset between 3–6 months, often misdiagnosed as colic
- Recurrent abrupt head and trunk flexion; arms and legs 'fling out', contraction held for few seconds. This distresses the baby, who usually cries.

Management
- The underlying aetiology (especially patients with symptomatic causes) and the delay in gaining seizure control correspond with the severity of the outcome.
- Admit immediately and do EEG the same day (to confirm hypsarryhthmia and burst suppression).
- Treatment: steroids (ACTH 20 IU IM daily for 10 days) or vigabatrin (increasing up to 120 mg/kg/day) (Table 7.2) ☆☆☆☆
- Vigabatrin is the first line recommended treatment for children with tuberous sclerosis and infantile spasms
- Neuro-metabolic and imaging investigations, particularly to exclude tuberous sclerosis
- Discuss management with a paediatric neurologist.

Severe myoclonic epilepsy
- Presents before 1 year of age with an atypical febrile convulsion.
- Later generalized tonic clonic events without fever; often neuro-regression.

Lennox-Gastaut syndrome
- Occurs independently or follows infantile spasms (West syndrome)
- Presents at about 2 years of age with drop attacks, myoclonic seizures and occasional generalized tonic clonic seizures.

Landau-Kleffner syndrome.
- Presents about 2 years of age in a previously normal child.
- Expressive and receptive language is lost over a few weeks.

When to request an EEG

Urgent EEG
- To exclude infantile spasms
- To exclude subclinical status.

Non-urgent EEGs
- After > 2 afebrile convulsions
- Suspicion of complex partial seizures
- Suspicion of an epilepsy syndrome
- If in doubt call the neurophysiology department and discuss the child to attain the optimal investigation (e.g. sleep study, prolonged recording).

When to treat epilepsy
- Two or more events occurring close enough to have an impact on the child's quality of life (usually within 3 months, but this depends on the effects of the events on the individual).

Treatment of epilepsy
This is summarized in Table 7.2.
- Initiate new anticonvulsants gradually, titrating up weekly.
- Monitor the patient for side effects, e.g:
  - Drowsiness (especially carbamazepine)
  - Liver dysfunction (sodium valproate),
  - Rash (carbamazepine, phenobarbitone)
  - Hyperactivity (phenobarbitone).
- Consider using phenobarbitone (< 5 mg/kg/day) for children with severe static encephalopathies, i.e. cerebral palsy. Aim to avoid episodes of status and provide the easiest regimen for the family to follow.
- For other epilepsies aim for one anticonvulsant only.
- Resistant seizure disorders may require 2-3 agents.
- Failure to attain seizure control with the first appropriately selected agent at the correct dose warrants referral to a paediatrician or paediatric neurologist.

When to stop treatment

- Generally after 2 years free of seizures (wean off over 6 weeks)
- Some types resolve sooner, e.g. related to TB granulomas, neurocystocercosis
- Some types are unlikely to resolve – these are most of the symptomatic epilepsies and severe syndromes.

Table 7.2 Medications for epilepsy

Medication	Dosage	Types of epilepsy	Comment
Acetazolamide	5 mg/kg 2 to 4 times/day	Focal/generalized	Usually second or third line, better for epilepsies due to channelopathies
ACTH	20–40 IU IM daily for 10 days	Infantile spasm	Monitor BP and for glycosuria. Increased risk of intercurrent infections
Carbamazepine	Start 5 mg/kg/day bd regimen. Increase weekly to 20 mg/kg/day	Focal – CPS Geralized – tonic	Warn of rash, stop drug immediately if occurs. Steven-Johnson can occur. Avoid with absence, myoclonic and drop attacks
Clobazam	0.5 mg–1 mg/kg/night	Generalized – drop attacks, myoclonus, Lennox-Gastaut syndrome	Usually additional agent. Associated with drooling, drowsiness and behavioural difficulties. Tolerance limits long-term effectiveness
Diazepam	0.3 mg/kg IV 2.5-10 mg rectal	Status epilepticus	See status protocol. Rectal dosage depends on patient age
Ethosuximide	15–50 mg/kg/day	Generalized – absence epilepsy	Alternative to sodium valproate for absence seizures
Gabapentin	35 mg/kg/day	Partial epilepsy	Second line agent. Also good for neuropathic pain

bd: repeat twice a day, tds: three times a day, CPS: complex partial seizure, IU: international units, IV: intravenous

Medication	Dosage	Types of epilepsy	Comment
Lamotrigine	0.2-5 mg/kg/day (when used with sodium valproate) 1-10 mg/kg/day (monotherapy)	Lennox-Gastaut syndrome. Intractable seizure disorders.	Good second line agents. Usually with sodium valproate. Often used in monotherapy (higher dose). Introduce over several months to reduce chance of rash. Stop immediately if rash
Levitiracetam	40 mg/kg/day	Partial or photosensitive epilepsy	New agent, may be very effective .
Lorazepam	50–100 µg/kg IV, rectal, sublingual	Status epilepticus	Good agent, long-acting, inexpensive
Nitrazepam	500 µg/kg bd	Infantile spasms	Occasionally for seizure control, also very good for hypertonia
Phenobarbitone	5 mg/kg/day oral 10-15 mg/kg IV	Neonatal seizures Status epilepticus	Exellent for emergency care. Useful for cerebral palsy. Not for absence and myoclonic seizures. Oral therapy often results in behavioural and learning difficulties
Phenytoin	5 mg'kg bd	Generalized tonic clonic seizures	Often for post-head injury and neonatal seizures. Difficult to maintain bioavailability. May cause gum hypertrophy
Sodium valproate	40 mg/kg/day	Generalized – absence, drop and myclonic	Give syrup tds. Slow release tablets bd. Crushed tablets also very good for infants
Topiramate	7 mg/kg/day	Partial and generalized	Titrate up slowly, watch for renal stones and weight loss

bd: repeat twice a day, tds: three times a day, CPS: complex partial seizure, IU: international units, IV: intravenous

Medication	Dosage	Types of epilepsy	Comment
Vigabatrin	40-150 mg/kg/day	Infantile spasms Structural malformations	First line for infantile spasms with tuberous sclerosis or cortical blindness. In older children risk of visual field defects, behavioural difficulties. Exacerbates absence and myoclonic epilepsy

bd: repeat twice a day, tds: three times a day, CPS: complex partial seizure, IU: international units, IV: intravenous

Epilepsy in the child with HIV on antiretroviral therapy ☆☆☆

- First line intervention sodium valproate, monitor liver function tests and avoid efavirenz
- Carbamazepine, phenobarbitone and phenytoin are associated with antiretroviral treatment failure and anticonvulsant drug toxicity and should be avoided.

Paroxysms

Reflex anoxic attacks

- Breath-holding attacks
- Common
- Toddler to 6 years
- Vagally mediated, usually triggered by crying or pain
- The child takes a deep gasp, stops breathing, becomes pale or blue with brief loss of consciousness
- Spontaneous recovery occurs and no neurological sequelae are evident.

Management:
- Exclude: sepsis, seizures, metabolic derangement, cardiac arrhythmias, Munchausen by proxy
- Reassurance (this is difficult with the first event, the parent often needs to have experienced several distressing episodes to accept this)
- Treat for iron deficiency anaemia.

Syncope (fainting)
- Common in adolescent girls but can affect all ages.
- Like reflex anoxic spells they are vagally mediated.
- Can be abrupt and easily confused with seizures.
- Exclude a long QT interval.

Benign paroxysmal vertigo
- Affects a toddler: pale, frightened, runs and clings to a carer and may vomit
- Lasts a few minutes, then child appears completely well
- Differential diagnosis: temporal lobe epilepsy, so do a sleep EEG.

Pseudoseizures
- Usually a diagnosis of exclusion
- Adolescent girls; dramatic rolling on the ground, random flinging of limbs, eyes closed
- Incontinence can occur
- A child with confirmed epilepsy also can have pseudoseizures
- Often a response to *abuse (often sexual)*.

Movement disorders
The following abnormal involuntary movements occur in childhood.

Ataxia
- It is critical to distinguish acute from chronic ataxia; the former needs prompt investigation.

Differential diagnosis
- Cerebellar dysfunction; associated with:
  - Posterior fossa tumour (acute)
  - Toxic (carbemazepine, phenytoin) (acute)
  - Post-infectious (e.g. varicella) (acute)
  - Metabolic mitochondrial (acute)
  - Ataxic cerebral palsy (chronic/static)
  - Neurodegenerative (chronic progressive).
- Encephalopathy associated with:
  - Pseudoataxia (poorly controlled epilepsy)
  - Encephalopathy
  - Hydrocephalus.
- Vestibular dysfunction

Tics

- Complex, stereotyped movements (motor tic) or utterances (verbal tic) that are sudden, brief and purposeless. Exacerbated by stress and disappear in sleep.
- *Tourette syndrome* is a combination of tics, attention deficit hyperactivity disorder (ADHD) and obsessive-compulsive behaviour. Methylphenidate may make the tics worse.

Athetosis

- Slow, writhing movements of limbs, associated with chorea or hypoxic-ischemic encephalopathy in patients with cerebral palsy.

Tremor

- Involuntary oscillatory movement with a fixed frequency
- Exclude hyperthyroidism.

Myoclonus

- Rapid muscle jerks, less frequent and severe in sleep but do not necessarily disappear.

Hemiplegia

Acute/sub-acute hemiplegia

Acute/sub-acute hemiplegia (also called a stroke) may occur due to arterial ischaemic events or cerebral sinovenous thrombosis. Incidence ranges from 2-6 per 100 000 children a year. History and clnical findings are very important as the preceding event such as a pyrexial illness or head injury will direct investigations and management. Any illness associated with hypotension can result in a focal brain lesion. In a child over 2 years of age with cyanotic congenital cardiac disease, hemiplegia is due to a brain abscess until proven otherwise. However, hemiplegias in otherwise well children are often idiopathic.

Differential diagnosis of stroke in childhood

Infective:
- Meningitis (especially TBM, *Haemophilus influenzae*)
- Encephalitis (especially herpes simplex)
- HIV – direct cause and secondary to opportunistic infections and vasculitis.

Haematological:
- Trauma
- Bleeding disorders (e.g. haemophilia, idiopathic thrombocytopenia)
- Malignancy, e.g. leukaemia, lymphoma
- Sickle cell disease.

Structural mass lesion:
- Tumour
- Abscess (embolic from cardiac lesion, dental or lung source)
- Granulomas (TB, neurocysticercosis)
- Arterio-venous malformation
- Sturge-Weber syndrome.

Vasculopathy:
- Tuberculous meningitis
- Systemic lupus erythematosis
- Takayasu's disease.

Post infectious/inflammatory:
- Acute disseminated encephalomyelitus
- Post varicella zoster infection
- Post mycoplasma infection.

Metabolic:
- Mitochondrial disorders
- Lipodystrophy.

Systemic:
- Hypertension
- Dehydration.

'Pseudo-strokes':
- Migraine
- Epilepsy – Todd's paresis.

Management
- Treat acute obvious exacerbating factors, e.g. dehydration
- Exclude active TB
- CT brain
- Blood film
- Exclude meningitis/encephalitis – CSF if safe
- Exclude features of HIV

- Exclude cardiac disease
- Screen for organomegaly
- Refer paediatrican/paediatric neurologist/paediatric neurosurgeon

Anticoagulation remains a contentious issue (✦☆☆☆): current guidelines recommend:
- Arterial ischaemic stroke:
  — Due to extra-cranial dissection or cardiogenic embolism – anticoagulation with heparin or warfarin
  — Other causes: antiplatelet therapy (Aspirin® – 2-5 mg/kg/day).
- Cerebral sinovenous thrombosis: anticoagulation even in presence of haemorrhagic venous infarction.

Chronic hemiplegia

- Refer electively for specialist opinion.
- *Congenital hemiplegia*: affected infants are usually diagnosed at about 5-6 months of age when the primitive reflexes resolve.

The floppy infant

Consider pathology from the brain to spinal cord to peripheral nerves to muscles. Differentiate between *central* or *peripheral* hypotonia.

Exclude: sepsis, endocrine diseases, syndromes e.g. Down's, metabolic abnormalities.

NB: The key to diagnosis is in differentiating between central and peripheral pathology.

Upper motor neuron (UMN)

- Cognitive impairment
- Brisk deep tendon reflexes
- Power retained despite hypotonia.

Lower motor neuron (LMN)

- Cognitively normal
- Absent or reduced deep tendon reflexes
- Weak and hypotonic.

Central hypotonia (UMN)

- Hypoxic ischaemic encephalopathy
- Intraventricular haemorrhage
- Congenital infection.

Investigations
- U/S head
- CT scan head
- Chromosomes
- CPK (some myopathies have central and peripheral pathology)
- Screening for congenital infections.

Peripheral hypotonia (LMN)
- *Spine – anterior horn cells*: spinal muscular atrophy (Werdnig-Hoffman type 1)
- *Peripheral nerves*: rarely affected in neonates
- *Neuromuscular junction*: congenital myasthenia gravis, botulism.
- *Muscle*

Investigations
- CPK
- SMA gene deletion
- NCS/EMG
- Refer to neurology, genetics, physiotherapy, speech therapy.

The weak child

Acute weakness
Central/systemic pathology:
- *Sepsis* and *dehydration*
- *Encephalopathy*
- *Cord lesion*: pain, sensory and motor levels, scoliosis
- *Spinal cord compression*: tumour, haematoma, infection (epidural abscess, TB, hydatid); surgical emergency – refer to neurosurgery.
- *Transverse myelopathy*: (check the bladder).

Management
These differentials will require neuroimaging (MRI brain/spine) and CSF in the stable child.

Anterior horn cell
- *Infective causes*: polio, enteroviruses, coxsackie.

Peripheral nerve

Guillain-Barré syndrome
Acute inflammatory demyelinating radiculo-polyneuropathy (AIDP).

Clinical features:
- Post–infection, rarely follows trauma, vaccination or anaesthetic.
- Evolving *distal* symmetrical weakness of 'glove and stocking' pattern, areflexia
- May present with initially painful muscles
- Pins and needles in the same distribution
- Normal consciousness
- Weakness progresses proximally for few days and can involve the respiratory muscles requiring ventilation support
- CSF protein is raised from the second week and the CSF should be acellular.

Management/investigations:
- Refer PICU: inability to talk, failure to protect the airway at rest or on eating, increase in use of accessory muscles
- Otherwise monitor in high care facility
- Blood pressure and pulse rate (autonomic dysfunction occurs)
- Refer paediatrician/paediatric neurologist
- CSF/NCS
- Physiotherapy
- Counselling: the child is often very frightened (remains aware)
- Analgesia (radicular pain is marked if the proximal lumbar roots are involved or at the time of re-innervation)
- Intravenous immunoglobulin (2 g/kg over 6 hours divided over 2 consecutive days) is indicated in those who are no longer ambulant or have airway compromise ☙ ☆ ☆ ☆ ☆
- The outcome is good; most recover fully.

Neuromuscular junction

Myasthenia gravis
- Rare in children
- History of fatigability in the proximal muscles, variable ptosis, occasionally ophthalmoplegia
- Refer to paediatrician/paediatric neurologist.

Botulism

The toxin blocks the neuromuscular junction resulting in complete paralysis.

Organophosphate poisoning

- Features: pin-point pupils, autonomic instability and paralysis
- Diagnosis is based on history, the above findings, anticholinestase levels and degree of reversibility with atropine.

Muscle

Dermatomyositis

- Pain (misery), proximal weakness and rash
- Diagnosis is reinforced by a raised creatinine kinase
- Refer paediatrician/paediatric neurologist.

Chronic weakness: proximal

Spinal muscular atrophy

This is caused by programmed cell death of a fixed number of anterior horn cells.

- Type 1: patients do not maintain functional head control or sitting
- Type 2: attain sitting but not walking
- Type 3: can ambulate but still have proximal weakness making an impact on their daily living.

Clinical features

- Tongue fasiculations, distal tremor, proximal weakness, reduced or absent reflexes
- Retained facial expression, no ophthalmoplegia and normal intellect
- Confirm diagnosis on PCR-DNA testing (deletion in the SMN gene on chromosome 5).

Management

- Refer to paediatrician/paediatric neurologist
- Physiotherapy
- Treat intercurrent illnesses aggressively and maintain nutrition
- Types 2 and 3 SMA can live well into adulthood if appropriately supported.

Myopathies

- Static muscle disorders, often evident at birth
- Improve with time, though full power is never attained
- Refer paediatrician/paediatric neurologist and physiotherapy.

Dystrophies

Duchenne muscular dystrophy

- X-linked recessive disorder (deficiency in muscle protein, dystrophin)
- Presents between 2 and 4 years of age with proximal weakness
- Typically occurs in boys
- Creatine kinase > 10 000 mmol/l
- Difficulty getting up stairs and off the ground (Gower sign); striking calf hypertrophy
- Delayed speech and subtle learning difficulties
- Progressive disorder – death between 15-30 years.

Management

- Maintain ambulation for as long as possible
- Physiotherapy
- Steroids while ambulant
- Cardiac monitoring
- Refer paediatrician/paediatric neurologist for assessment and genetic screening.

Chronic weakness: distal

Chronic inflammatory demyelinating polyradiculoneuropathy (CIDP)

- This is the chronic form of AIDP (CIDP remains in plateau state for > 1 month).

Charcot-Marie-Tooth (CMT)/hereditary motor sensory neuropathies

- Slowly progressive distal weakness and impaired sensation
- Foot drop, pes cavus, marked wasting of the hand small muscles results in clawing.

Management:

- Refer to a paediatrician/paediatric neurologist/physiotherapist.

Loss of skills: neuro-regression

When evaluating developmental delay establish whether the child has:
- *Static developmental delay*: some progress but remains behind peers
- *Neuro-regression*: loss of a previously acquired skill or plateauing in acquisition of skills.

Exclude:
- Child abuse
- Accidental poisoning
- Infection, especially HIV encephalopathy
- Post-ictal and poorly controlled seizure states.

Most neuro-metabolic and mitochondrial conditions cannot be cured but have genetic implications.

Management
Refer to a paediatrician.

Acute disseminated encephalomyelitis (ADEM)

Definition
This is a post-infectious immune-mediated disorder.

Suspect in cases of:
- Multifocal neurological signs
- Acute presentation
- CSF may have mild pleocytosis and raised protein.

Investigations
- Lumbar puncture (exclude meningitis/encephalitis)
- MRI brain/spine

Management
- High dose methylprednisone 30 mg/kg/day IV for 5 days
- Refer to paediatrician/paediatric neurologist
- Outcome good with appropriate supportive care.

Infections of the CNS

Meningitis
Suspect this in:

- *Newborn*: ceases to suck well, vomits, has recurrent apnoea, has temperature instability or seizures
- *Infant*: feverish, irritable, vomiting, seizures, full fontanelle
- *Toddler or child*: triad of headache, fever, vomiting.

NB: Signs of meningeal irritation (neck stiffness, Kernig and Brudzinski signs) are often absent in infants and small children.

Diagnosis
- Confirm by examination of cerebrospinal fluid (CSF)
- May be atypical in early tuberculous meningitis and partially treated bacterial meningitis
- After 48 hours, CSF features improve considerably in viral meningitis, but repeat LP not recommended unless diagnostic uncertainty
- In atypical patients (i.e. those with chronic and/or recurrent symptoms), especially if immuno-compromised, request India ink stain for cryptococcal infection.

NB: Rather obtain CT scan before LP if evidence of raised intracranial pressure or focal neurological signs .

Table 7.3 Normal CSF values

	Protein (g/l)	Glucose (mmol/l)	Chloride (mmol/l)	Cells/mm (per mm)
Normal (neonates)	0.2–1.5	Normal[1]	116–130	0–10 lymphocytes
Normal (older)	0.2–0.4	Normal[1]	116–130	0–5 lymphocytes
Aseptic viral	0.2–2.0	Normal[1]	Normal	20 to a few 100, mainly lymphocytes[2]
Tuberculosis	0.5–3.0	Moderately reduced	Very low, 100 or less	20–500, mainly lymphocytes[2]
Pyogenic	0.5–5.0	Reduced, may be absent	Normal, slightly reduced	50 to 1 000s, nearly all polymorphs

1 Normal CSF glucose concentration is about two-thirds of the blood glucose concentration.
2 In early stages, polymorphs may predominate.

Management

- *Viral meningitis*. Treatment is supportive. There is often dramatic relief of headache after LP. If diagnosis is doubtful, treat for bacterial and tuberculous meningitis.
- *Bacterial meningitis*. Start antibiotic treatment immediately after drawing blood for culture, as prognosis directly related to the length of time between onset of symptoms and treatment.
- Use broad spectrum agents until culture results and sensitivities are known.

Antibiotic therapy ☙ ☆ ☆ ☆ ☆

- *Neonates and infants under 3 months of age*: ceftriaxone 100 mg/kg daily or cefotaxime 50 mg/kg 6 hourly. Add ampicillin 50 mg/kg 6 hourly in high doses (for at least 48 hours until *Listeria* is excluded)
- *Infants over 3 months and children*: ceftriaxone or cefotaxime as above
- Review antibiotic cover with specific organism sensitivities. Antibiotics can be stopped after 7 days in meningococcal meningitis. In *Group B strep, S. pneumoniae* and *H. influenzae* continue treatment for 10–14 days and 21 days when Gram negative sepsis has been demonstrated.

Steroid therapy

- Remains controversial. Possibly reduces severity of long-term sequelae (particularly sensorineural deafness) ☺ ☆
- Dexamethasone IV 0.15 mg/kg 6 hourly for 2–4 days (in children > 2 months)
- Give immediately prior to or simultaneously with first antibiotic dose.

General measures

- Analgesics for conscious patients in pain
- LP need not be repeated in those with uncomplicated recovery
- Audiometry follow up after acute illness.

Table 7.4 Causes of meningitis

	Under 3 months	3 months – 2 years	2 years – adolescence
Bacterial	E. coli Group B Streptococci S. pneumonia* N. meningitidis* Listeria monocytogenes* H. influenzae*	H. influenzae S. pneumoniae N. meningitidis M. tuberculosis	N. meningitidis M. tuberculosis S. pneumoniae
Viral	Uncommon	Herpes virus Enterovirus Adenovirus Para/influenzae EB virus Mumps, measles, varicella, rubella	

* Less common

Complications

- Deteriorating level of consciousness.
  Assume cerebral oedema and treat accordingly while awaiting *urgent* CT scan (mannitol 0.25–0.5 g/kg IV slowly over > 30 minutes and general neuroprotective measures). Contact ICU. Check blood glucose and electrolytes.
- Seizures.
  Exclude additional electrolyte abnormality of hypoglycaemia as cause (correct if present). Treat aggressively with lorazepam 0.05 mg/kg–0.1 mg/kg followed by phenobarbitone 20 mg/kg IV. ☙☆☆
- Subdural effusions and empyema.
  Persistence of fever, vomiting, seizures, focal signs or unsatisfactory course after 72 hours of appropriate antibiotic therapy. Obtain urgent CT scan. Refer to neurosurgeon.
- Hyponatraemia.
  Occurs in 20% of patients with meningitis. Diagnose cause (SIADH, fluid shifts due to inflammation or cerebral salt wasting). Paired urine and serum electrolytes and osmolality. Consider hypertonic saline in severe symptomatic cases. ☙☆☆
- Hydrocephalus.
  Obtain urgent CT scan if clinical suspicion.

NB: All children with CT scan evidence of hydrocephalus should be discussed with the neurosurgeons.

Formal surgical drainage is necessary for non-communicating HCP hydrocephalus, and likely for communicating hydrocephalus not due to TBM.

In TBM, communicating hydrocephalus may respond to daily LPs and medical treatment with acetazolamide (100 mg/kg/day) and furosemide (1 mg/kg/day) in 3–4 divided doses. ☗ ☆ ☆

Long-term sequelae

- Children < 1 year at higher risk
- Intellectual disability/cerebral palsy
- Symptomatic epilepsy
- Chronic hydrocephalus
- Blindness or sensorineural deafness
- Behavioural problems.

TB meningitis (TBM)

See Chapter 9, Immunization and infections.

Suspect in:
- Child often < 5 years (but can occur at any age)
- Insidious onset over weeks
- Lethargy/irritability/weight loss
- Focal neurology /focal seizures suggest more advanced disease
- History of TB household contact.

Key investigations:
- CT brain with contrast (exclude hydrocephalus)
- Lumbar puncture (see Table 7.3)

See Chapter 9, Immunization and infections, for treatment guidelines.

Brain abscess and empyema

Suspect in:
- Raised ICP
- Localizing neurological signs
- Seizures (often focal)
- Underlying disease: pansinusitis, dental sepsis, chronic ear sepsis, cyanotic heart disease, infective endocarditis, trauma
- Fever not always present.

Diagnosis

- CT/MRI with contrast
- LP contra-indicated.

Management:

- Refer neurosurgical opinion
- Surgical drainage (may require several repeats)
- IV antibiotics for minimum 4–6 weeks (if excised) and consider 6–8 weeks if treated conservatively. Cefotaxime 200 mg/kg dly and metronidazole 7.5 mg/kg 8 hourly. ♦☆☆☆
- Diligent search for source of infection!

Encephalitis

This implies diffuse involvement of the brain parenchyma by an infectious agent. In many cases there is meningeal involvement as well. The spectrum of clinical severity ranges from mild headache and malaise to profound cerebral derangement with fatal outcome. Usually viral aetiology.

There are 2 forms:
- *Primary encephalitis*: direct viral invasion
- *Post infectious encephalitis*: presumed alteration in immune response.

Clinical presentation

- Severe headache, vomiting, fever, convulsions, delirium, depressed level of consciousness and focal neurological signs.

Aetiology

- *Primary*: Herpes simplex virus, other viruses as for meningitis (Table 7.4)
- *Post infectious*: measles, mumps, rubella, varicella, mycoplasma.

Diagnosis

- *CSF*: as for viral meningitis (Table 7.3) but may be normal. In suspected cases request PCR for specific virus
- *CT/MRI*: generalized cerebral oedema. In herpes encephalitis there is classically focal, temporal lobe swelling with tissue destruction later
- *EEG*: generalized background slowing. In herpes encephalitis there may be classically asymmetry, focal spikes and slowing over temporal lobes.

Management

- Herpes encephalitis: acyclovir 20 mg/kg 8 hourly (< 12 years) or 10 mg/kg 8 hourly (> 12 years) IV infusion over 1 hour. Treat for minimum 3 weeks and confirm patient well and CSF PCR negative for herpes virus

- Ceftriaxone or cefotaxime if clinical picture and CSF suggests partially treated bacterial meningitis
- Aggressive treatment of seizures as for meningitis
- Cerebral oedema: mannitol ☺☆ and neuroprotective measures
- Steroids contraindicated in viral encephalitis.

Neurocysticercosis

Occurs when the larval form of the tapeworm, *Taenia solium*, invades the CNS. It occurs in children who ingest ova shed in faeces of human carriers of adult tape worm. Neurocysticercosis occurs where sanitation is poor and water and soil is contaminated. It is endemic in South Africa.

Clinical presentation
- May be entirely asymptomatic
- Seizures (often focal or complex partial and may be prolonged)
- Raised intracranial pressure.

Diagnosis
- CT or MRI
- If a single granuloma is present, it should be distinguished from a tuberculoma.

Management
- Aim to clear gastrointestinal helminth infestation with albendazole 400 mg oral stat dose (> 2 years) or 200 mg (< 2 years).
- Calcific foci do not require anti-helminthic treatment.
- Recurrent seizures require management with appropriate anticonvulsant.
- Difficult to control seizures and multiple contrast enhancing lesions on CT brain may require a prolonged course of albendazole with steroid cover. This should be discussed with a paediatric neurologist. ☙☆

Cerebral malaria

Diagnosis
- Suspect if child has impaired consciousness and has been to a malaria-endemic region.
- Examine thick and thin peripheral blood smears for *P. falciparum* malaria parasites, or a rapid malaria antigen test if available. An initial negative result does not exclude malaria.

- Exclude other causes for encephalopathy (e.g. hypoglycaemia, meningitis).

Management

- Control seizures, correct hypoglycaemia, hypoxia, shock and anaemia.
- Use antimalaria drugs recommended for the region.
- Assess for evidence of neurological damage (visual, speech, hearing, and motor deficits) before discharge.

Recommended reading

1. Winner P. Pediatric headache. *Current Opin Neurol* 2008; 21:316–322
2. Bakola E, Skapinakis P, Tzoufi M, Damigos D, Mavreas V. Anticonvulsant drugs for pediatric migraine prevention: An evidence-based review. *Eur J Pain.* 2009;13(9): 893–901
3. Yoong, M, Chin, R.F.M, Scott, R.C, Management of convulsive status epilepticus in children. *Arch Dis Child Educ Prac Ed.* 2009; 94:1–9
4. Mackay, MT, Weiss, SK, Adams-Webber, T, et al. Practice parameter: medical treatment of infantile spasms: Report of the American Academy of Neurology and the Child Neurology Society. *Neurology* 2004; 62: 1668.
5. Pappachan,J, Kirkham,F. Cerebrovascular Disease and Stroke. *Arch Dis Child.* 2008; 93:890–898
6. Hughes RAC, Raphaël JC, Swan AV, van Doorn PA. Intravenous immunoglobulin for Guillian-Barré syndrome. *Cochrane Database of Systemic Reviews* 2006, Issue 1. Art. No.: CD002063.DOI
7. Tyler KL. Neurological infections: advances in therapy, outcome, and prediction. *Lancet Neurol* 2009; 8: 19–21
8. Fitch M, Abrahamian F, Moran G, Talan D. Emergency Department Management of Meningitis and Encephalitis. *Infectious Dis Clin North America.* 2008; 22:33–52, v–vi. Review
9. Schoeman J, Donald P, van Zyl L, Keet M, Wait J. Tuberculous hydrocephalus: comparison of different treatments with regard to ICP, ventricular size and clinical outcome. *Dev Med Child Neurol.* 1991; 33: 396–405

8 Renal problems

P. Gajjar, M. McCulloch

Urinary incontinence in children

This section will discuss functional disorders of enuresis and daytime urinary incontinence.

Enuresis

Definition

Enuresis is recurrent, spontaneous urination during sleep in children aged at least 5 yrs of age. By the age of 5, a child is normally able to void at will and to postpone voiding in a socially acceptable manner.
Nocturnal enuresis and daytime incontinence are common disorders of childhood and adolescence. Although most have a non-organic background, they may rarely be caused by structural or neurogenic anomalies.

Prevalence

- At 7 years of age enuresis affects 15–22% of boys and 7–15% of girls, with evidence of decreasing prevalence with age, leaving enuresis in approximately 1–3% of adults.
- There is a higher prevalence in boys than in girls by a ratio of 2:1.
- Severe wetting (wet 7 nights/week) is uncommon (0.3% boys at 7.5 years of age) with generally poor long-term resolution, particularly after 10 years of age.
- It is a hereditary disorder with an autosomal dominant pattern of inheritance. If either parent had enuresis the relative risk of enuresis in the child is 7.8; if both parents had enuresis the relative risk is 16.
- Children with developmental delay, mental retardation, ADHD and minor neurological dysfunction have a higher prevalence.

Factors contributing to enuresis

- Genetic
- Decreased arousal response to a full bladder
- Nocturnal polyuria.

- Small functional bladder capacity due to
  - Constitutionally small bladder
  - Bladder overactivity or other bladder dysfunction.
- Stressful life events.

Classification of enuresis

- Primary versus secondary:
  Primary enuresis: in a child who has previously been dry for less than 6 months.
  Secondary enuresis: in a child who has been previously dry for at least 6 months.
- Monosymptomatic versus non-monosymptomatic:
  Monosymptomatic enuresis (MNE): enuresis without any other lower urinary tract (LUT) symptoms.
  Non-monosymptomatic enuresis (NMNE): enuresis with other LUT symptoms, e.g. daytime incontinence, urgency, frequency, weak or intermittent stream, abdominal straining.
- Wet nights/week:
  Mild (< 3), moderate (3–6), severe (7).

Causes of secondary enuresis

- Urinary tract infection
- Constipation
- Diabetes mellitus
- Diabetes insipidus
- Psychological stress
- Chronic renal failure
- Late onset bladder dysfunction, neurogenic tethered cord
- Obstructive sleep apnoea.

Evaluation of enuresis

It is important to distinguish between monosymptomatic and non-monosymptomatic enuresis.

Thorough history:
- Enuresis profile (see classification).
  - Mild, moderate, severe
  - Primary, secondary
  - MNE/NMNE
    - Can child wake to any external or internal stimuli (poor arousability)?

- Is wetting copious and within first third of night (nocturnal polyuria)?
- Are there daytime LUT symptoms (bladder dysfunction)?
- Complications:
  - Bladder dysfunction
  - Recurrent urinary tract infections
  - Constipation
  - Obstructive sleep apnoea
  - Sickle cell disease
- Neurodevelopmental factors
- Child and family factors: psychosocial, family setting and level of motivation.

Physical examination:
- ENT examination looking for adenotonsillar hypertrophy
- Abdominal examination for palpable bladder and faecal loading
- Lumbar region of back (deformation, pigmentation, hair growth) in NMNE
- Neurological examination (tone and reflexes of the lower limbs, gait, anal tone, perineal sensation, abnormal buttock crease, etc.) in NMNE
- Urine dipsticks (glucose and leucocytes).

Frequency-volume chart:
This involves documenting the enuresis episodes, the time and volume of all intake and voidings over 2 days. This gives information about severity, drinking habits, bladder capacity (maximum voided volume should equal expected bladder capacity (EBC) = (age in years × 30 ml) + 30 ml) and voiding pattern.

Further investigations are only indicated if there is a suspicion of an underlying anatomic or neuropathic cause or in the case of initial treatment failure.

Management
- The first step in management is to educate the child and the family to demystify the condition and reassure the child and parents.
- General measures for all include:
  - Improved drinking by day (6–8 drinks regularly spaced) with regular voiding (5 times/day)
  - Last drink one and a half hours before bed
  - Always void before bed

- Remove pads/nappies and stop parents waking child up to go to toilet late at night
- Use star/reward charts.
- Primary monosymptomatic enuresis responds to general measures with either the enuresis alarm or desmopressin.
- Before primary nocturnal enuresis is treated, daytime symptoms must be actively identified and managed.
- Secondary causes must be managed and treated appropriately.

Treatment options

Enuresis alarms:
- Wakes child at night at onset of wetting
- A form of operant conditioning, teaching child to wake and void
- Useful in the older, motivated child with cooperative parents
- Requires several months of continuous use
- Up to 65% success rate with effective use of alarms
- With 29 to 69% risk of relapse on discontinuation of use.

Dry bed training:
- Positive reinforcement
- Daytime bladder training and rewards
- Waking routines throughout night
- Includes use of alarm
- Not shown to be more effective than alarm alone.

Desmopressin (DDAVP):
- Synthetic analogue of antidiuretic hormone
- Decreases nocturnal urine output
- Rapid onset of action
- Good for short or longer term use
- 18% of children have fewer wet nights compared to 2% on placebo
- 2.2 fewer wet nights per week
- Dose 0.2 mg (oral tablets) to be taken an hour after meals; no fluids to be taken for 8 hours after medication; dose can be increased to 0.4 mg
- Strict rule for administration: last drink 1 hour prior to medication and bed and no further fluid intake for the next 8 hours
- Minimal side effects (headache and gastrointestinal). Symptomatic hyponatraemia can occur if fluid intake rules not adhered to.

Imipramine:
- Tricyclic antidepressant

- Anticholinergic and antidiuretic properties
- Side effects: drowsiness, lethargy, agitation, cardiac arrhythmias. Often lethal in overdose, therefore warn parents to keep out of reach of young children.

Oxybutynin:
- Anticholinergic
- Useful in NMNE to decrease detrusor overactivity
- Dose 5 mg up to 3 times a day (if daytime wetting present) otherwise at night only in combination with desmopressin.

Children with primary MNE, no daytime wetting, no apparent psychological stressors and with supportive parents, have a good prognosis with use of either alarm or desmopressin. The combination of desmopressin and alarm improves the response rate from 46% (when using alarm alone) to 76%.

In treatment-resistant enuresis, the combination of desmopressin and an anticholinergic has been shown to be more efficacious in a randomised controlled trial.

Daytime incontinence

Figure 8.1 Classification of daytime incontinence

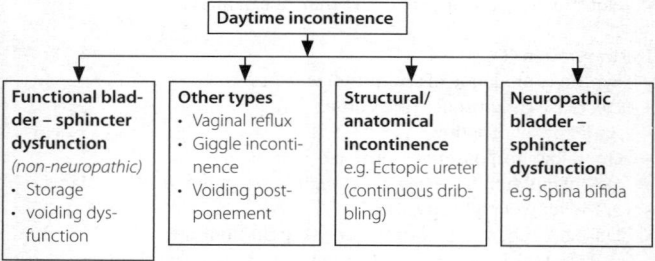

Evaluation of functional daytime urinary incontinence

Thorough paediatric history including:
- Onset
- Continuous or intermittent incontinence (constant dribbling suggests an anatomical cause such as ectopic ureter)

- Frequency, urgency, urge incontinence, post void incontinence (vaginal reflux), difficulty in initiating stream, fluctuating stream, abdominal straining, need to return to void shortly after voiding.
- Presence/absence of enuresis
- Bowel habit
- Urinary tract infections
- Renal tract anomalies
- Family history of renal, bladder dysfunction, spina bifida or maternal IDDM (sacral dysgenesis)
- Neurodevelopmental issues
- Child and family factors.

Assessment:
- Physical examination including blood pressure, abdominal palpation, genital examination, lumbar sacral spine and ankle deep tendon reflexes
- Urine dipstick
- Frequency-voiding chart (see above)
- Urinary tract ultrasound including post void residual volume (normal = 0 ml). Complete emptying occurs in overactive bladder but residuals are the norm in dysfunctional voiders
- Uroflowmetry to diagnose dysfunctional voiders (staccato/fractionated patterns suggest external sphincter overactivity)
- MRI spinal cord in suspected cases of spinal dysraphism
- MCUG/indirect nucleotide cystography
- Urodynamics if treatment resistance occurs or spinal dysraphism present.

Management of overactive bladder:
- Child-family education
- Bladder training (regular drinking 6–8 drinks equally spaced with 5 regular command voids)
- Treat constipation and treat/prevent urinary tract infections
- Anticholinergic medication
  - Oxybutynin (tablets or liquid)
    - 2.5–5 mg bd or tds (start low and build up slowly)
    - Side effects: constipation, dry mouth and eyes, skin rashes, heat intolerance, CNS irritability
    - Once daily slow release formulation available.
  - Tolterodine (tablets)
    - 1–2 mg bd

- Side effects similar to above but does not cross blood-brain barrier
- Once daily slow release formulation available.
— Desmopressin can be added at night to treat enuresis.

Management of dysfunctional voiding:
- Child-family education
- Treat constipation and treat/prevent urinary tract infections
- Bladder training
  — Regular fluid intake (6–8 drinks regularly spaced through day)
  — Regular voiding 5 times/day with
    - Relaxation of pelvic floor (correct seating)
    - Double voiding
    - Small doses of anticholinergics to diminish secondary bladder overactivity (full doses will worsen emptying and infections)
    - α-blockers (doxasozin) used by some
    - Clean intermittent catheterization.

Urinary tract infection (UTI)

- This is the second most common renal problem, affecting 3% of boys and 11% of girls with the majority recovering promptly with no long-term sequelae.
- A small minority, mainly the young infants, are at risk of developing long-term scarring. This is usually in association with an abnormally developed urinary tract.

Clinical presentation (is age dependent)
- Unexplained fever (> 38 °C),
- Non-specific features, including vomiting, abdominal pain, lethargy, irritability, malaise, FTT and jaundice.
- Specific features, including dysfunctional voiding, frequency, dysuria and haematuria, changes to continence and loin tenderness.

Diagnosis

This requires specimen collection, which is difficult in young infants.
- Use a urine bag attached to a *clean* perineum as a screening test.
- It is not a UTI if the Dipstix® test is normal.
- If it is abnormal, obtain a clean catch or suprapubic aspiration or catheter sample.

Table 8.1 Interpretation of urine Dipstix®

Urine Dipstix®	Diagnosis and management
Wbc +ve Nitrites +ve	Probable UTI – urine MC&S if high risk/past history – start antibiotics
Wbc +ve Nitrites –ve	May/may not be UTI – urine MC&S – management based on good clinical evidence of UTI – infection may be elsewhere
Wbc –ve Nitrites +ve	Possible UTI – urine MC&S – start antibiotics
Wbc –ve Nitrites –ve	UTI excluded – no urine to laboratory – look for other cause of fever

Wbc – White blood cells (leucocyte esterase)

- Send the urine for microscopy, culture and sensitivity (MC&S) as above.
- *E. coli* is the commonest organism cultured (usually resistant to amoxil and co-trimoxazole in Cape Town, South Africa). It is essential to know the antibiotic sensitivity of the organisms in your area.

Table 8.2 Management

Under 3 months old or very ill:	- Refer and admit for adequate fluid and nutrition - Check renal function - Start broad spectrum IV antibiotics: cefotaxime 25 mg/kg/dose 6 hourly, ceftriaxone 50 mg/kg/dose daily, or gentamicin 5–7.5 mg/kg/dose daily (monitoring levels) - Then according to urine culture results
Older children: acute pyelonephritis/upper UTI – temperature >38 °C, loin pain, vomiting	- Appropriate urine to lab - Oral antibiotics according to local sensitivities: amoxil/clavulanic acid 15 mg/kg/dose 8 hourly or cefuroxime 10 mg/kg/dose 12 hourly for 7 days. If ill: IV antibiotics for 48 hours (as above) then oral for 5 days
Older children: cystitis/lower UTI	- Oral antibiotic for 3 days e.g. nalidixic acid 25 mg/kg/dose 6 hourly - Review if still unwell after 48 hours

Antibiotic prophylaxis is NOT routine after first UTI as there is no evidence of prevention of recurrence or scars unless:

- Infant – use amoxil/clavulanic acid or cefuroxime under 6 weeks of age.
- Recurrent or atypical UTIs – use nalidixic acid 25 mg/kg/day or nitrofurantoin 2 mg/kg/day.

It is also safer to continue to give prophylaxis until the child has completed investigations of the urinary tract. ☆☆☆♦

Figure 8.2 Investigation of UTI ☆☆☆♦

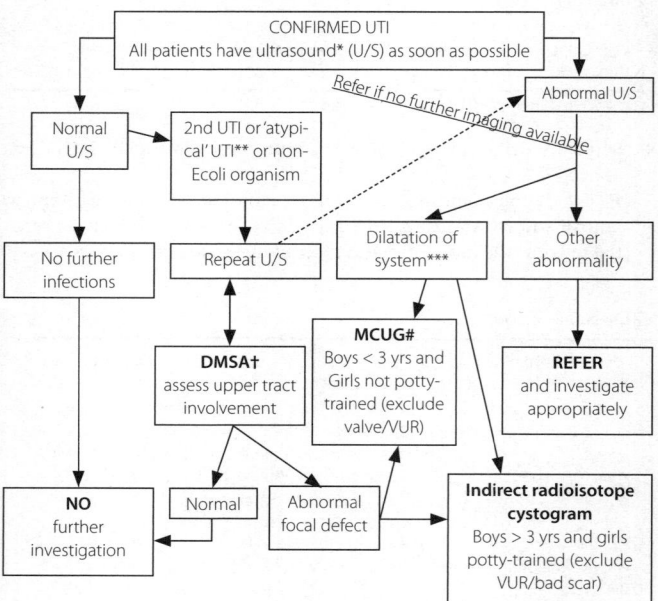

* Presumed reliable – 3rd trimester antenatal U/S not available in all patients
** Atypical = seriously ill/septicaemia, poor u/output, abdominal/renal mass, raised creatinine, poor response in 48 hrs
*** Dilated pelvis only – PUJ (pelvic-ureteric junction) obstruction need MAG3 isotope study
† DMSA in our setting best early as compliance better; if bad 'defect' proceed with investigations
\# MCUG not done while active infection, but as soon as infection cleared – remains on prophylaxis for procedure
High procalcitonin levels where available – validated predictor of renal involvement – useful screen for need for cystogram

✚ – *authors McCulloch/Gajjar/Sinclair/Nourse*

> *Practice points:*
> - All patients should have an ultrasound.
> - Any circumcised boy with a UTI must be investigated further.

Recurrent infections with a normal urinary tract

- These typically occur in girls aged 3 to 7 years and may be asymptomatic.
- Constipation with faecal loading is almost always present.
- Encourage fluid intake and regular voiding (by the clock if necessary).
- Pay attention to toilet hygiene and avoid bubble baths.
- Give 6 months empiric treatment with nalidixic acid or nitrofurantoin.
- Dysfunctional voiders may need oxybutinin for bladder stability.
- In boys with recurrent UTIs there may be benefit in circumcision.

An approach to haematuria

Haematuria is a common presenting symptom of renal and urinary tract disorders.

- It may or may not indicate serious underlying disease. It should be investigated urgently.
- Macroscopic haematuria may be
  - Symptomatic with: dysuria (UTI), renal colic (calculus), or loin pain (PUJ obstruction), or
  - Asymptomatic.

  Urinary tract infection is the commonest cause, e.g. haemorrhagic cystitis caused by adenovirus (that can last up to 6 weeks after the initial event).
- Asymptomatic microscopic haematuria may be detected incidentally or on family screening.
- Early consultation with a paediatric nephrologist is recommended if there is evidence of:
  - Impaired renal function
  - Proteinuria
  - Hypertension.

History and examination

- General symptoms of fever, lethargy, abdominal pain, oedema, dysuria, frequency of micturition, loin pain
- Pattern of the bleeding (beginning or end of stream more suggestive of bladder or urethral pathology)
- Red (local cause) versus tea coloured urine (more likely glomerular)

- History of a preceding sore throat, or recent URTI
- Skin rashes: impetigo, butterfly rash, purpuric or vasculitic rash
- Arthritis
- Easy bruising or delayed haemostasis
- Measure blood pressure and assess heart size
- Trauma to the back
- Abdominal mass
- Family history
  - Haematuria
  - Deafness
  - Sickle cell disease
  - Renal failure, including dialysis and renal transplant
  - Renal stones.

Figure 8.3 An approach to haematuria

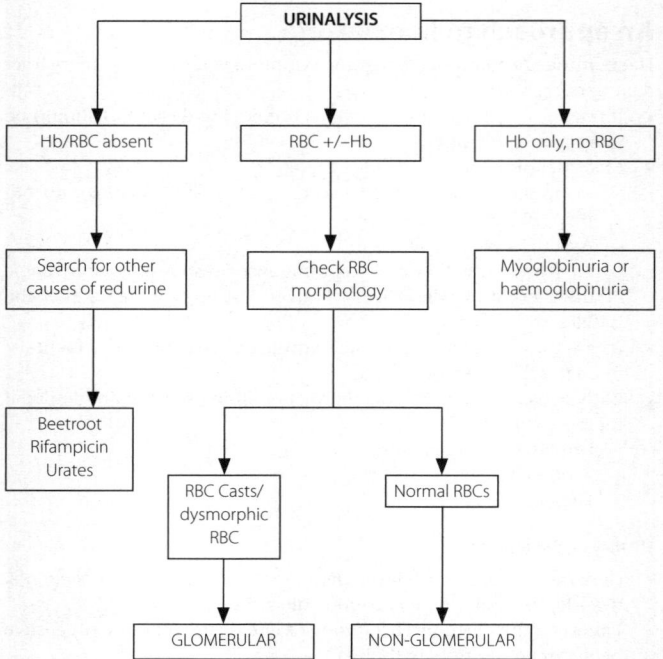

An approach to non-glomerular haematuria

Figure 8.4 An approach to non-glomerular haematuria

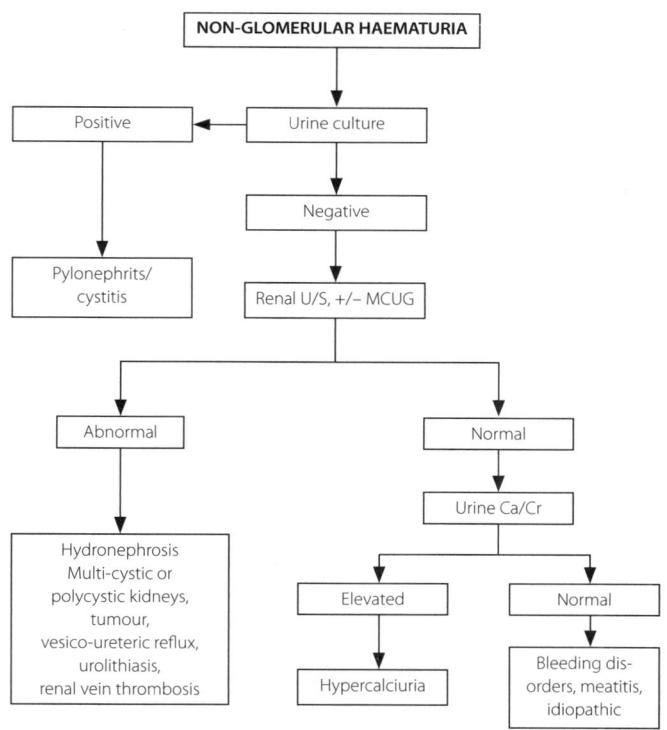

Glomerular haematuria

Causes

With a major clinical syndrome:
- Acute nephritis (post streptococcal) (*increased ASOT, anti-DNAse B, low C3*)
- IgA Nephropathy (Berger's disease) (*IgA deposits on immunofluorescence*)

- Haemolytic uraemic syndrome
- Interstitial nephritis
- Mesangiocapillary GN (MCGN) (*low C3*)
- Nephrotic syndrome.

With a typical hereditary or systemic syndrome:
- Henoch-Schönlein purpura
- Systemic lupus erythematosus
- Alport's (family history of deafness)
- Nail-patella syndrome
- Infective endocarditis.

Investigations
- Assess degree of proteinuria (urine protein/creatinine ratio)
- Check urine of parents and siblings for blood and protein
- Electrolytes, urea, creatinine, albumin
- Full blood count
- C3, C4
- ASOT/anti-DNAse B
- ANA, anti-ds-DNA
- IgA levels
- Hearing assessment
- Consider renal biopsy if:
  - Raised creatinine
  - Low albumin
  - Proteinuria
  - Family history
  - Hypertension.

Acute post-streptococcal glomerulonephritis (APSGN)

This usually occurs after a streptococcal throat or skin infection (impetigo in more than 50% of our cases), and occasionally following other infections. It is uncommon before the age of 2 years, and recurrences are rare.

Clinical presentation
Triad of, singularly or in combination:
- Macroscopic/microscopic haematuria (painless)
- Oligo-anuric renal failure
- Hypertension with severe fluid-volume overload and cardiac failure.

May be complicated by hypertensive encephalopathy with seizures and pulmonary oedema due to severe fluid overload. *This may occur with little or no oedema and only mild renal failure.*

Less common, but more serious glomerulonephritides (e.g. systemic lupus erythematosus (SLE), hepatitis B-associated nephropathy and HIV renal disease) may present similarly.

Investigations

- Urine dipstick: haematuria and proteinuria
- Urine microscopy: dysmorphic red blood cells and red cell casts are present.
- Urine culture: do this to exclude a urinary tract infection, if the dipstick is positive for leucocytes and nitrite.
- Renal function: measure plasma urea, creatinine, sodium, potassium, acid-base status, total protein and albumin.
- Evidence of recent streptococcal infection: do a throat or impetigo swab culture, ASOT and anti-DNAse B titres and C3 (reduced).
- Chest X-ray: for pulmonary congestion/oedema, cardiomegaly or pleural effusions if clinically indicated.
- ECG: for cardiac dysfunction or hyperkalaemia.

Management

Fluids:

- Restrict the fluid intake to that of output and monitor both accurately.
- If unsure start with 20 ml/kg/day for insensible losses.
- Check urine dipstick daily.
- Monitor blood pressure and treat hypertension with nifedipine, amlodipine or atenolol.
- Low salt diet (until resolution of fluid overload).

Drugs:

- Penicillin: orally for 10 days for streptococcal infection (or single IM injection of Benzathine benzylpenicillin). Will not change the course of the present episode but will treat the underlying cause. Long-term penicillin is unnecessary.
- Furosemide 1–2 mg/kg/dose PO 1–3 times per day is effective for fluid overload. Start with intravenous doses in severe cases (if gut is also oedematous). Furosemide decreases hospital stay.
- Diazepam PR or IV for seizures due to hypertension.

Pulmonary oedema

NB: This is life-threatening and requires immediate treatment.

- Sit the child up in bed and give oxygen.
- Restrict fluid and sodium intake to a minimum.
- Give furosemide 3–5 mg/kg/dose IV over 5–10 minutes to induce a diuresis and repeat 4–6 hourly when necessary.
- Morphine 0.05–0.1 mg/kg IV. Start with smallest dose.
- Intubation and ventilation may be needed.
- Urgent dialysis/filtration may be required to remove fluid, especially if the child is anuric, thus needs referral.

Indications for referral

- Rapidly deteriorating renal function
- Anuria
- Massive proteinuria, or persistent moderate proteinuria for more than 2 weeks
- Significant clinical or biochemical abnormalities for more than 2 to 4 weeks
- Persistent haematuria (macroscopic > 6 weeks or microscopic > 2 years).

Outcome

Clinical recovery usually occurs within a few weeks. Microscopic haematuria may persist for up to 2 years, but proteinuria should be minimal on an early morning urine collection.

Nephrotic syndrome

Definition

Nephrotic range proteinuria
Plasma albumin < 25 g/l

Clinical presentation

- Gradual onset of generalized oedema with ascites suggests minimal change nephrotic syndrome (MCNS).
- Macroscopic haematuria, renal failure and/or hypertension are indicative of glomerular disease other than MCNS.
- Secondary infection is common.

Investigation

Figure 8.5 Investigation of initial episode

✚ – Authors McCulloch/Gajjar/Sinclair/Nourse

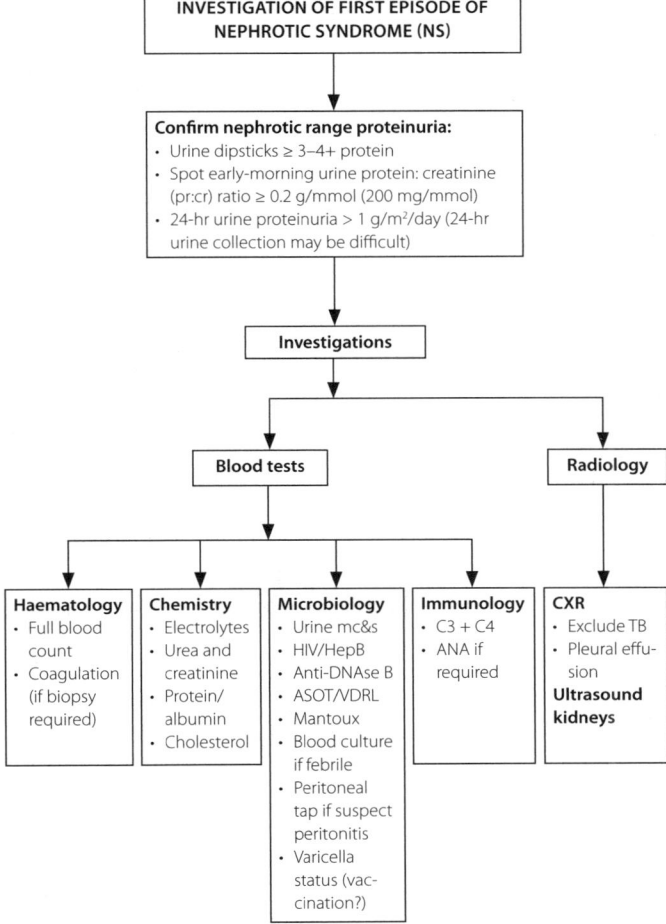

Treatment

Figure 8.6 Treatment of nephrotic syndrome

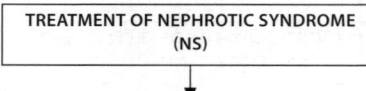

– Authors McCulloch/Gajjar/Sinclair/Nourse

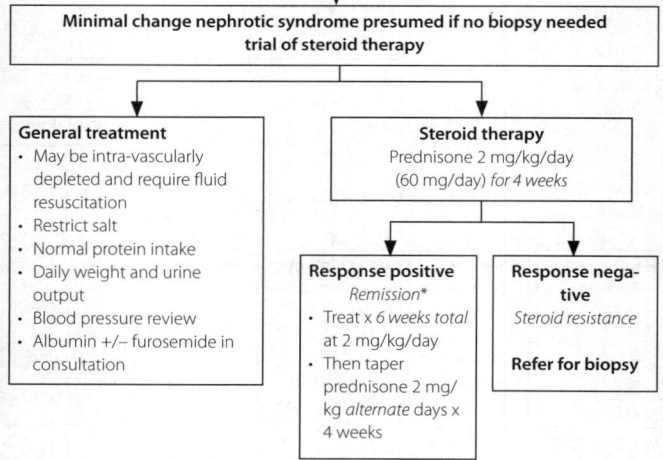

TREATMENT OF NEPHROTIC SYNDROME (NS)

Decision if needs renal biopsy – indications

- Age: under 6 months or over 10 years
- Macroscopic haematuria (persistent > 6 weeks)
- Persistent hypertension
- Hepatitis-B positive
- Low serum C3 and C4
- Steroid resistance
- Renal failure (excluding minor reversible pre-renal element seen in minimal change nephrotic syndrome)
- Clinical evidence of systemic disease, e.g. HIV, Henoch-Schönlein purpura, SLE, etc.

Minimal change nephrotic syndrome presumed if no biopsy needed trial of steroid therapy

General treatment
- May be intra-vascularly depleted and require fluid resuscitation
- Restrict salt
- Normal protein intake
- Daily weight and urine output
- Blood pressure review
- Albumin +/– furosemide in consultation

Steroid therapy
Prednisone 2 mg/kg/day (60 mg/day) *for 4 weeks*

Response positive
*Remission**
- Treat x *6 weeks total* at 2 mg/kg/day
- Then taper prednisone 2 mg/kg *alternate* days x 4 weeks

Response negative
Steroid resistance

Refer for biopsy

☆☆☆☆☆ Children in their first episode of steroid responsive nephrotic syndrome should be treated with prednisone for at least 3 months, as this significantly reduces the risk of relapse at 12–24 months.

* Remission = Urine dipstick neg/trace protein for 3 consecutive days or urine pr:cr ratio < 0.2 g/mmol

Management of oedema

- Patients with severe oedema may have a fluid-depleted intravascular compartment during relapse. Fluid restriction and aggressive diuretic therapy are therefore inappropriate.
- If peripheral perfusion is poor, give 20% albumin (5 ml/kg IV) over 3 hours.
- For severe oedema, if perfusion is good, give albumin (as above) mixed with furosemide 1–2 mg/kg.

> ***Practice point:***
> Do not give IV albumin to treat a low serum albumin.

The clinical indications for albumin are:
- poor perfusion
- severe oedema/ascites/pleural effusions
- severe intercurrent infections.

> ***Practice point:***
> Before giving albumin ensure that the urine output is adequate – if it is not, pulmonary oedema may be precipitated. Monitor carefully during infusion (i.e. blood transfusion protocol).

Amiloride has recently been shown to have diuretic benefit in nephrotic patients, but diuretics should *only* be used in consultation with renal specialists.

Relapses of nephrotic syndrome

Definitions:
- Relapse: defined as urine protein/creatinine ratio > 0.2 g/mmol, or 3–4 + proteinuria with oedema, following a remission.
- Frequent relapser: 2 or more relapses in 6 months or 4 or more within 1 year.
- Steroid dependence: 2 consecutive relapses during steroid therapy or within 14 days of stopping steroids.

Management:
- Start with prednisone 2 mg/kg/day (maximum 60 mg), until early morning urine clear for 3 consecutive days.
- Then taper slowly under renal team supervision:
  - Completely for initial relapse or
  - To low maintenance dose for the frequent relapser.
- Steroid dependant patients to be referred to the renal service for further evaluation and consideration of second line agents.

Acute renal failure

Causes
- Pre-renal: shock, hypovolaemia and dehydration from any cause may produce hypoperfusion of the kidneys. If not corrected, this will progress to acute tubular necrosis.
- Intrinsic: glomerulonephritides, acute tubular necrosis, haemolytic uraemic syndrome, septicaemia, pyelonephritis in infants, renovascular occlusion, myoglobinuria, nephrotoxins, acute-on-chronic renal failure, congenital renal anomalies.
- Post-renal: urethral obstruction, bilateral ureteric obstruction, obstruction of a single functioning kidney.

Clinical presentation
- History and clinical features of the underlying disease tend to dominate clinical findings.
- Anorexia, vomiting (due to uraemia)
- Fluid imbalance: intravascular depletion with dehydration, oedema, hypertension, and/or pulmonary oedema are common.
- The kidneys may be enlarged and even palpable.
- Persistent metabolic acidosis, presenting as tachypnoea in the absence of fluid overload or respiratory infection.
- Neurological signs, such as twitching, convulsions, disturbed level of consciousness, may be caused by uraemia or hypocalcaemia.
- Rash or arthropathy as markers of underlying systemic disease causing renal failure.

> *Practice point:*
> Anaemia, growth failure, rickets and small kidneys on ultrasound suggest chronic renal failure.

Investigations

All children should have:
- Urinalysis, microscopy and culture
- Urea, creatinine, sodium, potassium, acid-base
- Protein, albumin
- Urinary sodium, creatinine and urea, specific gravity
- Full blood count
- CXR:
  - Fluid overload
  - Heart size.
- Ultrasound kidneys and bladder:
  - Size
  - Echogenicity
  - Dilatation.

Children suspected of acute-on-chronic failure:
- Calcium, phosphate
- Parathyroid hormone.

Suspected haemolytic uraemic syndrome (HUS):
- FBC
- Smear (schistocyctes and fragmented RBCs)
- Reticulocyte count (↑)
- Haptoglobin (↓), LDH (↑)
- Blood culture
- Stool culture.

Major trauma/muscle injury:
- Urine and serum myoglobin
- Creatinine kinase.

Suspected urinary tract obstruction:
- DMSA
- Mag 3
- MCUG.

Suspected renal vein thrombosis:
- Doppler studies.

Management

- It is important to ascertain whether the patient has pre-renal or intrinsic renal failure. The fractional excretion of sodium can be useful for differentiating between the two.
- FeNa = uNa/uCr × pCr/pNa × 100
- FeNa < 1% in pre-renal failure; > 1% in intrinsic renal failure
- Record all intake and output.

Pre-renal failure

- Correct shock or dehydration: crystalloid fluid bolus 5–10 ml/kg, then reassess and repeat until circulation is restored. Reassess fluid balance hourly or more frequently. Central venous pressure is the best guide to fluid balance and cardiac status.
- Avoid potassium-containing fluids if there is a risk of hyperkalaemia. Add $NaHCO_3$ if necessary.
- If oliguria persists after correction of hypoperfusion, give furosemide 1–5 mg/kg IV over 5–10 minutes or mannitol 0.25–0.5 g/kg IV. Do not repeat mannitol unless there is a good diuretic response.
- Trial of low dose dopamine 1–3 mcg/kg/minute IV infusion – may have a beneficial effect in increasing urinary output, but does not affect renal function. ☆☆☺

Renal parenchymal failure

- Maintain homeostasis until normal renal function is restored. In acute tubular necrosis, recovery within 2 to 6 weeks is usual.

Post-renal failure

- Relieve any obstruction in the urinary tract.

Diet and caloric intake

- Ensure an adequate diet with high caloric intake.
- Dialysis may be required to permit adequate nutrition.

Fluid and electrolyte balance

- Record all intake and output. Regularly check fluid balance and weight and adjust intake.
- If in neutral fluid balance, restrict intake to total losses from all routes. If fluid-overloaded, restrict intake to less than output.
- Allow for insensible losses: 30 ml/kg/day for infants; 12 ml/kg/day for older children. Fever increases insensible loss. Also allow for gastrointestinal losses, which may be severe in diarrhoeal disease.

- Furosemide 1–10 mg/kg by slow IV injection may increase the urine volume (without increasing glomerular filtration rate).
- Aminophyllin 1 mg/kg infusion over 6 hours has been shown to increase urine output in diuretic dependant critically ill children. Side effects: nausea, vomiting, seizures, changes in heart rate and blood pressure. ☆☆☆◐
- Monitor blood pressure and treat pulmonary oedema if present (see *Nephritis*).

Hyperkalaemia

- The pulse may be slow and irregular.
- ECG: peaked T waves, prolonged PR interval. Ominous signs: P wave disappears, progressive widening of the QRS complex to a sine wave pattern, cardiac arrest.
- Plasma potassium > 8 mmol/l is life threatening. Commence stepwise treatment when plasma potassium is > 6.4–7.0 mmol/l (see Chapter 20, Fluids, electrolytes and acid-base).

Metabolic acidosis

- Partly correct with IV $NaHCO_3$ 8.4% 1–2 ml/kg if pH < 7.2 or standard bicarbonate < 12 mmol/l. Beware of fluid overload. Rapid correction may cause symptomatic hypocalcaemia. Consider IV calcium gluconate but not via same line.
- In ongoing renal failure, repeated correction or maintenance will be needed.

Hypocalcaemia and hyperphosphataemia

- Treat hyperphosphataemia with calcium carbonate, or aluminium hydroxide gel (if aluminium hydroxide used, it must only be short term).
- 10% calcium gluconate 1–2 ml/kg IV slowly for symptomatic hypocalcaemia or if plasma calcium concentration < 1.8 mmol/l.

Anaemia

There is a risk of hyperkalaemia, hypertension and fluid overload with blood transfusion.

- Correct anaemia with a slow transfusion of packed red cells, 10 ml/kg if the haemoglobin is < 6–8 g/dl or if there is active bleeding or severe haemolysis.
- Avoid blood transfusion if potential to progress to chronic renal failure and so require a transplant, unless haemodynamically unstable. The transfusion might sensitize the patient to donor antigens.

Seizures
- Diazepam 0.3 mg/kg and/or phenobarbitone 20 mg/kg (max 200 mg)
- Look for underlying cause: hypertension, uraemia, hypoglycaemia, hypocalcaemia, hyponatraemia or conditions unrelated to renal disease.

Medications
- Reduce the dosage of renally excreted drugs. Give usual loading dose, then normal dose at longer intervals, depending on severity of renal failure.
- Monitor plasma levels and adjust dosage intervals accordingly.
- Check package insert for guidance on dosage adjustment.

Indications for dialysis
- Severe oliguria or anuria unresponsive to aggressive diuretic therapy
- Severe fluid overload unresponsive to diuretics
- Uncontrollable hyperkalaemia > 7 mmol/l
- Uncontrollable metabolic acidosis with pH < 7.2
- To permit adequate nutrition or other therapy (e.g. coagulation support)
- Clinical uraemic syndrome with disturbed level of consciousness or convulsions
- Severe poisoning with a dialysable agent
- Inborn errors of metabolism, especially with hyperammonaemia.

Choice of renal replacement therapy
The choice of renal replacement therapy is individualized based on:
- Experience and availability in the individual unit.
- The patient's requirements for solute and fluid removal.
- Haemodynamic stability.

Acute peritoneal dialysis (for technique and principles: see Chapter 23, Procedures)
- The peritoneum has a greater surface area in proportion to body size in children, therefore is efficient in removing fluid and solutes.
- Access to the peritoneal cavity can be achieved through an acute Tenckhoff catheter placed at the bedside.
- Simple, inexpensive, yet effective. Does not require the expertise of a dialysis technician to facilitate.

Acute intermittent haemodialysis

Metabolic abnormalities and hypervolaemia can be corrected quickly.
- Need to achieve good vascular access; difficult in very young infants.
- Relative contraindications include haemodynamic instability and severe coagulopathy.
- Rapid ultrafiltration may produce hypotension and rapid shifts in blood urea predisposes to disequilibrium syndrome.
- Ideally should be run by a dialysis trained nurse or technician.

Continuous veno-venous haemofiltration and dialysis
- Blood is pumped by a blood pump from the patient via a central vein, through a haemofilter and returned to the patient. The passage of blood through the filter produces an ultrafiltrate.
- It allows renal replacement in children with low systemic blood pressure.

Chronic renal failure

- This causes profound alterations in body composition and results in impaired growth and development.
- Management is challenging and should be undertaken in consultation with a renal centre.
- Early detection and optimal management can prevent or delay the need for dialysis and transplantation.
- Serum creatinine alone may not accurately reflect kidney function and therefore the GFR should be estimated from the serum creatinine using prediction techniques, e.g.:
  - Counahan-Barrat formula: (simple)
    GFR (ml/min/1.73 m^2) = 40 × height (cm)/serum creatinine (umol/l), (the constant 40 may vary for different age groups e.g. constant for under 1 year of age: 2 weeks = 12, 3 months = 25, 6 months = 30 and 9 months = 35).

Risk factors
- Congenital renal tract abnormalities
- Glomerulonephritis
- Reflux nephropathy
- Familial kidney disease, e.g. polycystic kidney disease.

Management principles
Aim to slow down the rate of progression of end stage kidney disease. This is most effective when instituted early in the disease.

- Optimise nutrition: normal protein, low salt, adequate calorie diet.
- Monitor growth.
- Maintain acid-base status.
- Optimal management of renal osteodystrophy, by maintaining near-normal levels of calcium and phosphate and monitoring parathyroid levels.
- Blood pressure control: aim to get SBP < 95% for height.
- Reduce proteinuria with use of ACE inhibitors.
- Recognise anaemia as an early complication of CKD. Aim to keep Hb between 11–12 g/dl, using erythropoietin; also screen for iron deficiency.
- Avoid nephrotoxic drugs, such as NSAIDS, aminoglycoside antibiotics, and contrast agents.
- Provide psychosocial support.

The *South Africa Renal Society Guidelines* are available online at http://www.sa-renalsociety.org/CKD.

Hypertension

- *Measure blood pressure (BP) in every child* especially those with neurologic, cardiovascular or renal signs.
- Use an appropriate cuff:
  - Bladder width at least 40% of the arm circumference at a point midway between the olecranon and the acromion
  - Bladder length should cover 80 to 100 % of the circumference of the arm.
- Systolic BP is easy to measure and most management decisions can be made on this alone.
- When in doubt about hypertension monitor BP over 24 hours.

Proven hypertension

Definition: Systolic ± diastolic BP that is, on repeated measurements, ≥ 95th centile (using reference BP tables including centiles for gender, age and height, provided in the *Fourth Report on the Diagnosis, Evaluation and Treatment of High BP in Children and Adolescents*. Pediatrics 2004;114: 555–57).

The following formula correlated with the 95th centile for systolic blood pressure and measurements above this indicate hypertension:

- Upper limit of systolic BP = (age in years × 3) + 100 mmHg

NB: A BP 50% greater than the 95th centile constitutes a hypertensive emergency.

Clinical presentation

Hypertension may present with:
- Features of the primary disease or those of target organ damage, e.g. hypertensive encephalopathy, pulmonary oedema, renal disease or cardiac failure (in which case BP can be normal).
- Bizarre features such as facial palsy, pulmonary oedema, irritability, and unexplained vomiting, especially in young children.
- Heart failure, in which case blood pressure may be normal.

There has been a recent increase in adolescent essential hypertension related to the epidemic of childhood obesity.

All hypertension must be investigated – the majority of causes are renal or reno-vascular.

Table 8.3 Causes of secondary hypertension

Renal parenchymal	Dysplasia, chronic GN, reflux nephropathy, Wilms' tumour
Reno-vascular	Takayasu's, fibromuscular dysplasia
Cardiac	Coarctation of the aorta
Endocrine	Cushing's, Conn's, phaeochromocytoma
Central nervous system	Tumours, raised intracranial pressure

Investigation of hypertension

Step 1:
- Urine dipstick and analysis, urine protein/creatinine ratio
- Renal function
- FBC
- Ultrasound and dopplers of kidneys (note size)
- CXR/ECG/ECHO
- ESR and Mantoux (Takayasu's arteritis).

Step 2: (driven by previous findings)
- Renal
  - Plasma renin and aldosterone
  - DMSA scan
  - Multi-slice CT/MRI
  - Angiography with renal vein sampling
  - C3/C4/ASOT/Anti-DNAse B (nephritis suspected)
  - ANA/Anti-ds-DNA/ANCA (vasculitis suspected)
- Endocrine
  - Urinary catecholamines (HVA/VMA)
  - PTH/calcium

- Cortisol
- MIBG scan.
- Central
  - MRI/CT head.

Assess for end organ damage:
- Cardiac: CXR/ECG/ECHO
- Eyes: ophthalmology
- Renal: proteinuria, creatinine.

Management

Acute hypertension

Hypertensive crisis:
- Medical emergency with end organ decompensation:
  - ICU or high care setting
  - Frequent BP monitoring and neurological observations
  - *Reduce BP slowly because if there is established underlying hypertension, too rapid a fall in blood pressure can result in stroke or retinal or spinal cord infarction*:
    - ⅓ of total desired reduction in first 12 hrs
    - Next ⅓ over 12–36 hours
    - Last ⅓ over 36–72 hours.

Severe hypertension:
- BP is 20 mmHg above the 95th percentile
- Treat with oral agents.

Table 8.4 Drug therapy for severe hypertension

Drug	Dose	Route	Comments
Nifedipine (calcium channel blocker)	0.1–0.25 mg/kg 6 hourly	Sublingual/oral	Puncture capsule and instil contents under the tongue. Safe in acute onset hypertension. (May no longer be readily available)
Amlodipine (longer acting calcium channel blocker)	0.1 mg/kg 4–6 hourly/prn Maintenance of 0.1–0.2 mg/kg 12–24 hourly Max of 10 mg per dose	Oral	New recommendation for acute hypertension; can be dissolved in solution. Safer than nifedipine because amlodipine does not show negative inotropy

Drug	Dose	Route	Comments
Hydralazine (direct vasodilator)	0.1–0.2 mg/kg 0.4–1.5 mg/kg 6–8 hourly Max dose 50 mg	IVI, IMI oral	May be repeated in 10–30 minutes. Vomiting common with IV dose; BP may drop precipitously and tachycardia common; only use in fluid-overloaded patients
Labetalol	Load 0.25 mg/kg then 0.25–3 mg/kg/hour	Continuous IVI infusion	Titrate to lowest dosage. Requires dose monitoring; caution in heart failure and asthma
Sodium Nitroprusside	0.5–8.0 µg/kg/min	Continuous IVI infusion	Use in intensive care only. Effective in minutes. Short action. Check for thiocyanate and cyanide toxicity after 2–3 days. Protect from light
Furosemide	1–5 mg/kg 6–12 hourly	IVI or oral	Use if fluid overloaded. Infuse slowly to avoid ototoxicity

NB: When using IV antihypertensives, have a bag of normal saline connected to the infusion line via a 3-way tap. Give normal saline 5 ml/kg IV immediately if BP drops more than 10 mmHg below the desired level.

Chronic hypertension

- Monitor the BP over several weeks or months before starting drug therapy.
- Therapeutic lifestyle changes indicated for those with essential hypertension, including weight reduction, exercise and reduced salt intake.
- In choosing an antihypertensive agent consider:
  - Is the child hyper-, hypo- or normovolaemic?
  - Is the child in heart failure?
  - Is there a possibility of compromised cerebrovascular blood flow?
- *Aim for monotherapy.* Ideally once-a-day dosage promotes better compliance, although small children may need twice daily dosing due to increased metabolism of drugs. If control is not established gradually increase dosage over a few weeks to maximum before adding a second agent. Aim to achieve a normal blood pressure with the simplest regime and fewest side effects.

The ABC of anti-hypertensive drugs

Table 8.5 Anti-hypertensive drugs

ACEI: angiotensin-converting enzyme inhibitor (e.g. Captopril®, Enalapril®)	ACE inhibitors are indicated as first-line agents in glomerular disease associated with heavy proteinuria. They are *contraindicated* in renal artery stenosis. Work less well if patient fluid overloaded
β blocker: propanolol (short acting), atenolol, metoprolol (long acting)	β blockers can cause nightmares in children and interfere with school performance
Ca Channel blocker: nifedipine (short acting), amlodipine (long acting)	Amlodipine, which is dissolvable and thus titratable, is very useful even in young infants at 0.05–0.2 mg/kg/dose once daily (adult: 5–10 mg/day)
Diuretic: furosemide (loop), spironolactone (K^+ sparing), hydrochlorothiazide	Diuretics should be used in fluid overload states
Everything else: direct vasodilator (e.g. hydralazine) α blocker (e.g. prazosin, clonidine, minoxidil)	α blockers are better tolerated than hydralazine with less tachycardia; beware of dysrhythmias with clonidine; minoxidil causes salt and water retention and hypertrichosis

Recommended reading

1 Wright, A. Evidence-based assessment and management of childhood enuresis. *Paediatr Child Health*. 2008;18: 561-567.
2 Neveus T, von Gontard A, Hoebeke P, et al. The standardization of terminology of lower urinary tract function in children and adolescents: report from the Standardisation Committee of the International Children's Continence Society. *J Urol*. 2006;76:314-324.
3 NHS: National Institute for Health and Clinical Excellence. *Guideline for Diagnosis, treatment and long-term management of urinary tract infection in children.* http://www.nice.org.uk/cg54.
4 Thomson PD. *Approach to Haematuria*. Paediatric Refresher Course, UCT 2008.
5 Gulati S, Pena D. *Haematuria*. www.emedicine.com/ped/topics951.htm
6 Avner ED, Harmon W, Niaudet P. *Pediatric nephrology*. 5th ed. Philadelphia: Lippincott Williams & Wilkins. 2004.
7 Rees L, Webb N, Brogan P. *Paediatric nephrology*. Oxford. New York. Oxford University Press. 2007.
8 Webb NJA, Postlethwaite RJ. *Clinical paediatric nephrology*. 3rd ed. Oxford. New York. Oxford University Press. 2003.

9 Immunization and infections

K.I. Barnes, B. Eley, G. Hussey, J. Nuttall

Immunization

In South Africa the following vaccines are freely available at all public health clinics and are administered according to the following schedule:

Age of child	Vaccine	How and where given
At birth	BCG	Intradermal right deltoid region
	OPV (0)	Drops by mouth
6 weeks	OPV (1)	Drops by mouth
	RV (1)	Liquid by mouth
	Hep B (1)	Intramuscular, right thigh
	DTaP-IPV/Hib (1)	Intramuscular, left thigh
	PCV$_7$ (1)	Intramuscular, right thigh
10 weeks	Hep B (2)	Intramuscular, right thigh
	DTaP-IPV/Hib (2)	Intramuscular, left thigh
14 weeks	RV (2) *	Liquid by mouth
	Hep B (3)	Intramuscular, right thigh
	DTaP-IPV/Hib (3)	Intramuscular, left thigh
	PCV$_7$ (2)	Intramuscular, right thigh
9 months	PCV$_7$ (3)	Intramuscular, right thigh
	Measles (1)	Intramuscular, left thigh
18 months	Measles (2)	Intramuscular, right arm
	DTaP-IPV/Hib (4)	Intramuscular, left arm
6 years	Td	Intramuscular, left arm
12 years	Td	Intramuscular, left arm

* The first dose of the rotavirus vaccine should be given before 14 weeks of age. Rotavirus vaccine must *not* be administered after 24 weeks of age.

Key:
- BCG – bacille Calmette-Guérin
- OPV – oral polio vaccine
- RV – rotavirus
- Hep B – hepatitis B vaccine
- DTaP-IPV/Hib – diphtheria, tetanus, acellular pertussis, inactivated polio combined with *Haemophilus influenzae* type b
- PCV$_7$ – pneumococcal conjugate vaccine
- Td – Tetanus and reduced strength diphtheria

Additional vaccines

Additional vaccines are available but are not part of the national immunization programme.

Varicella vaccine

This live-attenuated vaccine is recommended after 12 months of age, with a repeat dose at 4–6 years of age. When given to leukaemic children in remission, sero-conversion and protection are slightly reduced and adverse reactions are more frequent. The safety and immunogenicity of varicella vaccine has been established in HIV-infected children with a CD4% > 15% and adolescents with CD4 ≥ 200 cells/mm^3. However, there are no efficacy studies. It may be effective post-exposure in susceptible children provided that it is given within 72 hours of exposure.

Measles, mumps and rubella

This can be used instead of the monovalent measles vaccine after the age of 1 year. A preschool booster is advisable.

Hepatitis A

Two doses of this inactivated vaccine are recommended after the age of 1 year. The second dose should be given at least 6 months after the first. Because of the high incidence of natural infection in early childhood and thus natural immunity, it is not recommended for routine use in developing countries. It is advised for travellers and may be of use in outbreak situations.

Influenza

This annually-updated trivalent inactivated vaccine is recommended for children with chronic lung, heart, or renal disease, diabetes, HIV infection, and for those on long-term salicylate (aspirin soluble) therapy. Ideally the vaccine should be given during March to provide adequate protection before the influenza season. The manufacturer's dosing instructions should be observed.

Meningococcal vaccine

Capsular polysaccharide vaccines are available against groups A, C, Y and W135. Although group A antigen can produce a weak immune response from the age of 3 months, the effectiveness of the vaccine under the age of 2 years is limited. The other serogroup capsular polysaccharides are poor immunogens under 2 years of age. In older children, protective antibody titres to capsular polysaccharides develop within a week and last for 1 to 3 years. Polysaccharide vaccines are used to control outbreaks of meningococcal disease and to protect travellers who are entering epidemic areas. Improved protein-conjugate monovalent (against group C) and tetravalent (against A, C, Y & W135) vaccines have been introduced in several countries and a search for effective B group vaccines is ongoing.

Typhoid

Two licensed vaccines are recommended for high-risk groups only. The Ty21a live-attenuated *Salmonella typhi* oral vaccine in an enteric-coated formulation is administered on alternate days for 3 doses. Alternatively a single parenteral dose of the Vi capsular polysaccharide vaccine results in 65–75% protection for 2 years. Information on the efficacy of both vaccines in infants is not available. Recently, a Vi conjugate vaccine (Vi-rEPA) was shown to be safe, immunogenic and conferred more than 90% efficacy in children aged 2–5 years.

Yellow fever

Children over the age of 6 months travelling to or from areas where yellow fever exists (outside South Africa) should be immunized with a single dose. Revaccination is required every 10 years for international travel.

Rabies

This human diploid cell vaccine is given to at-risk individuals. The *preexposure* schedule is 1 ml IM on days 0, 7, and 28 with boosters every 1 to 3 years depending on the level of exposure. The vaccine is also effective following a bite by a rabid animal (p. 265).

Adverse events

Vaccines are not entirely risk-free. Most side effects are minor and self-limited, including mild febrile reactions, irritability and pain or erythema at the injection site. Some vaccines have been associated with more serious side effects, e.g. paralytic polio following OPV and encephalopathy following whole cell pertussis vaccine. However these are extremely rare and do not preclude their use since their benefits outweigh risks. Effects that have incorrectly been ascribed to vaccines by the anti-vaccination lobby include autism (MMR), multiple sclerosis (HBV), diabetes (Hib) and sudden infant death syndrome (DPT). These allegations have been disproved.

HIV-infected children

The WHO recommends that children with HIV infection be immunized according to the normal schedule. WHO advised that BCG should not be administered to children with confirmed HIV infection. This recommendation has been difficult to implement in poor countries because of low HIV testing rates in young children and sub-optimal follow-up rates. For these reasons South Africa continues to administer neonatal BCG irrespective of HIV status.

BCG vaccination

The normal local reaction to BCG is a red indurated area 5–15 mm in diameter that appears 3 to 4 weeks after vaccination. A central crust may develop. This falls off leaving an ulcer that ultimately heals with a flat 3–7 mm scar.

Table 9.1 The spectrum of adverse BCG reactions

Local	Pain, ulceration, abscess, keloid formation
Regional	Lymphadenitis, suppurative lymphadenitis, fistulation
Disseminated	BCGosis, osteitis
Other	Erythema nodosum, lupus vulgaris, iritis

Disseminated BCG disease (BCGosis) is associated with HIV infection, and primary immunodeficiency diseases including severe combined immunodeficiency and genetic defects in the interferon-gamma pathway. HIV infection is also more frequently associated with local and regional complications. BCG adverse events develop in 6% of children after starting antiretroviral therapy, during immune recovery.

BCG lymphadenitis in immunocompetent children usually resolves spontaneously and requires no therapy. In the setting of HIV infection it is more likely to suppurate and/or fistulate. Rapidly enlarging or fluctuant glands should be managed with aspiration, or surgical incision and drainage. Pus should be sent for culture and speciation, to confirm that *Mycobacterium bovis* BCG is the causative organism. Local or regional disease in a thriving child does not require anti-mycobacterial therapy. Consider anti-mycobacterial therapy in patients with disseminated BCG disease, including children with systemic features suggesting dissemination, involvement of groups of nodes other than the right axillary nodes, and positive gastric washings or distant site cultures.

Initial anti-mycobacterial therapy may include both *M. tuberculosis* and *M. bovis* BCG cover (rifampicin 20 mg/kg/day, isoniazid 15–20 mg/kg/day, pyrazinamide 25–35 mg/kg/day, ethambutol 15–20 mg/kg/day or ethionamide 15–20 mg/kg/day plus ofloxacin 15–20 mg/kg/day). *M. bovis* BCG is naturally resistant to pyrazinamide. Once the BCG infection has been confirmed, therapy may be rationalized to 4 drugs. The duration of therapy is usually 6–9 months, but longer if severe immunodeficiency is present

Missed opportunities

These are likely to occur when immunizations are not offered at every contact or are denied because of inappropriate contra-indications or when one vaccine is given when more are indicated. Use every opportunity to immunize children, even those attending health facilities not designated as immunization centres. A lapse in the immunization schedule does not necessitate restarting the whole schedule. Give the remaining dose or doses irrespective of the intervening delay.

> *Practice point*
>
> If the child is well enough to be taken to a clinic, he/she is well enough to be immunized. Do not delay immunizations because of coughs or colds.

Precautions and contraindications

Egg allergy

Current measles and mumps vaccines (derived from chick embryo blast tissue culture) do not contain significant amounts of egg cross-reacting proteins. Children with egg allergy, even those with severe hypersensitivity, are at low risk for anaphylactic reactions. In addition, most allergic reactions to measles or MMR vaccine are due to other vaccine components, such as gelatin or neomycin. Therefore, children with egg allergy may be given MMR, mumps or measles vaccine routinely without prior skin testing.

As a precautionary measure, some experts recommend that those with a history of anaphylaxis should be observed for at least 90 minutes after administration of MMR, measles or rubella vaccine (in a setting where equipment for emergency treatment of anaphylaxis is immediately available).

Current influenza and yellow fever vaccine contain egg cross-reacting proteins and on rare occasions may induce allergic reactions. Those with a history of systemic anaphylactic symptoms should not receive influenza or yellow-fever vaccine in view of the risk of reaction and the likely need for repeated vaccination.

Immunosuppression

Children with malignant disease and those on cytotoxic drugs, prolonged high dose steroids or irradiation therapy should not be given live vaccines, i.e. BCG, measles, MMR, OPV. Defer vaccination for at least 3 months following cessation of therapy.

Pertussis vaccine

Anaphylaxis after DTP or DTaP, and encephalopathy within 7 days of DTP are absolute contraindications to further DTP or DTaP vaccination. The following adverse events are considered precautions because they have not been proven to cause permanent sequelae:
- Convulsions within 3 days of vaccination
- Persistent screaming for more than 3 hours
- Collapse or shock-like state (hypotonic-hyporesponsive episode) within 48 hours, or
- Fever above 40.5 °C within 48 hours.

A decision to withhold further doses of DTaP following these events should consider the pertussis exposure risk, and potential benefits and risks of pertussis vaccine. Further doses should be administered with adequate monitoring.

Previous plasma or immunoglobulin

Measles, mumps, and rubella vaccines should be deferred for 3 months following such administration. Other vaccines need not be withheld.

Conditions that do not contra-indicate immunization

These include:
- Minor illness with low grade fever (less than 38.5 °C)
- Diarrhoea
- Respiratory infections
- Malnutrition
- Breastfeeding
- Prematurity
- Family history of convulsions
- History of non-specific allergies, asthma, hay fever, rhinitis, eczema, or localized skin infections
- Allergy to antibiotics except anaphylactic reactions to neomycin or streptomycin (they are contained in some vaccines)
- Chronic diseases of the heart, lung, kidney or liver
- Static neurological disorders, such as cerebral palsy and Down's syndrome.

Children on topical, inhaled, short-term (less than 2 weeks) or low-dose maintenance steroid therapy for a non-immuno-suppressive condition can also be vaccinated.

Practical points

Intramuscular injections:
- Infants (<12 months): inject into mid antero-lateral aspect of the thigh (p. 531) using a 22–25-gauge needle with a minimum length of 25 mm.
- Older children: inject into deltoid (if muscle bulk adequate), or mid-antero-lateral aspect of thigh using a 22–25-gauge needle with a minimum length of 32 mm.

Subcutaneous injections:
- Give these into the thigh in infants and the deltoid in older children.

Simultaneous administration:
- Most vaccines can be given simultaneously. The exception is (but not absolute) yellow fever and cholera – give them 3 weeks apart. Preferably space vaccines that may cross-react, e.g. cholera and typhoid. Do not mix vaccines in same syringe unless so licensed.

Interchangeability of vaccines from different manufacturers:
- This is not a problem.

Storage and handling of vaccines (cold chain):
- Failure to adhere to recommended specifications renders vaccines impotent. Heat-sensitive products include OPV, yellow fever, measles. Vaccines that are sensitive to freezing include DPT, HBV, Hib, pneumococcal (PCV_7), and influenza. Keep them in a fridge at 2–8 °C. *Do not* place vaccines in a refrigerator door or freezer.

Passive immunisation:
- Measles (p. 259), rabies (p. 264), tetanus (p. 265), varicella zoster (p. 257)
- Hepatitis A: give household or day-care centre contacts immuno-globulin 0.02 ml/kg within 2 weeks of exposure. Although its efficacy has not been established, immunoglobulin may be given to infants of mothers who are jaundiced.
- Hepatitis B immunoglobulin (HBIG): newborns of mothers with acute or chronic hepatitis should be given HBIG within 12 hours of delivery; post-exposure prophylaxis should be administered to

household contacts of persons with acute hepatitis B infection if not fully immunized.

Bacterial and viral infections

Table 9.2 Incubation periods

Incubation period	Disease	Prodromal period	Isolation period
Short (1–7 days)	Cholera	Nil	Contact precautions for duration of illness
	Diphtheria	Nil	Until 3 throat swabs are negative (MC)
	Influenza	Nil	Until apyrexial and feeling better
	Meningococcal disease	Nil	2 days after start of treatment (MC)
	Scarlet fever	Nil	Until rash fades and desquamation starts
Intermediate (7–14 days)	Measles	3–7 days	5 days from start of rash
	Pertussis	Up to 21 days; usually 5–7 days	5 days after starting effective therapy or until 3 weeks after onset of paroxysms
	Polio	3–36 days	10 days (MC)
	Tetanus	Nil	Not required
	Typhoid	Nil	Until 3 consecutive stools are negative (MC)
Long (14–21 days)	Chickenpox	Nil to 2 days	Until lesions crusted, usually 5–7 days after the appearance of the rash
	Mumps	Nil to 1 day	Until swelling subsides (9 days)
	Rubella	Nil to 2 days	
15–40 days	Hepatitis A	2–5 days	7 days from onset of jaundice
60–180 days	Hepatitis B	2–5 days	Until no longer jaundiced

Note: Information in parentheses refers to when the patient may return to a teaching institution in terms of regulation R2438 (30 October 1987) of the 1977 Health Act. MC refers to submission of a medical certificate and figures refer to the number of days after which a patient may return to a teaching institution.

Table 9.3 Vesicular rashes during childhood

Disease	Organism	Distribution of rash	Complications
Chickenpox	Varicella-zoster virus	Trunk then periphery	Secondary infection, encephalitis, pneumonia
Eczema herpeticum	Herpes-simplex virus	Localized to areas of eczematous skin	Secondary infection
Hand, foot and mouth disease	Coxsackie A16 and enterovirus 71	Palms, soles, and mouth	Aseptic meningitis, encephalitis, paralysis
Herpes-simplex gingivostomatitis		Mouth and lips	Secondary infection, disseminated infection
Impetigo	*Streptococcus* and *Staphylococcus*	Periphery and face	Cellulitis, invasive infection, acute nephritis
Herpes zoster (shingles)	Varicella-zoster virus	Sensory nerve distribution — dermatomes	Recurrent episodes, disseminated disease
Monkeypox infection	Monkeypox virus	Trunk then periphery	Dissemination, encephalitis

Table 9.4 Erythematous infectious diseases

Disease	Cause	Prodome	Distribution of rash	Other features	Acute complications
Erythema infectiosum	Parvovirus B19	Unusual	Face (slapped cheeks), trunk, and limbs	Lace-like rash	Rarely polyarthritis, encephalitis Aplastic crisis in haemolytic/haemoglobinopathies and immunocompromise
Infectious mononucleaosis	Epstein-Barr virus	Fever and sore throat	Generalized	Accentuated with ampicillin & amoxicillin, adenopathy & splenomegaly	Haemolytic anaemia, thrombocytopaenia, hepatitis
Kawasaki syndrome	Unknown	Fever, sore throat, preceding respiratory illness	Generalized	Adenopathy, conjunctivitis, Changes of mucosae & peripheral extremities	Myopericarditis, urethritis, meningitis, diarrhoea, hepatitis, hydrops of gallbladder

Disease	Cause	Prodome	Distribution of rash	Other features	Acute complications
Measles	Rubeola virus	Fever, cough, conjunctivitis, Koplik spots	Face, trunk, limbs – confluent	Rash pigments and desquamates	Pneumonia, croup, eye complications, diarrhoea
Meningococcal disease	*Neisseria meningitidis*	Unusual	Variable	Classically petechiae or purpura, maculopapular rash may precede purpura	Shock, meningitis
Roseola infantum	Herpes 6 virus	High fever, irritability	Trunk, face	As the rash appears the fever subsides	Febrile convulsions
Rubella	Rubella virus	Mild fever	Face, trunk, limbs – discrete	Adenopathy, arthralgia/arthritis	Rare – encephalitis, thrombocytopaenia
Scarlet fever	Group A β-haemolytic Streptococcus	Fever and sore throat	Face then generalized – punctate erythema	Circumoral pallor, strawberry tongue	Myocarditis, nephritis, rheumatic fever, reactive arthritis
Toxic shock syndrome	*Staphylococcus aureus* (TSST–1)	Unusual	Diffuse macular erythoderma	Hypotension, chills, headache, myalgia, conjunctival hyperaemia, strawberry tongue	Renal failure, coma, diarrhoea, hepatitis
Viral exanthema	Coxsackie and echoviruses	Variable	Variable	Headache, myalgia	Meningitis, encephalitis, pneumonia, diarrhoea

Chickenpox

This is usually a mild disease (vesicular rash) but may cause life-threatening dissemination, particularly in immunocompromised children (Tables 9.2 and 9.3).

Treatment

- Acyclovir for immunocompromised patients, 20 mg/kg 4 times day for 5 days orally; or 500 mg/m^2 every 8 hours for 7 days intravenously for severely immunocompromised patients or those with disseminated disease
- Topical therapy: calamine lotion
- Post-exposure prophylaxis: varicella-zoster immune globulin (VZIG) should be administered within 96 hours of exposure, particularly in immunocompromised contacts (use manufacturer's dose), or varicella vaccine within 72 hours of exposure. VZIG is recommended for newborns whose mothers develop varicella from 5 days before to 2 days after birth.

Cholera

This acute, usually water-borne, infection is caused by V*ibrio cholerae*. It is characterized by profuse watery diarrhoea (rice-water stools) that lead to dehydration and hypovolaemic shock. Without treatment the case-fatality rate of severe cholera is 50%. The diagnosis can be confirmed by stool culture.

Treatment

- Vigorous fluid replacement and correction of electrolyte and acid-base imbalance (see Chapter 20, Fluids, electrolytes and acid-base).
- WHO does not advocate routine antibiotic treatment nor post-exposure prophylaxis.
- Basic sanitation and hygiene when properly applied should control cholera. Mass oral vaccination is a promising strategy for controlling infection in refugee settings.

Diphtheria

The major virulence factor is an exotoxin produced by *Corynebacterium diphtheria*.

Respiratory tract infection results in pseudomembrane formation that may involve the nasal passages, the palate and the larynx, and may be complicated by paralysis of the palate and the oropharynx. Direct skin involvement causes a scaly rash or ulceration.

Complications include progression to respiratory failure, myocardiopathy (beginning after 10 days with arrhythmias, shock, or heart failure) or motor neuropathy (beginning from the third week with palatal, ocular, pharyngeal, respiratory muscles or limb involvement).

The diagnosis is made on clinical features and bacterial culture of pseudomembrane or lesions.

Treatment

- Penicillin G (aqueous crystalline, 100 000 – 150 000 units (U)/kg/day in 4 divided doses intravenously or aqueous procaine, 25 000–50 000 U/kg/day intramuscularly, maximum 1.2 million U) or erythromycin (40 mg/kg/day, maximum 2 g/day) for 14 days.
- Give antitoxin 40 000–120 000 U (depending on severity) intravenously as soon as possible. Antitoxin, an equine-derived product, is in short supply, and may be arranged through the National Institute of Communicable Diseases, Johannesburg. Antitoxin can cause severe reactions in those sensitized to horse serum products. Before intravenous administration, sensitivity to horse serum should be performed. Apply 1 drop of 1:1000 dilution of antitoxin in saline to the volar aspect of the forearm and puncture the underlying skin with a sterile needle. A positive test is a wheal with surrounding erythema of ≥ 3 mm, read at 15–20 minutes.
- Isolate the child until 2 daily consecutive throat swabs are negative, after completion of antibiotic therapy.
- Prophylaxis: close, especially household, contacts during the previous 7 days: give a single diphtheria booster plus either a single dose of Benzathine penicillin G (600 000 U if < 30 kg or 1.2 million U for larger children) or erythromycin for 7 days.

Kawasaki syndrome

This is an acute, febrile, self-limiting, exanthematous, multi-system disease of unknown aetiology (Table 9.4). 80% of cases occur before the age of 5 years. Approximately 20% of untreated patients develop coronary artery aneurysms.

Diagnosis is based on the presence of specific clinical features:
- Fever persisting for at least 5 days (mandatory) plus 4 of the following 5 features:
  - Changes in peripheral extremities (erythema and/or oedema of palms and soles; during the later stages periungual desquamation) or perineal area
  - Polymorphous exanthema
  - Bilateral conjunctival injection
  - Changes in lips and oral cavity (red fissured lips, strawberry tongue, injection of oral and pharyngeal mucosa)
  - Cervical lymphadenopathy.

In the presence of coronary artery involvement and fever, fewer than 4 of the remaining 5 criteria are sufficient.

Treatment

- IVIG (2 g/kg administered over 10–12 hours) during first 10 days of illness reduces risk of aneurysms to < 5%. ☆☆☆☆◐
- Aspirin (30–50 mg/kg/day in 4 divided doses) for the first 2 weeks, then low-dose aspirin (3–5 mg/kg/day) for a further 6–8 weeks. ☆☆☆☆◐

Follow-up echocardiography at 6–8 weeks and ongoing cardiology review if aneurysms persist.

Measles

Clinical features

The prodrome typically lasts for 3 to 4 days and is characterized by high fever, coryza, conjunctivitis, cough and Koplik spots, i.e. white macular 1-mm lesions on the buccal mucosa. Maculopapular rash (initially discrete and later confluent) begins at the end of the prodrome. It appears behind the ears and then spreads to the rest of the body (Table 9.4). The rash fades after day 5 and the skin then desquamates. The infectious period extends from the prodrome until about 5 days after appearance of the rash.

Complications include:
- Pneumonia, a major cause of death, may be due to measles but is usually due to secondary adenovirus, herpes virus, or bacterial infections. Croup can be life threatening and diarrhoeal disease is frequently debilitating. Other complications include otitis media, corneal ulceration and rarely, acute encephalitis, nephritis, myocarditis, hepatitis and ileocolitis. Recovery may be prolonged (weeks or months) and is characterized by failure to thrive, recurrent infections and persistent pneumonia and diarrhoea.
- Subacute sclerosing panencephalitis (SSPE) is a rare complication, usually occurring 3–12 years after the acute infection, and characterized by progressive behavioural and intellectual deterioration and bizarre neurological symptoms. CSF measles antibody titres are excessively high.

Diagnosis

- This is based on clinical signs: it can be confirmed serologically. All children with suspected measles should have serological screening performed through the national surveillance programme (consult local infection control or diagnostic laboratory personnel for details).

Treatment and prophylaxis

- There is no specific therapy.
- Vitamin A orally (daily dose: 50 000 IU if < 6 months old, 100 000 IU if 6–11 months old, 200 000 IU if > 12 months old) on 2 successive days, significantly reduces morbidity and mortality. ☆☆☆☆☙
- Acyclovir 20 mg/kg 4 times/day for 5 days orally is recommended for herpes stomatitis and for post-measles croup due to herpes virus infection.
- Susceptible children may benefit from human anti-measles immunoglobulin (0.25 ml/kg IM and 0.5 ml/kg for those who are immunocompromised to a maximum of 15 ml) if given within 1 week of exposure.

Meningococcal septicaemia

This is a fulminating infection with high mortality caused by the Gram-negative diplococcus, *Neisseria meningitidis*. Although less common than meningococcal meningitis, meningococcal septicaemia (meningococcaemia) is associated with greater mortality.

Clinical features

Suspect meningococcaemia in a child with fever > 39 °C who has 2 or more of the symptoms in this triad:
- Altered mental state: irritability, confusion, convulsions, stupor, coma, meningism, bulging fontanelle. These features are caused by cerebral oedema (p. 213) from endotoxin.
- Circulatory shock: prolonged capillary filling time, tachycardia, hypotension, gallop rhythm. Hypovolaemia is the main cause of shock and the gallop rhythm signifies impaired myocardial contractility.
- Purpura: skin purpura or conjunctival purpura are classical manifestations of a generalized vasculitis. Conjunctival purpura consists of well-defined bright-red spots 1–2 mm in size. Skin purpura are 3–5 mm in size with margins that are initially ill-defined. The spots do not bleed when punctured (haemorrhagic infarcts). At the start they may be erythematous or maculopapular but soon evolve to purplish-black. In fulminant cases purpura may be sparse or absent.

Circulatory shock and coning from cerebral oedema cause death. Intravascular coagulation with arteriolar thrombosis may result in infarction with extensive skin loss, compartment syndromes, and gangrene of the limbs.

Diagnosis

- Do not do any investigations until you have commenced antibiotics and resuscitated the patient from shock.
- Do not perform a lumbar puncture at any time. It may precipitate coning.
- Diagnosis may be confirmed by blood culture.
- Intracellular Gram-negative diplococci can be observed on microscopy of skin scrapings from purpuric lesions.

Treatment

Treatment takes precedence over all investigations. Start treatment immediately when clinical findings suggest meningococcaemia.

Primary care
- *No shock:* establish IV access if possible. Give IV or IM Penicillin G 100 000 U/kg or ampicillin 50 mg/kg or ceftriaxone 100 mg/kg.
- If clinical features of meningitis are present, dexamethasone 0.4 mg/kg twice daily for 2 days. Administer dexamethasone 5–10 minutes before the first dose of antibiotics.
- *Shocked:* first, obtain either IV or intraosseous vascular access (see p. 526). Give bolus injections of normal saline or Ringer's lactate IV till the pulses are easily felt.
- Do not transport shocked children – resuscitate first.
- Give oxygen by facemask and maintain blood pressure during transfer.

Hospital care
Admit to ICU all children who are clinically shocked or who have serum bicarbonate < 20 mmol/l on arrival.
- Antibiotics: Penicillin G 400 000 U/kg/day in 4 divided doses (max 12 million U/day) or ceftriaxone 100 mg/kg/day (max: 4 g/day) for 5–7 days.
- *Shock*: monitor BP every 15 minutes until it remains stable. Maintain systolic BP above 100 mmHg to preserve cerebral perfusion. Do not use peripheral vasodilators.
- *Cerebral oedema*: this is invariably present. To maintain cerebral perfusion pressure maintain BP > 100 mmHg and do not use agents which may drop the BP.
- *Gangrene*: in the presence of generalized vasculitis, hypotension predisposes to arterial thrombosis. Give heparin 200 U/kg IV followed by 20 U/kg/hour until BP is stable. Limb compartment

syndromes require urgent surgery. Use morphine analgesia (p. 512) if gangrene is present.

- *Renal function*: catheterize the bladder if shock is present. Urine output should be 1–2 ml/kg/hour. Initially use 0.45% sodium chloride in 5% dextrose 80 ml/kg/day. Adjust the volume, electrolyte and glucose content as necessary. The syndrome of inappropriate antidiuretic hormone secretion sometimes occurs on day 3 or 4. Suspect it if fluid balance is positive and urine SG exceeds 1012. Restrict IV fluid but continue oral feeds (liquid diet).
- *Acid-base status*: give bicarbonate only if metabolic acidosis is due to renal failure.
- *Electrolytes*: hyponatraemia must be corrected (p. 476) otherwise it will aggravate cerebral oedema. Avoid hypokalaemia (p. 477) and correct hypocalcaemia (p. 477) if necessary.
- *Gut*: paralytic ileus is common. Empty the stomach by suction and leave an adequately sized (minimum 10F) naso-gastric tube in place to drain gastric secretions. Feeding tubes are inadequate for drainage.
- *Lungs*: assisted ventilation is indicated if oxygen saturation cannot be maintained above 90%.
- *Skin and eyes*: monitor skin lesions and treat disrupted areas as for burns. Apply methylcellulose drops to eyes and keep them closed if the child is in a coma.

Post-exposure prophylaxis

Any of 3 possible chemoprophylactic treatments may be given.

Table 9.5 Post-exposure prophylaxis for meningococcal disease

Drug	Paediatric dose (< 12 years)	Adult dose	Route	Duration
Ceftriaxone	125 mg	250 mg	IM	Single dose
Ciprofloxacin	10 mg/kg	500 mg	PO	Single dose
Rifampicin	10 mg/kg twice daily	600 mg twice daily	PO	2 days

- Prophylaxis is recommended for household contacts and close contacts in day-care centres and hostels. Hospital contacts need treatment only if contact has been close and intense, e.g. mouth-to-mouth resuscitation or intubation.
- School and work contacts generally do not need prophylaxis.
- Close pregnant contacts should receive a single dose of ceftriaxone.

Pertussis

This is caused by *Bordetella pertussis*. *B. parapertussis* may cause a similar clinical infection.

Clinical features

A catarrhal stage is followed by paroxysmal cough, which is characterized by whooping, cyanosis and apnoea. Infants and older children may present with non-classical symptoms. Complications include: persistent cough (100-day cough), convulsions due to hypoxaemia or encephalopathy, pneumonia and atelectasis.

Diagnosis

Absolute lymphocytosis is characteristic during late catarrhal and paroxysmal stages.

Organism identification is constrained by the low sensitivity of available tests, i.e. culture of deep nasopharyngeal aspirate (NPA) by immediate inoculation on special media or direct fluorescent antibody testing of NPA.

Differential diagnosis includes paroxysmal cough due to *Chlamydia trachomatis*, tuberculous lymphadenopathy and viral infections.

Treatment

- Hospitalize infants and those with severe disease. If given during the catarrhal stage, erythromycin 50 mg/kg/day in 4 divided doses for 14 days may eradicate the infection and prevent relapse. It has no ameliorating effect later.
- There is no evidence that glucocorticosteroids, salbutamol or sedation are beneficial. ☆☆☆☆☞
- Severe paroxysms have been managed with chlorpromazine 2 mg/kg/dose every 4 hours (starting dose) in hospitalized children. The dose may be increase progressively by 1 mg/kg/day until the cough is controlled, then continue at that level every 8 hours. Maximum single dose 100 mg. Reduce dose slowly over 3 to 4 weeks to avoid a relapse. ☆
- Children with severe paroxysms associated with frequent and prolonged de-saturation should be considered for controlled mechanical ventilation until paroxysmal spells resolve, to prevent the development of hypoxic brain damage.
- Patients are non-infectious after 5 days of erythromycin. Although the usefulness of chemoprophylaxis has not been well demonstrated, a 14-day course of erythromycin for all household and other close contacts may be beneficial.

Poliomyelitis

About 1% of individuals infected with polio virus develop clinical disease.

Clinical features
- Abortive poliomyelitis: this presents with fever, pharyngitis, and headache.
- Non-paralytic poliomyelitis: this presents as a viral meningitis and resolves within a week.
- Paralytic poliomyelitis: the hallmark is an asymmetrical lower motor neurone flaccid paralysis. Respiratory failure, mild hypertension, gastric dilatation or melaena are important complications.

Diagnosis
- This is clinical, and confirmation is by culture of the polio virus from the faeces, throat, and rarely CSF. Obtain 2 stool specimens, at least 24 hours apart, for polio virus culture from all suspected cases.

Treatment
- Strict bed-rest is necessary in the week following paralysis. Intensive physiotherapy after 7 to 10 days. Frequent assessment for paralysis of the muscles of respiration and the need for ventilatory support.
- Notify all suspect cases of poliomyelitis. The current WHO definition of a suspect case is *'any child under 5 years of age with acute flaccid paralysis (including Guillain-Barré syndrome) for which no other cause can be identified or a paralytic illness at any age when poliomyelitis is suspected.'*

Rabies

The rabies virus is transmitted by a bite from a rabid domestic or wild animal.

Clinical features
- Incubation period: generally 10–90 days but ranges from 4 days to 7 years.
- Prodromal period: 2–10 days, characterized by non-specific febrile illness.
- Neurological stage: characterized by intense anxiety, agitation, confusion, hydrophobia, progressing to high fever, confusion, disorientation, paralysis and generalized convulsions.
- Coma stage: during this phase autonomic instability, hypotension arrhythmias and hypoventilation develop, progressing rapidly to death.

Post-exposure prophylaxis

This is indicated following an unprovoked attack by an animal in an endemic area. It may be stopped if the animal remains healthy after 10 days, or if an immunofluorescent test for the virus in the animal's brain is negative.

Wash the bite wound thoroughly with soap and water.

Human rabies immunoglobulin (HRIG) 20 IU/kg body weight – inject as much as possible around the wound; the remainder should be given intramuscularly away from the lesion. Any excess immunoglobulin from the open vial may be run into the wound after cleansing.

Human diploid cell vaccine, intramuscularly in the deltoid region on days: 0, 3, 7, 14, and 28.

Treatment

The infection is invariably fatal. Treatment is supportive. Control or elimination of dog rabies will prevent > 95% of human infections

Tetanus

This is caused by tetanospasmin, a neurotoxin produced by *Clostridium tetani*.

Clinical features

Tetanus is characterized by muscle rigidity and painful muscle spasms. In newborns, infection arises following umbilical stump contamination, and presents within the first week with inability to suck, trismus, rigidity, spasms and convulsions. Susceptible older children usually acquire infection following contamination of wounds and present with muscle rigidity and spasms or rarely with local or cephalic tetanus.

Treatment

- Admit to an intensive care unit (ICU).
- Neutralize unbound toxin with human anti-tetanus immunoglobulin (HTIG): newborn 500 U IM, children 2 000 U IM.
- Local wound care, including surgical debridement is essential.
- Give penicillin 100 000 U/kg/day in 4 divided doses or metronidazole 30 mg/kg/day in 4 divided doses for 10–14 days.
- Control spasms and rigidity: diazepam (usually) 0.1–0.2 mg/kg intravenously every 4–6 hours. In uncontrolled spasms phenobarbitone and chlorpromazine may be used. However, neuromuscular blocking agents such as pancuromium or vecuronium in an ICU setting are preferable.
- Severe cases will need tracheostomy and ventilatory support.

- Control fluid and electrolyte balance. Provide adequate nutrition and nurse in quiet environment because sensory stimuli aggravate muscle spasms.

Prevention

- In countries where the elimination target (< 1 case per 1 000 live births at district level) has not been achieved, WHO recommends a targeted campaign: all women of child-bearing age should be immunized with 3 doses of dT (with an interval of 4 weeks between dose 1 and 2, and at least 6 months between doses 2 and 3). Two further boosters are needed for long-term protection. Furthermore, clean deliveries should be promoted.
- In developing countries, pregnant women with an inadequate or unknown immunization history should receive 2 doses of the tetanus toxoid vaccine 4 weeks apart. Every effort should be made to complete the recommended series of 5 immunizations in these women.
- Incompletely immunized children with severe wounds, prophylactic HTIG (75 U if under 5 years, 125 U for children aged 5 to 10 years, and 250 U for those over 10 years old) and complete immunization schedule.
- Incompletely immunized children with clean, minor wounds should be given tetanus toxoid.
- After recovery from tetanus complete immunization schedule as the disease does not confer immunity.

Tick bite fever

Definition

Six tick-borne rickettsial spotted fevers are known to occur in sub-Saharan Africa. African tick bite fever (ATBF) caused by *Rickettsia africae*, an aerobic Gram-negative obligate intracellular bacterium, commonly occurs in southern Africa. *Amblyomma hebraeum*, a tick of large ruminants is the principal vector and reservoir of *R. africae* in southern Africa.

Clinical features

At the site of inoculation, an eschar develops, consisting of a central black crust surrounded by a red halo, and associated with regional lymphadenopathy. *Amblyomma hebraeum* readily bites humans, frequently causing multiple eschars. However, the eschar is not always found and may be hidden, for example in the scalp. After an incubation of 5–7 days, a prodrome ensues comprising of malaise, fever, headache, nightmares and myalgia. After 3 days the generalized rash (involving palms and soles) appears, which may be maculopapular or vesicular. ATBF is usually a mild disease with no reported fatalities. Uncommon complications include myocarditis, encephalitis, thrombocytopenia, thrombosis, renal failure and pneumonitis.

Diagnosis

The classical clinical triad of fever, eschar and generalized rash occurs in 50–75% of patients. Laboratory confirmation is usually by serological tests. The Weil-Felix agglutination test, although widely used in South Africa, is obsolete.

Treatment

Doxycycline remains the treatment of choice. For children > 8 years: oral doxycycline 4 mg/kg/day in 2 divided doses on day 1, then 2 mg/kg/day in 2 divided doses for a further 7–10 days. For children < 8 years: oral doxycycline 4 mg/kg/day in 2 divided doses for 2 days, then erythromycin 40 mg/kg/day in 4 divided doses for a further 7 days. In children with encephalitis administer intravenous chloramphenicol 50 mg/kg/day in 4 divided doses for 7–10 days

Sexually transmitted infections

The causes of vaginal discharge in children include poor hygiene, foreign bodies, pinworms, irritants such as bubble bath, deodorants and detergents used to wash under garments, indigenous bacterial vaginosis, *Candida* species, and sexually transmitted infections including *Neisseria gonorrhoeae*, *Chlamydia trachomatis*, *Trichomonas vaginalis* and *Gardnerella vaginalis*.

Diagnosis

In the presence of a vaginal discharge, an aspirate or pus swab should be sent for microscopy and culture, and serological tests requested for syphilis and HIV.

Treatment

Table 9.6 Treatment of sexually transmitted infections

Indigenous bacterial vaginosis	Metronidazole orally 22.5 mg/kg/day in 3 divided doses for 7 days, plus amoxicillin orally 90 mg/kg/day in 3 divided doses for 7 days
Candidiasis	Nystatin cream apply 8 hourly for 7 days OR 1% clotrimazole cream applied intravaginally for 7 days OR 2% miconazole cream applied intravaginally for 7 days
Gonorrhoea	Ceftriaxone intramuscularly as a single dose < 25 kg: 125 mg > 25 kg: 250 mg
Chlamydia trachomatis	< 8 years: erythromycin orally 50 mg/kg/day in 4 divided doses for 14 days > 8 years: doxycycline orally 100 mg twice daily for 7 days OR Erythromycin for 14 days
Trichomonas vaginalis or *Gardnerella vaginalis*	Young children: metronidazole orally 22.5 mg/kg/day in 3 divided doses for 7 days Adolescents: metronidazole 2 grams as a single dose
Syphilis	Early disease: Benzathine penicillin G 50 000 U/kg IM as a single dose (maximum dose 2.4 million units) Syphilis present for more than 1 year: Benzathine penicillin G intramuscularly 1.2 million units, weekly for 3 doses

Tuberculosis

Definitions

Tuberculosis is caused by *Mycobacterium tuberculosis* complex group of organisms. The clinical disease spectrum is broadly divided into *pulmonary TB* and *extrapulmonary TB*.

Multi-drug resistant (MDR) TB: resistance to at least isoniazid (INH) and rifampicin (RIF).

Extensively drug resistant (XDR) TB: resistance to INH, RIF, any fluoroquinolone and at least one second-line injectable agent (kanamycin, amikacin or capreomycin)

Pre-XDR-TB: resistance to INH and RIF, plus any fluoroquinolone or at least one second-line injectable agent (kanamycin, amikacin or capreomycin).

Clinical features

- The primary infection is silent and is contained in over 85% of cases. It may be diagnosed fortuitously when the child presents with another problem or as a contact of an adult with pulmonary TB.
- Signs of hypersensitivity may be present, such as mild fever and tiredness or, less commonly, erythema nodosum, pleural effusion, phlyctenular conjunctivitis or reactive (Ponçet) arthritis.
- The symptoms of a 'simple' primary complex (cough, wheezing or stridor) are caused by compression of the bronchial tree by large lymph nodes.
- If the disease progresses, symptoms are more severe. Documented weight loss or failure to thrive, longstanding fever, lassitude and persistent unremitting cough are usually present.
- The disease is more likely to progress in children under 2 years of age who experience heavy and repeated exposure and/or in children whose immune responses are depressed by malnutrition or infection (e.g. HIV or measles).
- Infection may spread to any organ in the body along the lymphatics or via the bloodstream. Signs include:

Enlarged neck lymph nodes with/without draining sinus	Signs of pericardial effusion
Enlarged liver and spleen	Arthritis
Enlarged mesenteric nodes and peritonitis	Gibbus/paraparesis due to TB spine
Chronic ear discharge	TB meningitis or convulsions from tuberculoma
Cold abscess formation	Sterile pyuria (TB kidney)

- Large pleural effusions and adult-type, cavitary PTB are more common in older children and adolescents.

> ***Practice point:***
>
> BCG vaccine partly protects against miliary TB and TB meningitis but does not provide much protection against PTB in young children

Diagnosis

The isolation of mycobacteria on culture is far less common in children than in adults because of the difficulty in obtaining suitable specimens (e.g. sputum) and the paucity of TB bacilli. Frequently a presumptive diagnosis has to be made from the history, clinical findings, tuberculin skin tests, chest radiology and special investigations.

History
Being suspicious is halfway to the diagnosis. Always enquire about possible contacts in the home. Think of TB when there is:
- Weight loss or failure to gain weight
- A cough lasting longer than 2 weeks, especially with a wheeze or stridor
- Enlarged (often matted) lymph nodes, liver or spleen.

Tuberculin skin test (TST)
The TST is administered by the Mantoux method, using the volar aspect of the left forearm:
- Use 2 tuberculin units (2 TU) of the RT23 strain.
- Inject 0.1 ml of 2 TU purified protein derivative (PPD) RT23 just beneath the skin with the needle bevel facing upwards. This should produce a skin weal 6–10 mm in diameter.
- Read the test at 48 to 72 hours. Measure the transverse diameter of palpable induration only. Record the result in millimetres of induration, not as reactive/positive.

Interpretation:
- Diameter of induration ≥ 5 mm is positive in HIV-infected children and severely malnourished children (marasmus/kwashiorkor)
- Diameter of induration ≥ 10 mm is considered positive in all other children, irrespective of prior BCG vaccination.

Causes of false-negative TST:
- Incorrect administration
- Incorrect interpretation of test
- Improper storage of tuberculin
- Viral infections, e.g. measles and varicella
- Vaccinated with live viral vaccines (within 6 weeks)
- Malnutrition and low protein states
- Bacterial infection, e.g. typhoid, leprosy, pertussis
- Immunosuppressive therapy, e.g. glucocorticosteroids
- Primary immunodeficiency diseases

- Diseases of lymphoid tissue, e.g. Hodgkin's disease, sarcoidosis, lymphoma, leukaemia
- Severe TB.

Causes of false-positive TST:
- Incorrect interpretation of test
- BCG vaccination
- Infection with non-tuberculous mycobacteria.

Chest radiography
Radiographic changes suggestive of TB include:
- Persistent opacification in the lung together with enlarged hilar or subcarinal lymph nodes
- Compression of the airways due to diseased lymph nodes
- Miliary pattern, particularly in HIV-uninfected children
- Persistent opacification after a course of antibiotics
- Isolated pleural effusion.

Culture diagnosis
Obtain 2 or 3 consecutive early-morning sputum specimens (or gastric washings in infants) for microscopy and culture. Neutralize the acid in gastric washings with bicarbonate before sending the specimen to the laboratory. Where possible, a single sputum sample collected by the induced sputum method following saline nebulization should replace conventional sputum collection for microscopy and culture.

Interferon-gamma release assays
These tests are generally not useful in high TB prevalence settings. The exception is HIV-infected children, where interferon-gamma release assays are more sensitive than TST for diagnosing TB, but a negative interferon-gamma release assay result does not exclude TB.

Table 9.7 Investigation of extrapulmonary TB

Site	Diagnostic approach
Peripheral lymph nodes	Fine needle aspirate or biopsy (p. 541)
TB meningitis (TBM)	Lumbar puncture for opening pressure measurement, biochemical analysis, microscopy and culture, CT scan, air encephalogram to determine whether hydrocephalus is communicating
Miliary TB	Chest radiograph, lumbar puncture (to test for TB meningitis)
Pleural effusion	Chest radiograph, pleural tap for biochemical analysis, microscopy and culture
Abdominal ascites	Abdominal ultrasound, ascitic tap for biochemical analysis, microscopy and culture
Osteoarticular TB	Radiographs, joint tap and or synovial biopsy
Pericardial TB	Cardiac ultrasound, pericardial tap
Chronic ear discharge, especially in HIV-infected children	Pus swab for microscopy and TB culture

Diagnostic certainty

M. tuberculosis frequently causes paucibacillary disease in children; culture confirmed disease is less common than in adult TB cases. Therefore, the strength of TB diagnosis can be classified according to the following criteria:

Definite TB
Isolation of *M. tuberculosis* on culture of sputum, gastric washings, CSF or tissue from a site that is normally sterile, e.g. bone marrow, lymph node or other tissue.

Probable TB
Symptoms or signs consistent with TB plus 2 or more of the following: known TB contact, TST ≥ 10 mm, acid fast bacilli on microscopy, chest radiograph findings consistent with PTB or CSF findings ± CT scan findings consistent with TBM, and a good response to treatment.

Possible TB
Symptoms or signs consistent with TB plus 1 of the following: known TB contact, TST ≥ 10 mm, chest radiograph findings consistent with PTB or CSF findings ± CT scan findings consistent with TBM, and a good response to treatment

Treatment and prophylaxis

Table 9.8 TB drug dosing chart for children < 8 years of age (2010)

Body weight (kg)	Uncomplicated TB disease (Primary TB)		Complicated TB disease (excluding TB meningitis/miliary TB)			TB meningitis or miliary TB			Body weight (kg)
	Intensive phase 2 months	Continuation phase 4 months	Intensive phase 2 months		Continuation phase 4 months	Single phase of treatment 6 months			
	RHZ dissolvable tablets 60/30/150 mg (scored)	RH dissolvable tablets 60/30 mg (scored)	RHZ dissolvable tablets 60/30/150 mg (scored)	E tablets 400 mg (un-scored)	RH dissolvable tablets 60/30 mg (scored)	RH dissolvable tablets 60/60 mg (scored)	Z tablets 500 mg (scored)	Eto tablets 250 mg (scored)	
2–2.9	½	½	½	Use Eto ¼	½	Use RHZ (60/30/150) ½ + H ¼		¼	2–2.9
3–3.9	1	1	1		1	Use RHZ (60/30/150) 1 + H ½)			3–3.9
4–4.9				¼				½	4–4.9
5–5.9									5–5.9
6–6.9	1½	1½	1½		1½	2	½		6–6.9
7–7.9						2½		¾	7–7.9
8–8.9				½					8–8.9
9–9.9	2	2	2		2	3	¾		9–9.9
10–11.9						4			10–11.9

H = Isoniazid, R = Rifampicin, Z = Pyrazinamide, E = Ethambutol, Eto = Ethionamide

Uncomplicated TB disease in children = new smear negative pulmonary TB, or mild forms of extrapulmonary TB e.g. lymphadenitis, pleural effusion

Complicated TB disease in children = new smear positive pulmonary TB, or extensive parenchymal/cavitatory lung disease, or extrapulmonary TB (excl. TB meningitis or miliary TB), or patients with severe immunosuppression from HIV disease.

Body weight (kg)	Uncomplicated TB disease (Primary TB)		Complicated TB disease (excluding TB meningitis/miliary TB)				TB meningitis or miliary TB Single phase of treatment 6 months			Body weight (kg)
	Intensive phase 2 months RHZ dissolvable tablets 60/30/150 mg (scored)	Continuation phase 4 months RH dissolvable tablets 60/30 mg (scored)	Intensive phase 2 months RHZ dissolvable tablets 60/30/150 mg (scored)	E tablets 400 mg (un-scored)	Continuation phase 4 months RH dissolvable tablets 60/30 mg (scored)		RH dissolvable tablets 60/60 mg (scored)	Z tablets 500 mg (scored)	Eto tablets 250 mg (scored)	
12–12.9	2½	2½	2½	½	2½		4	¾		12–12.9
13–13.9										13–13.9
14–14.9	3	3	3	¾	3		5	1	1	14–14.9
15–16.9										15–16.9
17–19.9	4	4	4	1	4		6	1¼	1½	17–19.9
20–24.9								1½		20–24.9
25–29.9	5	5	5	1¼	5				2	25–29.9
30–35.9	6	6	6	1½	6			2	2¼	30–35.9

H = Isoniazid,   R = Rifampicin,   Z = Pyrazinamide,   E = Ethambutol,   Eto = Ethionamide

Uncomplicated TB disease in children = new smear negative pulmonary TB, or mild forms of extrapulmonary TB e.g. lymphadenitis, pleural effusion

Complicated TB disease in children = new smear positive pulmonary TB, or extensive parenchymal/cavitatory lung disease, or extrapulmonary TB (excl. TB meningitis or miliary TB), or patients with severe immunosuppression from HIV disease.

Table 9.9 TB drug dosing chart for children ≥ 8 years of age

Body Weight (kg)	All forms of TB disease (excl. MDR-TB)			Body Weight (kg)
	Intensive phase 2 months	Continuation phase 4 months		
	RHZE tablets 150/75/400/275 mg	RH tablets 150/75 mg	RH tablets 300/150 mg	
30–37	2	2		30–37
38–54	3	3		38–54
55–70	4		2	55–70
≥ 71	5		2	≥ 71
H = Isoniazid, R = Rifampicin, Z = Pyrazinamide, E = Ethambutol				

Drug-susceptible TB

Regimens and drug doses for drug susceptible TB depend on the type of TB, age and HIV status (Tables 9.8 and 9.9).

All TB drugs should be given once daily 7 days per week. The use of appropriate fixed-dose combination drugs is strongly encouraged. For children experiencing persistent vomiting associated with taking the TB medication, consider dividing the dose and administering twice daily, particularly ethionamide. Drug doses should be adjusted on a monthly basis according to the current weight of the patient.

Supplemental pyridoxine (12.5 mg in children and 25 mg in adults, daily) is recommended particularly in malnourished patients and those receiving antiretroviral therapy (p. 307).

Duration of therapy

The duration of therapy for drug-susceptible TB is generally 6 months. In HIV-infected children, some experts extend the duration of treatment to 9 months. Re-evaluation of TB/HIV co-infected children for treatment response is important if a 6-month treatment regimen is used.

Corticosteroids

Prednisone 2 mg/kg/dose increasing to 4 mg/kg/dose in severe TB (maximum dose 60 mg) orally daily for 4 weeks then tapered over 2 weeks is added to the treatment regimen for patients with TBM, pericardial TB, airway obstruction due to mediastinal lymphadenopathy and miliary TB.

Drug-resistant TB

For INH mono-resistant TB, an 8–9-month course of RIF, pyrazinamide and ethambutol is recommended. A flouroquinolone (usually ofloxacin) should be added in the presence of extensive disease. If an INH-resistant patient fails to respond to treatment or if INH mono-resistance is discovered late in the course of drug-susceptible therapy, do not add a single drug to the failing regimen. Instead add 2 or 3 effective drugs to the regimen and continue treatment for 8–9 months after the first negative culture.

MDR-TB, pre-XDR-TB and XDR-TB should be treated under the direction of a TB specialist. The drug regimen for MDR-TB should include 4–7 drugs to which the isolate is susceptible. High-dose INH (15–20 mg/kg) should be added to the treatment regimen. Daily therapy should be administered without interruptions over weekends. After the intensive phase the injectable agent is usually discontinued. The optimal duration of therapy is not known. A long course of therapy is required, extending 12–18 months beyond the time of bacteriological conversion.

Table 9.10 Drug doses for multi-drug resistant TB

Drug	Daily dose (mg/kg)	Maximum daily dose
First line agents		
Isoniazid	15–20	400 mg
Pyrazinamide	25–40	2.0 grams
Ethambutol	20–25	2.5 grams
Injectable anti-TB agents		
Aminoglycosides		
Amikacin	15–30*	1.0 gram
Kanamycin	15–30	1.0 gram
Capreomycin	15–30	1.0 gram
Fluoroquinolones		
Ofloxacin	15–20	800 mg
#Ciprofloxacin	30–40 (2 divided doses)	2.0 grams
Levofloxacin	7.5–10	750 mg
Moxifloxacin	7.5–10	400 mg
Oral bacteriostatic agents		
Ethionamide	15–20	1.0 grams
Terizidone	10–20	750 mg
Para-aminosalicylic acid (PAS)	150 (2–3 divided doses)	8–12 grams
Anti-TB agents not for routine use in MDR-TB		
Linezolid	20 (2 divided doses)	1 200 mg
Amoxycillin/clavulanate	30–45 (3 divided doses)	4 grams
Clarithromycin	30 (2 divided doses)	1 000 mg

* Amikacin administered daily for 1st month, then 3 times weekly, intramuscularly
\# Ciprofloxacin is generally not recommended, but may be useful in young children

Isoniazid preventive therapy

A 6-month course of INH (10 mg/kg/day) is indicated following drug-susceptible TB exposure in all children less than 5 years of age, and all HIV-infected children irrespective of age. It is important to exclude active TB disease before starting preventive therapy. ☆☆☆

Table 9.11 Dosing of isoniazid preventive therapy

Mass (kg)	2–2.4	2.5–4.9	5–7.4	7.5–9.9	10–19.9	20–24.9	≥25
Daily dose (tablets)	¼	½	¾	1	2	2½	3

1 tablet = 100 mg INH

Chemoprophylaxis after drug-resistant exposure (children < 5 years of age or HIV-infected children):
- Exposure to INH mono-resistant TB: rifampicin 15–20 mg/kg/day for 4 months. ☆
- Exposure to MDR-TB: INH (15–20 mg/kg/day) plus ethambutol (20–25 mg/kg/day) or ethionamide (15–20 mg/kg/day), plus ofloxacin (15–20 mg/kg/day) for 6 months. ☆☆
- Exposure to pre-XDR-TB or XDR-TB: INH 15–20 mg/kg/day for 6 months. ☆

> ***Practice point:***
>
> Careful follow-up of all drug-resistant childhood contacts for a minimum of 12 months is essential (WHO recommends 2-year follow-up).

Typhoid fever

This is caused by *Salmonella typhi*. Humans are the only host and natural reservoir. Transmission is via the faecal-oral route.

Clinical features include diarrhoea, pneumonia, unexplained fever, acute abdomen, meningitis, jaundice and splenomegaly. Constipation and rose spots are rare. 10–15% will develop severe disease. Complications include gastrointestinal bleeding, perforation, septic shock and disseminated intravascular coagulopathy.

Diagnosis

While the organism may be cultured from stool, urine and bone marrow, blood culture remains the method of identification. The optimal time for recovering the organism is after 7–10 days of fever. The Widal test may assist diagnosis.

Treatment

Uncomplicated disease: ceftriaxone 50 mg/kg/day or ciprofloxacin 7.5–10 mg/kg/dose 12 hourly for 7–10 days. For severe disease requiring hospitalization the duration of therapy should be extended to 14 days. Chronic carriage may be cured by a prolonged course of ciprofloxacin.

Isolate until 3 consecutive stools are negative for the organism after therapy.

Common parasitic diseases

Clinical parasitology is restricted to those protozoan (single-celled) and metazoan (multi-celled) organisms that use human beings as a host.

Protozoa

Cryptosporidium parvum

Clinical features

Watery diarrhoea, cramps and vomiting, but may be asymptomatic. Self-limiting: duration < 3 weeks in immunocompetent; may cause chronic severe diarrhoea in immunocompromised and rarely causes pulmonary, biliary tract or disseminated infection.

Diagnosis

Oocysts on stool microscopy (make specific request for *C. parvum* on repeated stools).

Treatment

Azithromycin may result in clinical improvement but is not effective in eradicating infection. Nitazoxanide is not routinely available in South Africa. Chronic cryptosporidiosis is an indication for antiretroviral therapy in HIV-infected patients.

Entamoeba histolytica

Clinical features

Asymptomatic (non-invasive intestinal infection), colitis (diarrhoea progressing to bloody dysenteric stools, lower abdominal pain, fever), caecal ameboma, extraintestinal disease (abscess formation in liver, lungs, pericardium, brain, skin, genitourinary tract).

Diagnosis

Trophozoites or cysts in stool or biopsy specimens; serologic tests; imaging (ultrasound and CT scan).

Treatment:

Metronidazole 15 mg/kg/dose 8 hourly PO for 10 days.

Giardia intestinalis

Note: previously *Giardia lamblia*

Clinical features

Asymptomatic, acute watery diarrhoea, chronic diarrhoea with malabsorption, iron-deficiency anaemia.

Diagnosis

Trophozoites or cysts, or immunofluorescent antibody or enzyme immunoassay tests on stool specimens or duodenal aspirates.

Treatment

Metronidazole 5 mg/kg/dose 8 hourly PO for 5 days. Alternatively, according to age as a single dose for 5 days: 1–3 years of age 500 mg, 3–7 years of age 600–800 mg, 7–10 years of age 1 g.

Isospora belli

Clinical features

Prolonged, foul-smelling watery diarrhoea, abdominal pain, anorexia, weight loss, vomiting. Usually self-limiting in immunocompetent patients, may be life-threatening in immunocompromised patients.

Diagnosis

Oocysts on stool microscopy or duodenal aspirates; visualisation of parasite in small intestine biopsy specimens.

Treatment

Trimethoprim (as co-trimoxazole) 5 mg/kg/dose 6 hourly PO for 10 days; prolonged treatment (3 weeks or more) and prophylaxis may be required in immunocompromised patients.

Toxoplasma gondii

Clinical features

Congenital infection is asymptomatic at birth in majority; subsequent development of visual impairment, learning disabilities or mental retardation months to years later is common. Symptomatic congenital infection may present at birth with rash, lymphadenopathy, hepatosplenomegaly, jaundice, hydrocephalus, microcephaly, chorioretinitis and seizures.

Acquired infection is usually asymptomatic; non-specific flu-like symptoms and signs may be present. Ocular disease may follow congenital or acquired infection. Reactivated infection in the immunocompromised patient may present with encephalitis, pneumonitis or systemic disease.

Diagnosis

Serologic tests; *T. gondii* PCR; fundoscopy and brain imaging.

Treatment

Standard treatment is pyrimethamine + sulfadiazine. Alternatives include clindamycin + pyrimethamine, clarithromycin + pyrimethamine, and atovaquone. Co-trimoxazole is the preferred treatment in HIV-infected adults but this has not been studied in children. Expert consultation is recommended.

Trichomonas vaginalis

Clinical features

Asymptomatic, or frothy grey-green vaginal discharge, vulvovaginal pruritis.

Diagnosis

Identification of motile flagellated parasite on microscopy.

Treatment

Metronidazole 1–3 years of age: 50 mg 8 hourly; 3–7 years of age: 100 mg 12 hourly; 7–12 years 100 mg 8 hourly PO for 7 days; > 12 years of age: 2 g as a single dose.

Malaria

Definition
Malaria is a common cause of childhood morbidity, mortality and failure to thrive in the tropics, with sub-Saharan Africa carrying the greatest burden of this disease. There are 5 *Plasmodium* species that cause malaria in humans: *P. falciparum*, *P. vivax*, *P. ovale*, *P. malariae* and very rarely, *P. knowlesi*. Almost all deaths and severe disease are caused by *P. falciparum*, which accounts for over 90% of infections in Africa.

Diagnosis
- Suspect malaria in a child with fever or a history of fever who resides in or has travelled to a malaria endemic area. Children with *P. falciparum* infections may deteriorate rapidly, because of delayed diagnosis or inappropriate treatment. A high index of suspicion is most important for prompt diagnosis.
- Clinical features are non-specific. A definitive diagnosis should be made promptly using a blood smear or a rapid malaria antigen test. An initial negative result does not exclude malaria.

Clinical features
- Symptoms and signs usually present 7–21 days after the bite of an infected mosquito, but may be delayed in those taking malaria prophylaxis or certain antibiotics. Fever is usual, but often intermittent.
- A young child may present with fever, lethargy, poor feeding, vomiting, diarrhoea and cough.
- An older child may have 'flu-like' symptoms – fever, rigors, headache, tiredness and myalgia and, less often, abdominal pain, diarrhoea, loss of appetite nausea, vomiting and cough.

It is important to differentiate between uncomplicated malaria and severe malaria. It is easy to underestimate severity of disease.

A patient with *uncomplicated malaria*:
- Is alert
- Is able to take oral medication
- Is able to sit, stand or walk unaided (appropriate for age)
- Has no evidence of organ dysfunction either clinically or on laboratory tests and has a parasite count of less than 5%.

The most frequent manifestations of *severe malaria* are:
- A depressed level of consciousness ranging from confusion to coma, which may be due to the infection or to hypoglycaemia, acidosis, hyponatraemia or convulsions.
- Prolonged or repeated convulsions.
- Metabolic acidosis and breathing difficulties: tachypnoea may be due to pyrexia, anaemia, cardiac failure, chest infection or brainstem dysfunction (deep breathing suggests acidosis with serum lactate > 5 mmol/l, bicarbonate < 15 mmol/l).
- Severe anaemia (Hb < 5 g/dl): occurs mostly in areas of intense malaria transmission and is due to haemolysis and/or bone marrow dysfunction.
- Hypoglycaemia (blood glucose < 2.2 mmol/l).
- Hyper-parasitaemia: asexual parasite counts exceed 4% (other indications of severe malaria seen on peripheral blood smear are *P. falciparum* schizonts or the presence of malaria pigment in more than 5% of neutrophils).
- Jaundice, bleeding, acute renal failure and acute respiratory distress syndrome (ARDS) are less common in children than adults.

Treatment

Treat malaria cases promptly with the most effective drug regimen available.

Uncomplicated *falciparum* malaria:
- In non-malaria endemic areas, treatment should ideally be initiated in hospital.
- The recommended treatment for uncomplicated *P. falciparum* malaria in children weighing > 5 kg is oral artemether-lumefantrine (Table 9.12). Administer each dose with high fat food or drinks such as milk; a minimum of 1.2 g fat is needed per dose to ensure adequate absorption.
- Artemisinin-based combination therapy (ACT) improves cure rates, clears parasites rapidly, delays resistance and reduces malaria transmission. ☆ ☆☆☆☆
  (WHO 2006, WHO 2009, http://www.doh.gov.za/docs/facts-f.htm)
- If artemether-lumefantrine is not promptly available or for infants weighing < 5 kg, give supervised oral quinine. Add clindamycin or, in children > 8 years, doxycycline, before discharge. (Table 9.12). Clindamycin may be given intravenously for children < 15 kg where accurate oral dosing is impossible (given a dose of 10 mg/kg 12 hourly with a 150 mg capsule).

- Although the principle of treating malaria with a combination of effective antimalarials is sound, 7–10 days of quinine monotherapy can be used in infants for whom an appropriate dose of clindamycin or artemether-lumefantrine is unavailable. Quinine is poorly tolerated and adherence is seldom achieved unless treatment is directly observed.
- If oral intake is unreliable (e.g. repeated vomiting) start treatment with quinine by slow intravenous infusion or intramuscular injection until able to tolerate oral medication (Table 9.12).

Additional measures:
- If a patient vomits within 30 minutes of receiving oral antimalarial medication, give an additional full dose. For vomiting 30–60 minutes after the dose, give an additional half dose. For repeated vomiting, treat with parenteral quinine or artesunate (Table 9.12).
- Paracetamol provides symptomatic relief and reduces vomiting. Avoid aspirin compounds and non-steroidal anti-inflammatory drugs.
- Fluid loss is commonly underestimated in the febrile, vomiting, sweating child. Ensure an adequate intake.
- Monitor for and treat hypoglycaemia. Quinine increases the risk.

Effective treatment of uncomplicated malaria would result in:
- A clinical response within 2 days.
- Fever resolution (and at least a 75% decrease in the initial parasite count) within 3 days.

Consider drug resistance, non-compliance or an additional diagnosis if clinical or parasitological response is poor.

Severe malaria:
- Death from severe malaria may occur within hours of admission, so it is essential that therapeutic concentrations of antimalarial drugs are achieved as soon as possible. Most deaths and cases of severe malaria result from late diagnosis or a delay in effective treatment. If parasitological confirmation of malaria is not readily available, make a blood film and start treatment on the basis of the clinical diagnosis.
- Treat patients with severe malaria in an intensive or high care unit.

Intravenous quinine (Table 9.12):
- Treat children with severe malaria promptly with a quinine *loading dose*. The risks (arrhythmias, hypoglycaemia) associated with a loading dose of quinine are much lower than those of insufficient treatment.

- The loading dose should be reduced only if there is clear evidence of adequate pre-treatment before presentation. Halve the loading dose (and monitor ECG) if the patient has definitely received quinine (more than 40 mg/kg in the previous 2 days), or mefloquine or halofantrine (within 24 hours).
- The loading dose can be omitted in children who have no features of severe malaria but who need parenteral treatment because of repeated vomiting.
- After 8 hours, start the maintenance quinine dose.
- After the second day of parenteral quinine treatment, if there is no clinical improvement or in acute renal failure, reduce the maintenance doses of quinine given by infusion by one-third to avoid accumulation.
- Following initial parenteral treatment, once the patient can tolerate oral therapy, it is essential to continue and complete treatment with an effective oral antimalarial (7 days quinine or 3 days artemether-lumefantrine).
- If intravenous quinine is unavailable, or considered unsafe (as the rate flow cannot be controlled), give intramuscular quinine (a full 6-dose course of artemether-lumefantrine or oral quinine to complete 7 days treatment) divided between anterior thighs, not the buttock to avoid sciatic nerve injury.

Intravenous and rectal artesunate (Table 9.12):
- Parenteral artesunate should be used in preference to parenteral quinine if available, following evidence of a 22.5% reduction in in-hospital mortality among African children treated with IV or IM quinine. Artesunate was well tolerated with less post-treatment hypoglycaemia. ☀☆☆☆☆
- Rectal administration of artesunate as pre-referral treatment has been shown to reduce mortality by 50% in children who take > 6 hours to reach a centre where they can receive parenteral treatment. ☀☆☆☆☆

Monitoring:
- Regularly check core temperature, respiratory rate, blood pressure, level of consciousness and other vital signs.
- Measure parasite density, blood glucose and haemoglobin concentrations, and where possible, blood urea and creatinine, electrolytes and acid-base status.
- Record state of hydration, intake and output accurately.
- Monitor blood glucose 4–6 hourly, especially during quinine therapy.

Management of complications

Hypovolaemia/shock (p. 463):
- Fluid resuscitation (p. 465) may be needed. Hypovolaemia can result in shock, metabolic acidosis and renal failure.
- Avoid fluid overload as it can precipitate fatal pulmonary oedema.

Decreased level of consciousness:
- Identify and treat any correctable cause of altered consciousness: hypoglycaemia, acidosis, shock, seizures, hyperpyrexia.
- Bacterial meningitis is an alternative possible diagnosis, even with parasitaemia. Antibiotic cover should be given for possible meningitis until a lumbar puncture can safely be performed.
- Avoid dexamethasone and mannitol.

Convulsions (p. 192):
- Identify and treat any correctable cause of convulsions: hyperpyrexia, hypoglycaemia, acidosis or another metabolic disturbance.
- Treat convulsions with standard anticonvulsant drugs (p. 192).
- Avoid prophylactic anticonvulsants.

Metabolic acidosis:
- A severe metabolic acidosis (p. 470) is ominous and needs urgent treatment by correcting hypovolaemia (p. 463), dehydration (p. 466), anaemia or hypoglycaemia.
- Avoid routine use of bicarbonate.

Severe anaemia (p. 394):
- Indications for a blood transfusion:
  - Any patient whose Hb is less than 8–10 g/dl (PCV 24–30) should be considered for transfusion in the presence of shock, acidosis, coma, cardiac failure and pneumonia requiring oxygen.
  - The decision to transfuse a stable patient must be made on a case by case basis depending on the patient's age and the presence or absence of co-morbidities
- Give whole blood, ± additional fluid replacement if severe anaemia is associated with shock, acidosis or hypovolaemia.
- In cardiac failure, use packed cells and transfuse slowly.

> ***Practice point:***
>
> Transfusion thresholds may vary from centre to centre according to the safety and availability of blood products. WHO, for example has set the threshold for transfusing stable malaria patients at only 4 g/dl.

Hypoglycaemia (p. 473):
- Measure blood glucose initially in all patients with severe malaria, and monitor regularly in children with any change in neurological function (e.g. convulsion, confusion, coma) to exclude hypoglycaemia as a cause.

Secondary infections:
- Have a low threshold for early administration of broad-spectrum antibiotics for nosocomial infections, aspiration pneumonia or septicaemia (especially non-typhoid *Salmonella*) that may complicate severe malaria.

Plasmodium vivax, Plasmodium ovale, and *Plasmodium malariae* infections:
- In sub-Saharan Africa, these comprise < 10% of infections and are rarely associated with severe disease.
- The majority are sensitive to chloroquine (Table 9.12).
- In mixed infections which include *P. falciparum*, or if there is doubt about the species treat the acute attack as for uncomplicated *P. falciparum* malaria (p. 282).
- In *P. vivax* or *P. ovale* infections, add primaquine phosphate (Table 9.12) after the acute attack, to eradicate the latent liver stage that causes relapses. Primaquine is contraindicated in infants and G6PD deficiency.

Table 9.12 Dosage guidelines for the treatment of malaria

Drug	Dosage		
Artemether - lumefantrine 1 tablet contains artemether 20 mg plus lumefantrine 120 mg. Administer with fat-containing food/milk to ensure adequate absorption	Weight	Give a dose stat, then again after 8 hours and then twice daily for the following 2 days	Total course
	5 – < 15kg	1 tablet	6 tablets
	15 – < 25kg	2 tablets	12 tablets
	25 – < 35kg	3 tablets	18 tablets
	> 35 kg	4 tablets	24 tablets

- Wear long-sleeved, light coloured clothing when outdoors.
- Apply DEET-containing insecticides to exposed skin (not for infants < 3 months old).
- Treat clothes with permethrin.

Use chemoprophylaxis when there is a significant risk of malaria. Children are at particular risk and can progress to severe malaria rapidly. Weigh the risk of adverse drug reactions against the possibility of acquiring malaria.
- The 3 recommended prophylactic options (Table 9.13) are equally effective, although mefloquine resistance is emerging in South East Asia (Thai-Cambodian and Thai-Burmese borders). Resistance to medication is increasing and up-to-date international recommendations can be obtained on www.who.int or www.cdc.org
- Full compliance is essential but no prophylactic regimen is 100% effective. Urge parents to seek immediate medical advice should an exposed child develop fever or a 'flu-like' illness.

Table 9.13 Dosage guidelines for chemoprophylaxis

	Mefloquine 1 tablet = 250 mg	Atovaquone-proguanil 1 paediatric tablet = 62.5 mg atovaquone plus 25 mg proguanil	Doxycycline 1 tablet = 50 or 100 mg
Dosing regimen	Dose *weekly*, starting 1 week before entering the area, once weekly while in the area, and once weekly for *4 weeks* after the last possible exposure to malaria	Dose *daily*, starting 1–2 days before exposure, continued daily during exposure and for *7 days* after the last possible exposure to malaria	Dose *daily*, starting 1–2 days before entering the area, continuing daily while in the area, and daily for *4 weeks* after the last possible exposure to malaria
Weight			
< 5 kg	Contraindicated	Contraindicated	Contraindicated
5–10 kg	62.5 mg (1/4 tablet)	Contraindicated	Contraindicated
11–20 kg	62.5 mg (1/4 tablet)	1 paediatric tablet	Contraindicated
21–30 kg	125 mg (1/2 tablet)	2 paediatric tablets	Contraindicated
31–45 kg	187.5 mg (3/4 tablet)	3 paediatric tablets (31–40 kg body weight)	50 mg (if > 8 years)
> 45 kg	250 mg (1 tablet)	1 adult tablet [250 mg atovoquone + 100 mg proguanil] (> 40 kg body weight)	100 mg

Drug	Dosage
Quinine (parenteral) 1 ampoule (1 ml) usually contains 300 mg quinine dihydrochloride. Quinine doses are usually prescribed as salt (10 mg of salt = 8.3 mg of base)	*Loading dose:* quinine dihydrochloride salt 20 mg/kg, diluted in 5–10 ml/kg body weight of 5% normal saline by IV infusion over 4 hours. *Maintenance dose:* 10 mg/kg quinine dihydrochloride salt (diluted in 5–10 ml/kg body weight of a dextrose-containing solution infused over 4–6 hours) 8 hourly until the patient can take oral quinine (usually by 48 hours).
Quinine (oral) 1 tablet usually contains 300 mg quinine sulphate	10 mg/kg 8 hourly for 7 days. Tablets may be crushed with banana, jam or chocolate syrup
Doxycycline (use with quinine) 1 tablet contains 50 or 100 mg doxycycline	Not for children under 8 years old 4 mg/kg stat, then 2 mg/kg daily for at least 7 days or until negative smears
Clindamycin (use with quinine) 1 tablet usually contains 150 mg clindamycin	10 mg/kg 12 hourly or 5–7 mg/kg 8 hourly for 7 days
Chloroquine (use only to treat *P. vivax*, *P. ovale* or *P. malariae*)	*Daily dose*: 10 mg/kg on day 1, followed by 5 mg/kg 6–8 hours later and 5 mg/kg once daily on days 2 and 3 1 tablet usually contains 150 mg chloroquine base. The concentration of chloroquine per 5 ml varies in different brands of the syrup
Primaquine 1 tablet usually contains 26.3 mg primaquine phosphate = 15 mg primaquine base	0.25–0.3 mg base/kg daily for 14 days following standard treatment Contraindicated in children < 1 year old and in G6PD deficiency

Table adapted with permission from the Malaria Update 4th Edition (2000), edited by Annoesjka Swart of the Medicines Information Centre, University of Cape Town.

Prevention

Use preventive measures, particularly between dusk and dawn, as the mosquito responsible for malaria transmission feeds during this time:
- Stay in dwellings with screened windows and doors.
- Use insecticide coils and sprays.
- Sleep under insecticide (permethrin)-impregnated bed-nets.

Metazoa

Platyhelminths (flatworms)
Cestodes (tapeworms)
Taenia and *Hymenolepis* species

Clinical features

Taeniasis and *Hymenolepiasis* (adult tapeworm infection): mild gastrointestinal symptoms including diarrhoea, nausea and abdominal pain. *Cysticercosis* (larval stage of *Taenia solium*): depends on location and number of pork tapeworm cysts and host response. Most commonly in brain (seizures, behavioural disturbances, hydrocephalus) but also spinal column, eye.

Diagnosis

Adult tapeworms: proglottids or ova in faeces or perianal region, species identification possible. Neurocysticercosis based on imaging studies (CT, MRI); serological tests.

Treatment

Adult tapeworm: albendazole > 2 years of age: 400 mg, < 2 years of age: 200 mg PO as a single dose. Alternative is praziquantel 5–10 mg/kg/dose PO as a single dose, or niclosamide > 6 years of age: 2 g PO as a single dose, 2–6 years: 1 g, < 2 years 500 mg.

Calcified cysticercosis cysts do not respond to cysticercocidal treatment. For patients with imaging evidence of live or inflamed parenchymal cysts, treat with albendazole 15 mg/kg/day (maximum 800 mg) in 2 divided doses for 2 weeks, together with corticosteroids and anticonvulsant medication. There is a risk of developing reactive cerebral oedema and treatment is best undertaken in hospital with expert advice and supervision.

Echinococcus species

Clinical features

Humans only suffer the larval stage which develop into *hydatid cysts* – slow-growing mass lesion(s) in various organs including liver, lungs, kidney or spleen.

Diagnosis

Cystic space-occupying lesions on imaging studies (X-ray, ultrasound, CT); serologic tests, eosinophilia (non-specific).

Treatment

Surgery in combination with albendazole 15 mg/kg/day (maximum 800 mg) in 2 divided doses for 28 days, repeated for 3 cycles with intervals of 14 days.

Trematodes (flukes)
Schistosomiasis

Clinical features

Transient, pruritic papular rash (*cercarial dermatitis/swimmer's itch*); 1–2 months after exposure an acute illness with fever, malaise, cough, rash, abdominal pain, nausea, lymphadenopathy, mucoid bloody diarrhoea and hepatomegaly may occur (*Katayama fever*).

Chronic disease symptoms relate to worm burden and inflammation/fibrosis secondary to egg deposition in tissues. Portal or pulmonary hypertension, abdominal pain, bloody diarrhoea, spinal cord involvement, dysuria, haematuria, bladder infections and fibrosis may occur.

Diagnosis

Characteristic eggs on microscopy of concentrated stool specimens or biopsy of rectal mucosa (*Schistosoma mansoni*), examination of filtered urine (egg excretion usually peaks between 12 noon and 3 pm) or bladder biopsy for eggs (*S. haematobium*), serologic tests; eosinophilia (non-specific).

Treatment

Praziquantel 20 mg/kg/dose 8–12 hourly PO for 1 day. Re-treatment may be required.

Nematodes

Ancylostoma caninum/braziliense (dog and cat hookworms)

This is the usual cause of cutaneous larva migrans, also known as sandworm infection.

Clinical features

Pruritic reddish papules at site of skin entry, intensely pruritic serpiginous tracks as larvae migrate through the skin a few millimetres to a few centimetres a day. May continue for a few weeks or months but is self-limiting.

Diagnosis

Clinical diagnosis; eosinophilia may occur.

Treatment

Usually self-limiting; albendazole > 2 years of age: 400 mg, < 2 years of age: 200 mg daily PO for 3 days.

Ancylostoma duodenale, Necator americanus (hookworm)

Clinical features

Stinging or burning of skin (usually feet) at site of larval penetration of skin followed by pruritis and a papulovesicular rash for 1-2 weeks. Pneumonitis is uncommon. Colicky abdominal pain with diarrhoea and eosinophilia can develop 4-6 weeks after exposure. Frequently asymptomatic. Chronic infection may result in anaemia, hypoproteinaemia and oedema secondary to blood loss.

Diagnosis

Characteristic eggs on stool microscopy (8-12 weeks after infection).

Treatment

Albendazole > 2 years of age: 400 mg, < 2 years of age: 200 mg PO single dose or mebendazole 100 mg twice daily for 3 days or 500 mg PO single dose (> 5 years of age).

Ascaris lumbricoides (roundworm)

Clinical features

Frequently asymptomatic, non-specific gastrointestinal symptoms may occur. Acute transient pneumonitis (Loeffler's syndrome) associated with fever and eosinophilia may occur during larval migration phase. Intestinal or biliary obstruction and peritonitis may occur.

Diagnosis

Characteristic eggs on stool microscopy; adult worms may be passed from the rectum, nose or mouth in vomitus.

Treatment

Albendazole or mebendazole as for *A. duodenale/N. americanus*.

Enterobius vermicularis (threadworm/pinworm)

Clinical features
Pruritis ani. Rarely, urethritis, vaginitis, salpingitis or pelvic peritonitis may occur.

Diagnosis
Visualization of adult worms in the perianal region or in the stool. Transparent adhesive tape can be applied to perianal skin to collect eggs, the tape applied to a glass slide and examined microscopically.

Treatment
Albendazole or mebendazole as for *A. duodenale/N. americanus* and repeat after 2 weeks.

Strongyloides stercoralis

Clinical features
Frequently asymptomatic. Transient pruritic papules at site of skin penetration (usually feet) by larvae. Larval migration may produce pneumonitis with cough and blood-streaked sputum. Non-specific intestinal symptoms, malabsorption, transient pruritic urticarial skin lesions in perianal or lower abdominal region. Disseminated strongyloidiasis may occur in immunocompromised patients, especially related to corticosteroid treatment (not common in AIDS).

Diagnosis
Characteristic larvae on microscopy of stool or duodenal aspirate; larvae may be found in sputum in disseminated disease; eosinophilia (may be only manifestation of infection).

Treatment
Albendazole > 2 years of age: 400 mg, < 2 years of age: 200 mg twice daily PO for 7 days.

Toxocariasis (visceral larva migrans)

Clinical features
Depends on number of larvae ingested and degree of allergic response. Frequently asymptomatic, history of pica, fever, hepatomegaly, cough, anaemia, ocular symptoms (endopthalmitis or retinal granulomas). Rarely pneumonia, myocarditis, encephalitis.

Diagnosis

Enzyme immunoassay, hypereosinophilia and hypergammaglobulinaemia.

Treatment

Albendazole > 2 years of age: 400 mg, < 2 years of age: 200 mg twice daily PO for 5 days or mebendazole 100 mg twice daily for 5 days or 500 mg PO single dose (> 5 years of age).

Trichuris trichiura (whipworm)

Clinical features

Abdominal pain, bloody mucoid diarrhoea, iron deficiency anaemia, growth retardation, rectal prolapse (heavy infections).

Diagnosis

Characteristic eggs on stool microscopy.

Treatment

Albendazole or mebendazole as for *A. duodenale/N. americanus* and repeat after 2 weeks.

> *Practice point:*
>
> Treatment of intestinal nematodes is recommended in children > 1 year of age. There is limited data in infants and rare reports of convulsions. In cases where the worm infection is assessed as causing significant interference with nutritional status and development treatment of infants may be justified.

Statutory notifiable diseases

In South Africa notifiable conditions are divided into 2 sub-categories: (1) conditions that require immediate notification, telephonically or by fax within 24 hours followed by written notification within 5 days (marked with an asterisk), and (2) conditions requiring written notification, within 7 days of diagnosis

During an outbreak of a notifiable disease, all cases must be reported immediately, by telephone, email or fax, to the designated local health officer.

Priority reporting: All cases of MDR and XDR TB must be reported to the department of health within 24 hours.

- *Acute flaccid paralysis
- *Anthrax
- ˜Brucellosis
- *Cholera
- ˜Congenital syphilis
- *Crimean-Congo haemorrhagic fever, other haemorrhagic fevers of Africa
- ˜Diphtheria
- *Food poisoning
- ˜*Haemophilus influenzae* type b infections
- *Lead poisoning
- ˜Legionellosis
- ˜Leprosy
- ˜Malaria
- *Measles
- *Meningococcal infection
- ˜Paratyphoid fever
- *Plague
- ˜Poisoning from agricultural stock remedies
- *Poliomyelitis
- *Rabies (specify whether human case or human contact)
- ˜Rheumatic fever
- ˜Tetanus
- ˜Tetanus neonatorum
- ˜Trachoma
- ˜Tuberculosis (primary, pulmonary and extrapulmonary)
- *Tuberculosis (MDR and XDR)
- *Typhoid fever
- ˜Typhus fever (lice-borne and ratflea-borne)
- ˜Viral hepatitis A, B, non-A, non-B, and unspecified
- ˜Whooping cough
- *Yellow fever

10 HIV infection

J. Nuttall

Prevention of vertical transmission

This is the most important and effective means to prevent HIV infection in children and must be supported at every opportunity. Measures to reduce vertical transmission include antiretroviral prophylaxis, safe obstetric practices, delivery by caesarean section and exclusive breastfeeding or exclusive formula feeding of HIV-exposed infants. All HIV-infected pregnant women require effective antiretroviral prophylaxis to prevent HIV transmission to the infant; many HIV-infected pregnant women require triple antiretroviral therapy for their own health.

In line with World Health Organization (WHO) recommendations, current South African guidelines are:

1 Rapid initiation of lifelong antiretroviral therapy in all pregnant women with:
   - CD4 count ≤ 350 cells/mm^3 or
   - WHO stage 3 or 4 disease, irrespective of gestational age.

   Infants born to HIV-infected women receiving antiretroviral therapy for their own health should receive daily nevirapine (NVP) (15 mg, or 10 mg if birth weight < 2.5 kg) from birth until 6 weeks of age, irrespective of infant feeding choice.

2 All HIV-infected pregnant women who do not meet these antiretroviral therapy eligibility criteria should receive:
   - Zidovudine (AZT) 300 mg orally 12 hourly starting from as early as 14 weeks gestation (second trimester) or as soon as possible when women present late in pregnancy, in labour or at delivery.
   - At onset of labour/rupture of membranes (or 2-4 hours before caesarean section), NVP 200 mg single oral dose and continue AZT 300 mg orally every 3 hours until delivery.
   - Post delivery of infant, the mother should receive tenofovir (TDF) (300 mg) and emtricitabine (FTC) (200 mg) single oral dose.
   - Infant receives once daily NVP (15 mg, or 10 mg if birth weight < 2.5 kg) from birth until 6 weeks of age, irrespective of infant feeding choice. Breastfeeding infants who test HIV PCR negative at 6 weeks of age continue once daily NVP for the duration

of breastfeeding (6 weeks to 6 months: 20 mg/day; 6 months to 9 months: 30 mg/day; 9 months until end of breastfeeding: 40 mg/day).

The decision to breast or bottle feed is made on an individual basis, accompanied by comprehensive counselling and assessment of whether exclusive formula feeding is available, affordable, accessible, sustainable and safe. Mixed feeding (breastmilk plus other fluids or solids) poses a greater risk for HIV infection than exclusive breastfeeding ☆☆☆☆☘. HIV-infected women who decide to breastfeed must be supported so that they can do so exclusively for 6 months, introduce appropriate complementary foods thereafter and continue breastfeeding for the first 12 months of life. Breastfeeding mothers whose infants are confirmed to be HIV-infected should be encouraged to continue breastfeeding for the first 2 years of life.

Diagnosis

In ideal circumstances, PMTCT programmes would identify all HIV-exposed infants by identifying all HIV-infected pregnant women. HIV-exposed infants should be tested for HIV infection at 4-6 weeks of age and all HIV-infected infants should routinely be assessed for antiretroviral therapy.

In reality, the uptake of HIV testing among pregnant women is relatively low and many HIV-exposed infants are not identified through their mothers or may miss HIV testing at 4-6 weeks of age.

> **Practice point:**
>
> HIV testing of infants and young children should be considered at each contact with the health care system, including immunization visits, nutritional clinic visits, and during intercurrent illnesses.

Clinical manifestations

There may be no clinical evidence to suggest HIV infection, particularly in infants and very young children, or there may be a diverse range of symptoms and signs involving any or all systems and overlapping with the clinical features of other common childhood illnesses. Table 10.1 gives some examples that should alert the clinician to the need for HIV testing.

Table 10.1 Conditions that should prompt HIV testing in children

Clinical signs and conditions common in HIV-infected children, but uncommon in uninfected children
Generalized lymphadenopathy (other than inguinal)
Bilateral painless parotid swelling
Persistent or recurrent fever
Hepatosplenomegaly
Persistent generalized dermatitis not responding to treatment
Persistent or recurrent oral candidiasis
Herpes zoster (single dermatome)
Severe bacterial infections especially if recurrent
Neurologic dysfunction
Clinical signs and conditions common in HIV-infected children but also common in ill uninfected children
Anaemia
Chronic ear infection
Persistent or recurrent diarrhoea
Severe pneumonia
Tuberculosis
Bronchiectasis
Failure to thrive
Marasmus
Clinical signs and conditions more specific to HIV infection
Pneumocystis jirovecii pneumonia (PCP)
Oesophageal candidiasis
Extrapulmonary cryptococcosis
Invasive salmonella infection
Lymphoid interstitial pneumonitis (LIP)
Herpes zoster affecting several dermatomes
Kaposi sarcoma
Rectovaginal or rectovesical fistula

HIV testing

- Definitive diagnosis of HIV infection:
  — In children > 18 months of age antibody testing is used to detect the presence of HIV antibodies
  — In children < 18 months of age virologic testing is carried out using DNA polymerase chain reaction.
- Antibody testing, including the rapid antibody test, is also used in children < 18 months of age with unknown HIV status in order to identify HIV-exposed children (HIV antibody may be present but may originate from the mother or from the child) who will require further virologic testing.

(continued on page 300)

298 Handbook of Paediatrics

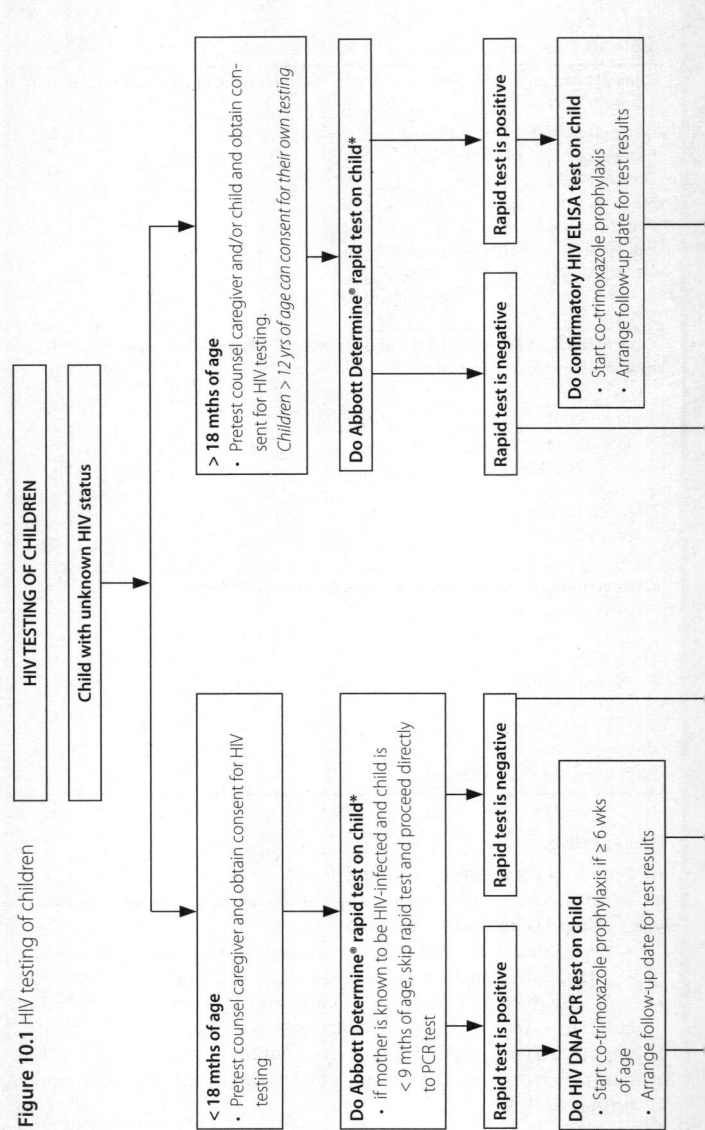

Figure 10.1 HIV testing of children

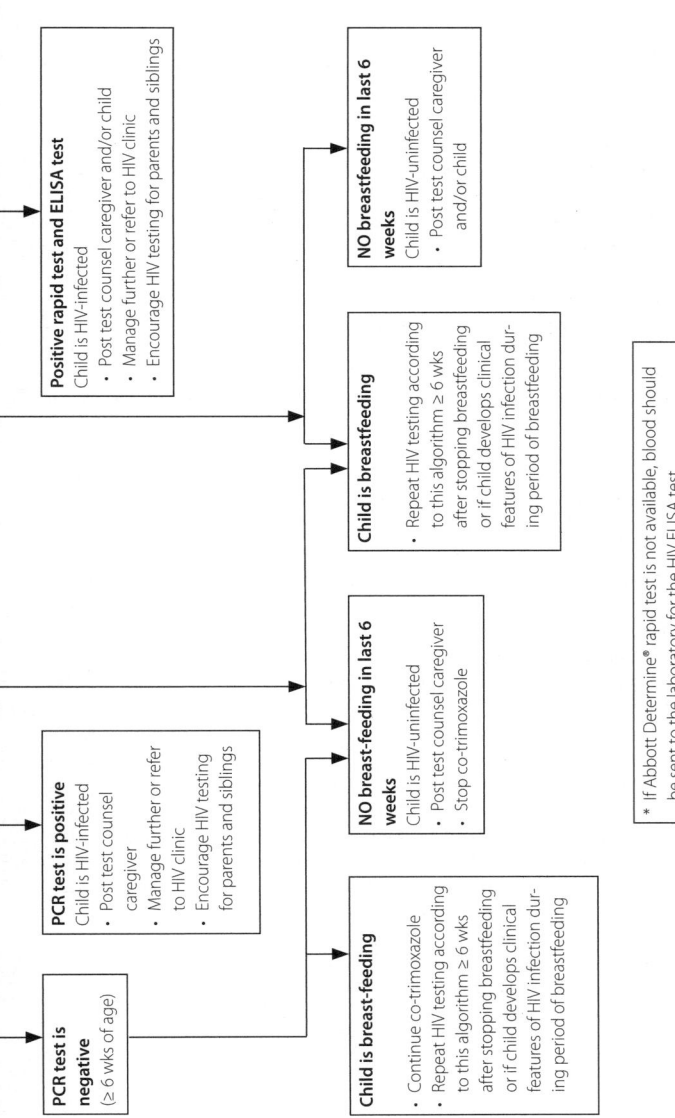

- At present, the only HIV rapid test found to be adequately sensitive in this age group is the Abbott Determine® HIV 1/2 test ☆☆☆✤. If this test is not available, blood should be sent to the laboratory for the HIV ELISA test.
- Antibody testing may be useful to identify children from the age of 9–12 months or older who are known to be HIV-exposed (history of maternal HIV infection or previous testing) and who no longer have maternally-derived HIV antibody in their bodies (sero-reversion) and are therefore HIV-uninfected and do not require further virologic testing (provided there has been no breastfeeding in the preceding 6 weeks and no future breastfeeding).
- The HIV DNA PCR test is most accurate from ≥ 6 weeks of age. If the test is done at < 6 weeks of age and is negative, then it should be repeated when the child is ≥ 6 weeks. It is good practice to confirm the HIV status of HIV exposed children with an HIV ELISA Determine® rapid test at 18 months of age.
- If HIV is strongly suspected clinically and the rapid test is negative, an HIV DNA PCR test (< 18 months) or HIV ELISA test (≥ 18 months) should be sent to the laboratory.

Pre- and post-test counselling of the caregiver, family and where indicated of the child undergoing testing, is an important component of HIV testing. The importance of HIV testing, testing procedures, and the immediate and longer term implications and anticipated psychological reactions to a positive or negative test result should be discussed. In South Africa, consent for HIV testing in children is included in the Children's Act of 2005.

- *Children < 12 years of age* (unless they are of sufficient maturity to understand the benefits, risks, and social implications of the test results themselves) require the consent of their parent or primary caregiver (i.e. does not have to be legal guardian, but the person who cares for the child) but all children should be provided with age-appropriate information prior to HIV testing.
- Children ≥ 12 years of age can provide consent to be tested; they must also provide written consent if it is necessary to disclose their test result to anyone else.
- Whoever consents must receive pre- and post-test counselling by an appropriately trained or experienced person.

Selected clinical problems

Bacterial pneumonia

Bacterial pneumonia is common. The major pathogens are *Streptococcus pneumoniae, Haemophilus influenzae* type b, *Staphylococcus aureus* and gram negative bacteria. *S. pneumoniae* is the commonest. Empiric antibiotic therapy for pneumonia should therefore be broad spectrum, i.e. ampicillin plus gentamicin or a 2nd or 3rd generation cephalosporin. For ambulatory therapy, amoxicillin 30 mg/kg/dose 8 hourly for 5 days is the first line agent.

Pneumocystis pneumonia (PCP)

Symptoms include tachypnea, fever, dyspnea and cough. Infants < 6 months of age are especially at risk and have an acute, severe illness characterized by prominent and progressive hypoxia and increasing respiratory difficulty. The chest radiograph usually shows a diffuse interstitial pattern, which progresses to alveolar opacification, but any CXR pattern may occur. Definitive diagnosis requires identification of *P. jirovecii* from lower respiratory tract secretions such as bronchoalveolar lavage (BAL) or induced sputum with immunofluorescence or other staining.

There is a high mortality rate and early treatment is essential. Treat with intravenous co-trimoxazole (preferred) 10 mg/kg loading dose followed by 5 mg/kg/dose 6 hourly for 21 days. Oral treatment, loading with 20 mg/kg and then 10 mg/kg/dose 6 hourly can be used if intravenous therapy is not feasible or if disease is mild. A dose of 5 mg/kg/dose 6 hourly can be used as oral step-down treatment after clinical improvement occurs with IV therapy. Prednisone should be added early (within 48 hours of co-trimoxazole) in hypoxic children – a recommended regime is prednisone 2 mg/kg for 5–7 days with tapering doses over 10–14 days or until the child is no longer hypoxic.

Prevention of PCP is a most important and effective intervention if initiated in HIV-exposed infants from 4–6 weeks of age. Oral co-trimoxazole is the most effective prophylactic agent (see section on prophylaxis).

Viral pneumonia

Respiratory viruses are more likely to result in pneumonia than bronchiolitis. Cytomegalovirus (CMV) pneumonia is common, especially in severely immunosuppressed infants. Diagnosis depends on blood PCR for CMV and isolation of CMV from a respiratory tract specimen. Treatment is with ganciclovir/valganciclovir for 4–6 weeks, and initiation of antiretroviral therapy.

Tuberculosis

Clinical features may overlap with other HIV-associated lung diseases. May present with acute pneumonia. Attempt to make a microbiological diagnosis (gastric washings, induced sputum or sputum for TB smear, culture and drug sensitivity testing). Obtain sputum culture and drug sensitivity results of known TB contacts of child. In severely immunosuppressed children or smear positive children, use a 4 drug regimen (rifampicin, isoniazid, pyrazinamide, ethambutol) for 2 months followed by a 2 drug regimen (rifampicin, isoniazid) for 4–7 months depending on clinical and radiological response to treatment. There are important drug-drug interactions between antiretroviral therapy and TB therapy that may require adjustment of drugs and/or doses (see section on Antiretroviral therapy and anti-TB therapy, p. 309).

Other HIV-associated lung disease

Lymphoid interstitial pneumonitis (LIP)

May co-exist with pneumonia or TB and complicate the diagnosis of these conditions. No specific treatment but usually responds well to antiretroviral therapy. If airway obstruction or hypoxia is present, prednisone 1–2 mg/kg/dose once daily may be helpful. If there is a good response to steroids, then a prolonged course of 4–6 weeks of tapering doses may be needed.

Chronic lung disease

May result from multiple previous respiratory tract infections of various causes or develop in time as part of immune decline due to HIV. Treatment is directed at current infective exacerbations and limitation of progressive damage and bronchiectasis. Antiretroviral therapy is indicated.

Malignancy (e.g. lymphoma, Kaposi's sarcoma)

May present as non-resolving clinical and radiological features. Referral for further imaging and tissue diagnosis is indicated.

Haematological conditions

Anaemia and thrombocytopaenia

Aetiology may be multifactorial, including HIV-associated bone marrow suppression, autoimmune, mineral and micronutrient deficiencies, recurrent or chronic infection, bone marrow infiltration with infection or malignancy, and antiretroviral-associated. Initial empiric treatment and referral for further investigation including bone marrow biopsy may be indicated if poor response. Variable response to initiation of antiretroviral therapy.

Neurological manifestations

HIV encephalopathy
Often presents in infancy with developmental delay or loss of milestones, impaired brain growth and motor deficits. This is an indication for antiretroviral therapy. Prevention and some reversibility may be anticipated with early treatment.

Seizures
Aetiology may be multifactorial. There may be important drug-drug interactions between antiretroviral therapy and anticonvulsant therapy that may require adjustment of drugs and/or doses.

CNS infections
Bacterial and tuberculous meningitis, and various viral causes of encephalitis occur at all ages. Cryptococcal and parasitic infections are more common in older children and adolescents.

Prophylaxis

Co-trimoxazole (trimethoprim plus sulfamethoxazole)
- All HIV-exposed infants and children < 18 months of age should receive co-trimoxazole, starting from 4–6 weeks of age and continued until HIV infection can be excluded (negative PCR test ≥ 6 weeks of age in non-breastfed children OR negative PCR test ≥ 6 weeks after the last breastfeed in breastfed infants).
- All HIV-infected children < 12 months of age should receive co-trimoxazole regardless of clinical stage or CD4 count.
- For HIV-infected children > 12 months of age, co-trimoxazole is recommended for all symptomatic children (WHO clinical stage 2, 3 or 4) or children with CD4 < 25%.
- Children > 5 years of age should receive co-trimoxazole according to adult recommendations (any WHO clinical stage plus CD4 count < 200 cells/mm^3 OR WHO clinical stage 3 or 4 irrespective of CD4 count).

- For co-trimoxazole intolerant patients, an alternative is dapsone 2 mg/kg/day (maximum daily dose 100 mg) or 4 mg/kg/week.
- Discontinuation of co-trimoxazole may be considered in the context of antiretroviral therapy-associated immune reconstitution: children > 18 months of age and who have been receiving antiretroviral therapy for at least 6 months with CD4 > 15% on 2 successive occasions 3–6 months apart.

Table 10.2 Co-trimoxazole prophylaxis dosing schedule for children (WHO, 2009)

Weight / age of child	Once daily dose Oral suspension (40 mg trimethoprim + 200 mg sulfamethoxazole/5 ml) or single-strength tablet (80 mg/400 mg)
< 5 kg /< 6 mths	2.5 ml
5–< 14 kg/6 mths–5 yrs	5 ml or ½ tablet
14–< 30 kg/6–14 yrs	10 ml or 1 tablet
≥ 30 kg/> 14 yrs	2 tablets

Isoniazid

- HIV-infected children of any age who are in close contact with an adult or adolescent with pulmonary TB should be screened for TB infection and disease. Remember to assess if the source case might have drug-resistant TB.
- Take a careful history of symptoms suggestive of TB, including unremitting cough that is not improving and has been present for more than 21 days, fever > 14 days without another obvious cause, weight loss or failure to thrive.
- Examine the child for signs suggestive of pulmonary or extrapulmonary TB.
- Perform a Mantoux skin test and chest X-ray.
- If there is clinical or radiological evidence suggestive of TB and/or the Mantoux skin test is positive (≥ 5 mm diameter of induration in the setting of HIV), the child should whenever possible have further investigations directed at bacteriological confirmation of TB. These include sputum (by expectoration or by induced sputum techniques), gastric aspiration and other relevant samples such as lymph node aspiration or biopsy. Thereafter TB therapy should be initiated.

- If there is no clinical or radiological evidence suggestive of TB disease and regardless of the Mantoux skin test result, the child should receive isoniazid preventive therapy (IPT). Current recommendations are for 6 months IPT.
- An HIV-infected child of any age with a positive Mantoux skin test and no clinical or radiological evidence of TB disease and no known TB contact should receive IPT.

Table 10.3 Dosing for isoniazid preventive therapy (IPT) in children

BodyWeight (kg)	Daily isoniazid (INH) 100 mg tablet
2–2.4	¼
2.5–4.9	½
5–7.4	¾
7.5–9.9	1
10–19.9	2
20–24.9	2½
≥ 25	3

Vaccination

- HIV-infected infants and children should receive vaccinations according to the national Expanded Programme on Immunization (EPI).
- HIV-infected infants receiving BCG vaccination at birth are at increased risk of developing BCG adverse events including local or regional adverse events (BCG adenitis) as well systemic or disseminated BCG disease. Current local recommendations are that BCG vaccination should continue to be administered at birth to all infants, regardless of HIV exposure until programmatic conditions necessary, for the implementation of selectively delayed BCG vaccination in HIV-exposed infants exist.
- Annual influenza vaccination is strongly recommended

Clinical staging and immunological assessment

Table 10.4 Clinical staging of HIV for infants and children with established HIV infection (WHO, 2006)

STAGE ONE
Asymptomatic
Persistent generalized lymphadenopathy
STAGE TWO
Unexplained persistent hepatosplenomegaly
Papular pruritic eruptions
Extensive wart virus infection
Extensive molluscum contagiosum
Recurrent oral ulcerations
Unexplained persistent parotid enlargement
Lineal gingival erythema
Herpes zoster
Recurrent/chronic upper respiratory tract infection (otitis media, sinusitis, otorrhoea)
Fungal nail infections
STAGE THREE
Unexplained moderate malnutrition not adequately responding to standard therapy
Unexplained persistent diarrhoea ($\geq$ 14 days)
Unexplained persistent fever (> 37.5 °C, > 1 month)
Persistent oral candidiasis (after first 6 weeks of life)
Oral hairy leukoplakia
Acute necrotizing ulcerative gingivitis/periodontitis
Lymph node tuberculosis
Pulmonary tuberculosis
Severe recurrent bacterial pneumonia
Symptomatic lymphoid interstitial pneumonitis (LIP)
Chronic HIV-associated lung disease incl. bronchiectasis
Unexplained anaemia (< 8 g/dl), neutropaenia (< 0.5 $\times 10^9$/l), or chronic thrombocytopaenia (< 50 $\times 10^9$/l)

STAGE FOUR
Unexplained severe malnutrition
Pneumocystis pneumonia
Recurrent severe bacterial infections (excl. pneumonia)
Chronic herpes simplex infection (oral or skin for > 1 month, or visceral at any site)
Extrapulmonary tuberculosis
Kaposi sarcoma
Oesophageal candidiasis (or candida of trachea, bronchi or lungs)
Central nervous system toxoplasmosis outside neonatal period
HIV encephalopathy
Cytomegalovirus infection (retinitis or another organ outside neonatal period)
Extrapulmonary cryptococcosis including meningitis
Any disseminated endemic mycosis
Chronic cryptosporidiosis (with diarrhoea)/isosporiasis
Disseminated non-tuberculous mycobacteria infection
Cerebral or B-cell non-Hodgkin lymphoma
Progressive multifocal leukoencephalopathy (PML)
HIV-associated cardiomyopathy or nephropathy
Acquired HIV-associated rectovaginal fistula

Immunological assessment

- CD4 counts are used to assess the immunological status of a patient with HIV infection.
- In young children, absolute CD4 counts are more age-dependent and variable than %CD4 (percentage of lymphocytes which are CD4+), but may be falsely elevated if absolute lymphopenia is present. Therefore both absolute and %CD4 count should be assessed.
- The recommended CD4 thresholds for starting antiretroviral therapy in children are indicated in Table 10.5 (indications for starting antiretroviral therapy in children with confirmed HIV infection).

Antiretroviral therapy

Indications

There are a number of different guidelines with differing recommendations on when to start antiretroviral therapy in children. These include

World Health Organization (WHO) 2008 revision, National Institutes of Health USA 2009, Paediatric European Network for Treatment of AIDS (PENTA) 2009, Department of Health South Africa, 2010 revision.

> **Practice point:**
>
> There has been recent broad consensus that antiretroviral therapy is recommended for all infants (< 12 months of age) regardless of clinical status, CD4 count or viral load. There is greater urgency to initiate antiretroviral in infants < 6 months of age.

Recommendations differ on when to start treatment in children > 12 months of age.

Table 10.5 Indications for starting antiretroviral therapy in children with confirmed HIV infection (SA DOH guidelines 2010 and Southern African HIV Clinicians Society, 2009)

Age of child	Clinical stage	CD4 criteria
< 1 year	All infants	Any CD4 count
1–5 years	WHO stage 3 or 4	CD4 ≤ 25% or absolute CD4 < 750 cells/mm^3
> 5 years	WHO stage 3 or 4	CD4 < 350 cells/mm^3

Preparation

- Antiretroviral therapy is advocated as continuous lifelong treatment. Long-term adherence to treatment remains one of the strongest predictors of a successful outcome.
- Identification and preparation of the child's primary caregiver is of utmost importance. In older children and adolescents, a degree of responsibility for taking medication rests with the child him/herself.
- Issues around disclosure of the child's HIV status to the child him/herself, to other family and household members and friends, and eventually to sexual partners, must be addressed.
- Preparation varies according to the individual needs of the patient and their family or caregiver situation and includes psychological counselling and support as well as practical education in the administration of medications to the child. This usually requires a number of counselling and education sessions before or at the time of starting treatment and regular intermittent support thereafter.

Recommended first-line treatment regimens (treatment naïve patients)

Table 10.6 Recommended first-line treatment for treatment naïve patients (SA DOH guidelines 2010 and Southern African HIV Clinicians Society, 2009).

Children < 3 years of age at start of treatment
Abacavir + lamivudine + lopinavir/ritonavir
Alternative: Stavudine + lamivudine + lopinavir/ritonavir

Children > 3 years of age and > 10 kg body weight at start of treatment
Abacavir + lamivudine + efavirenz
Alternative: Stavudine + lamivudine + efavirenz

Antiretroviral drug doses

A practical approach to antiretroviral drug dosing is by using a standardized weight-based chart, provided for antiretroviral drugs currently available in the South African public sector. (Refer to Antiretroviral Drug Chart on next double-page spread.)

Antiretroviral therapy and anti-TB therapy

- All children with suspected or definite TB should undergo HIV testing. TB should always be considered during the clinical follow-up of children with HIV infection.
- Children with HIV/TB co-infection are classified as HIV clinical stage 3 (pulmonary or lymph node TB) or stage 4 (extrapulmonary TB).
  - All infants (< 12 months of age) with HIV-TB co-infection should receive concurrent antiretroviral and anti-TB therapy.

> *Practice point:*
>
> All children with HIV/TB coinfection are eligible for antiretroviral therapy.

Table 10.7 Antiretroviral Drug Dosing Chart for Children (2011)

Target dose	Stavudine (d4T)	Lamivudine (3TC)	Zidovudine (AZT)	Didanosine (ddI)	Abacavir (ABC)
	1 mg/kg/dose TWICE daily	4–6 mg/kg/dose TWICE daily	240 mg/m²/dose TWICE daily	90–120 mg/m²/dose TWICE daily	8 mg/kg/dose TWICE daily
Available formulations	Sol. 1 mg/ml Caps 15, 20, 30 mg	Sol. 10 mg/ml Tabs 150 mg (scored)	Sol. 10 mg/ml Caps 100 mg Tabs 300 mg (not scored)	Tabs 25, 50, 100 mg (dispersible in at least 30 ml water) Caps 250 mg EC	Sol. 20 mg/ml Tabs 300 mg (not scored)
Weight (kg)					
<3	Consult with a clinician experienced in paediatric ARV prescribing				
3–3.9	6 ml	3 ml	6 ml	avoid	3 ml
4–4.9					
5–5.9	7.5 mg: open 15 mg capsule into 5 ml water: give 2.5 ml & discard rest			2 × 25 mg tabs (am & pm)	
6–6.9		4 ml	9 ml	1 × 50 mg + 1 × 25 mg tabs am; 2 × 25 mg tabs pm	4 ml
7–7.9	10 mg: open 20 mg capsule into 5 ml water: give 2.5 ml & discard rest				
8–8.9			1 cap		
9–9.9					
10–10.9	15 mg: open 15 mg capsule into 5 ml water	6 ml		1 × 50 mg + 1 × 25 mg tabs (am and pm)	6 ml
11–11.9					
12–13.9					
14–16.9	20 mg: open 20 mg capsule into 5 ml water	½ tab	2 caps am; 1 cap pm	2 × 50 mg tabs am; 1 × 50 mg + 1 × 25 mg tabs pm	8 ml
17–19.9					
20–24.9		1 tab am; ½ tab pm	2 caps	2 × 50 mg tabs (am and pm)	10 ml
25–29.9	30 mg	1 tab	1 tab	1 × 100 mg tab + 1 × 25 mg tab twice daily OR 1 × 250 mg EC cap once daily	1 tab
30–34.9					
35–39.9					
>40					

*Children 14–24.9 kg may also be dosed with LPV/rtv 200/50 mg tabs as follows: 1 tab twice daily
Children 25–34.9 kg may also be dosed with LPV/rtv 200/50 mg tabs as follows: 2 tabs am; 1 tab pm

Chapter 10: HIV infection

Efavirenz (EFV)	Nevirapine (NVP)	Lopinavir/ ritonavir (LPV/rtv)	Ritonavir boosting (RTV)	Co-trimoxazole	Multi-vitamins	Target dose
y weight band ONCE daily	150 mg/m²/ dose *TWICE daily (after once daily lead in)	300/75 mg/m²/dose LPV/rtv TWICE daily	** ONLY as booster for LPV/ rtv when on Rifampicin TWICE daily	ONCE daily	ONCE daily	
aps 50, 200 mg Tabs 50, 200, 600 mg (not scored)	Sol. 10 mg/ml Tabs 200 mg (scored)	Sol. 80/20 mg/ml Tabs 200/50 mg, 100/25 mg	Sol. 80 mg/ml	Sol. 40/200 mg/5 ml Tabs 80/400 mg (scored)	Sol. Tabs (B Co)	Available formulations
						Weight (kg)
neonates (< 28 days of age) and infants weighing < 3 kg				2.5 ml	2.5 ml	< 3
Dosing < 10 kg not established	5 ml	1 ml	**1 ml			3–3.9
		1.5 ml	**1.2 ml			4–4.9
				5 ml OR ½ tab		5–5.9
	8 ml					6–6.9
						7–7.9
						8–8.9
						9–9.9
100 mg cap/tab	10 ml	2 ml twice daily OR 100/25 mg tabs: 2 tabs am, 1 tab pm	**1.5 ml		5 ml	10–10.9
						11–11.9
						12–13.9
200 mg cap/ tab + 2 x 50 mg cap/tab	1 tab am; ½ tab pm	2.5 ml twice daily OR 100/25 mg tabs: 2 tabs twice daily	**2 ml	10 ml OR 1 tab		14–16.9
						17–19.9
		3 ml twice daily OR 100/25 mg tabs: 2 tabs twice daily	**2.5 ml			20–24.9
x 200 mg caps/ tabs	1 tab	3.5 ml twice daily OR 100/25 mg tabs: 3 tabs twice daily	**3 ml			25–29.9
		4 ml twice daily OR 100/25 mg tabs: 3 tabs twice daily		2 tabs	1 tab	30–34.9
600 mg tab		5 ml twice daily OR 200/50 mg tabs: 2 tabs twice daily	**4 ml			35–39.9
						> 40

- Anti-TB therapy takes priority over antiretroviral therapy but the optimal timing of antiretroviral initiation in HIV-infected children presenting with TB is unknown.
  - The risk of delayed antiretroviral therapy in children with HIV/TB co-infection is HIV disease progression and a poor response to anti-TB therapy.
  - Concurrent or early initiation of antiretroviral therapy within days to weeks of starting TB treatment may increase the risk of immune reconstitution inflammatory syndrome and have an impact on toxicity and adherence, and drug interactions may affect antiretroviral treatment efficacy.
  - Most guidelines recommend antiretroviral initiation 2–8 weeks after starting TB treatment. Infants < 1 year, extrapulmonary TB, and multi-drug resistant (MDR) or extensively drug resistant (XDR) TB are criteria for more urgent initiation of antiretroviral therapy (generally within 2 weeks of starting TB treatment).

Rifampicin is a potent inducer of the cytochrome p450 enzyme system and thereby increases the rate of metabolism of the NNRTI and PI groups of antiretroviral drugs. This may result in reduced serum concentrations of these drugs, in particular lopinavir and nevirapine, and predispose to HIV treatment failure and viral resistance mutations.

Table 10.8 Combining antiretroviral and anti-TB regimens

Antiretroviral and rifampicin-based TB treatment combinations
Currently recommended:
2 NRTIs + efavirenz (children > 3 years or > 10 kg body weight)
2 NRTIs + lopinavir/ritonavir with additional ritonavir*
NOT currently recommended:
2 NRTIs + nevirapine
2 NRTIs + lopinavir/ritonavir
2 NRTIs + 'double-dose' lopinavir/ritonavir
3 NRTI regimens

* To provide lopinavir:ritonavir in a 1:1 concentration (see dosage chart for prescribing details)

Monitoring

- Check adherence to treatment: 2 weeks after starting therapy and at each clinic visit thereafter
- Clinical review: after 1 month and then 1–3 monthly. Monitor growth (weight, length) and neuro-developmental progress
- FBC at baseline and at months 1, 2 and 3 if starting on a zidovudine-based regimen.
- ALT at baseline if starting a nevirapine-based regimen, if develops rash or jaundice on a nevirapine-based regimen, and at baseline and monthly in patients on antiretroviral and TB treatment
- CD4 count (absolute and percentage): baseline, then 3–6 monthly
- Viral load: baseline, then 3–6 monthly
- Annual lipid profile in those on protease inhibitors.

Drug toxicity

- Consider whether the event is likely to be due to antiretroviral agents or to other medication, intercurrent infection, immune reconstitution inflammatory syndrome (IRIS) or HIV disease progression.
- Assess severity using grading tables and consider whether there is a need to interrupt antiretroviral therapy.
- Severe or life-threatening events, e.g. pancreatitis, severe hepatitis/hepatic failure, hypersensitivity reactions including abacavir hypersensitivity, and severe rashes, including Stevens-Johnson syndrome, lactic acidosis: *discontinue all antiretrovirals temporarily.* Manage the medical event then reintroduce antiretrovirals using a modified regimen.
- For less severe/non-life-threatening toxicity, interruption of an NNRTI-containing regimen should incorporate a strategy (e.g. inclusion of lopinavir/ritonavir for 10 days) to cover the prolonged plasma half-life of NNRTI drugs in order to reduce the development of resistance to NNRTIs.
- Mild or moderate events: can usually continue antiretrovirals. Evaluate and monitor more frequently. Single drug substitution may occasionally be necessary.

Table 10.9 Drug toxicity and substitution

Drug	Toxicity	New drug
Stavudine	lactic acidosis	abacavir or zidovudine
	lipoatrophy	
	peripheral neuropathy	
	pancreatitis	
Zidovudine	anaemia/neutropenia	stavudine or abacavir
	lactic acidosis	abacavir
	gastrointestinal intolerance	stavudine or abacavir
Abacavir	hypersensitivity	zidovudine
Efavirenz	persistent severe central nervous system disturbance	nevirapine
	pregnancy risk or early pregnancy	
Nevirapine	hepatitis	efavirenz
	severe hypersensitivity	lopinavir/ritonavir
	severe rash	

Treatment failure and changing therapy in children on antiretroviral therapy

Virological failure usually precedes CD4 count decline or clinical disease progression. Intercurrent infections and immunizations may temporarily decrease the CD4 count or elevate the viral load, and these tests should be deferred or repeated one month later. Antiretroviral therapy should not be changed on the basis of a single viral load or CD4 result. Immune reconstitution inflammatory syndrome (IRIS) should be considered as a cause of paradoxical clinical deterioration during the first 3–6 months after starting antitetroviral therapy.

Sustained high level adherence to the prescribed medication is the most important factor determining the success of an antiretroviral regimen.

> *Practice point*
>
> In any patient with a detectable viral load on antiretroviral treatment, adherence to medication should be carefully evaluated and support provided.

Depending on the age of the child, this includes assessing the caregiver and child's ability to demonstrate correct preparation, accurate dosing and administration of medication on time; tolerance including problems with vomiting or spitting out medications and whether appropriate supervision is occurring. Supportive measures include counselling of the caregiver and/or child, identification of secondary caregivers from within the family to assist with directly observed therapy, feedback of laboratory results in response to interventions such as pillboxes and reminder techniques such as alarms or cellphones. Where relevant, disclosure of HIV status to the child and/or other caregivers must also be addressed. Adherence must be optimized before changing therapy.

Table 10.10 Viral load monitoring and recommended response (Modified from SA DOH guidelines, 2010)

Viral load (VL) copies/ml	Response	
< 400	6–12 monthly VL monitoring and routine adherence support	
400–1000	Repeat VL in 3–6 months Step-up adherence support if VL still 400–1 000	
> 1 000	Step-up adherence support Repeat VL in 3-6 months	Repeat VL < 400 Return to routine 6–12 monthly VL monitoring
		Repeat VL 400–1 000 Continue step-up adherence and repeat VL in 3–6 months
		Repeat VL > 1 000 despite stepped up adherence support Further management depends on current regime and treatment history
Repeat VL > 1 000	Child on a NNRTI-based regimen • Switch to second-line therapy only if adherence is > 80%, otherwise improve adherence and repeat VL test in 3–6 months Child on a PI-based regimen: • It is very difficult to fail a PI-based regimen unless the child received an unboosted PI (e.g. ritonavir alone) in the past. Only switch to second-line therapy if adherence is > 80%, otherwise improve adherence and repeat VL test in 3-6 months • If never received an unboosted PI and adherence is > 80% consider drug resistance testing if available and change to second line if VL > 5 000. (If 1 000–5 000 reinforce adherence and repeat VL test in 3–6 months) • If child received an unboosted PI in the past, do resistance testing if available and change to second line if VL > 1 000	

Patients with poor CD4 count responses despite virological suppression and those failing treatment with second-line or subsequent regimens should be discussed with an expert. Although still very expensive and frequently unavailable in the public sector, appropriate indications for viral genotype testing include children on PI-based regimens with non-suppressed viral load despite good adherence, children with non-suppressed viral loads who received unboosted PI regimens (e.g. ritonavir) in the past and infants infected despite maternal antiretroviral therapy before the infant starts antiretroviral therapy. Genotype results should be interpreted in conjunction with a detailed treatment-history and expert advice should be obtained.

Second line treatment

Table 10.11 Second line treatment currently available in the South African public sector

First-line regimen		Second-line regimen options	
NRTI backbone	Third drug	NRTI backbone	Third drug
Stavudine + lamivudine	Lopinavir/ritonavir	Abacavir + didanosine*	Efavirenz or nevirapine
	Nevirapine or efavirenz		Lopinavir/ritonavir
Zidovudine + lamivudine	Lopinavir/ritonavir	Abacavir + didanosine*	Efavirenz or nevirapine
	Nevirapine or efavirenz		Lopinavir/ritonavir
Abacavir + lamivudine	Lopinavir/ritonavir	Zidovudine + didanosine*	Efavirenz or nevirapine
	Nevirapine or efavirenz		Lopinavir/ritonavir

* If available, genotype resistance testing is advisable before switching patients who are failing therapy on a lopinavir/ritonavir-based regimen in order to design an effective NRTI backbone for second-line therapy.

Post exposure prophylaxis (PEP)

If HIV uninfected at baseline, PEP should be started as soon as possible after exposure. Counselling, information and support should be provided to all individuals after possible HIV exposure. Specific advice may be required for pregnant or breastfeeding women and information on safe sex precautions.

Laboratory monitoring is to exclude acquisition of infection and for those given PEP to monitor toxicity. HIV testing should be performed at

Figure 10.2 Antiretroviral post-exposure prophylaxis for the sexually assaulted child

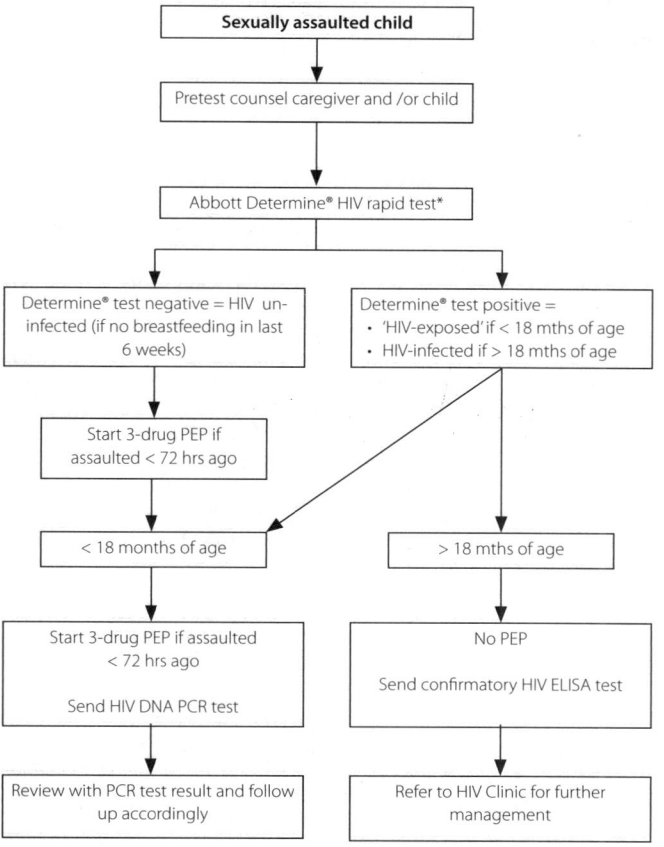

the time of the exposure and again at 6 weeks, 3 months and 6 months after exposure. Full blood count should be done at baseline and at 2 and 4 weeks as zidovudine can cause anaemia and neutropenia.

Sexually assaulted children

Standard 3 drug PEP is AZT+3TC+lopinavir/ritonavir taken *for 28 days* (dose according to weight bands in chart). Post-exposure prophylaxis (PEP) starting > 72 hours after assault is not recommended. Screening and follow-up for hepatitis B and syphilis is also required.

Occupational exposure

- This includes health care workers as well as children in hospital or attending clinics
- Standard prophylaxis comprises zidovudine + lamivudine twice daily orally for 28 days.
- The addition of lopinavir/ritonavir twice daily orally for 28 days may be considered for high-risk injuries, including deep percutaneous sharps injuries, percutaneous exposure involving a hollow needle that was used in a vein or an artery, visible blood on the sharp instrument involved in a percutaneous injury, patients with terminal AIDS, seroconversion illness, or high viral load.
- If the source patient is on antiretroviral therapy and failing treatment, an HIV specialist should be consulted about appropriate prophylaxis.
- Review the need to continue prophylaxis when the HIV result of the source patient is known

Recommended reading

1 *Guidelines for antiretroviral therapy in children – November 2009 version. Southern African HIV Clinicians Society.* South Afr J HIV Med. 2009; issue 36. Available at http://www.sahivsoc.org
2 *Report of the WHO technical reference group, paediatric HIV/ART care guideline group meeting, April 2008.* Available at http://www.who.int/hiv/pub/paediatric/WHO_Paediatric_ART_guideline_rev_mreport_2008.pdf
3 *WHO case definitions of HIV for surveillance and revised clinical staging and immunological classification of HIV-related disease in adults and children.* World Health Organization, 2006. Available at http://www.who.int
4 *Guidelines for the use of antiretroviral agents in paediatric HIV infection. 2009.* Available at http://aidsinfo.nih.gov/ContentFiles/PaediatricGuidelines.pdf
5 *Post-exposure prophylaxis guideline. Southern African HIV Clinicians Society.* South Afr J HIV Med. 2008; issue 35. Available at http://www.sahivsoc.org
6 *Guidelines for the management of HIV in children.* 2e. 2010. National Department of Health, South Africa. Available at: http://www.sanac.org.za/resources/art-guidelines.

11 Asthma, allergic problems and immunodeficiency

B. Eley, M. Klein, C. Motala

Asthma

Diagnosis

Any child with chronic persistent/recurrent wheeze with or without cough (due to bronchoconstriction) triggered by multiple factors, including viral infections, allergens, irritants (pollution), exercise and sudden emotional changes (e.g. crying, laughing) that responds to an inhaled bronchodilator must be diagnosed as asthmatic. Features supporting the diagnosis are a family or personal history of atopy, nocturnal cough, exercise-induced cough and/or wheeze and seasonal variation in symptoms. Allergy is often the main trigger of asthma in children. Early sensitization, severe atopy and synergistic interaction between atopy and infections are risk factors for uncontrolled and severe asthma. Cough variant asthma is a rare form of asthma that presents with cough but no wheeze and no evidence of airway obstruction on spirometry.

Children older than five years

A careful history and physical examination, together with objective evidence of reversible airflow obstruction after administration of a short acting beta agonist (an increase in $FEV_1 > 12\%$ or in PEF > 15% after 10 minutes) will, in most instances, confirm the diagnosis. Monitoring symptoms and PEF using a diary card is also useful for making the diagnosis; diurnal PEF variability > 20% is highly suggestive of asthma. Conditions that need to be considered when the diagnosis of asthma is uncertain are listed in Table 11.1.

Table 11.1 The differential diagnosis of asthma in children older than 5 years

Hyperventilation syndrome and panic attacks
Vocal cord dysfunction
Upper airway obstruction and inhaled foreign bodies
Other forms of obstructive lung disease (e.g. bronchiolitis obliterans)
Non-respiratory causes of symptoms (e.g. left ventricular failure)

Children five years and younger

The diagnosis of asthma in early childhood is challenging and has to be based largely on *clinical judgment* (assessment of symptoms and physical findings). Since the use of the label 'asthma' for wheezing in children has important clinical implications, it must be distinguished from other causes of persistent and recurrent wheeze (Table 11.2). It should be remembered that most wheezing young children do not have asthma.

Table 11.2 The differential diagnosis of asthma in children 5 years and younger

Infections	Recurrent respiratory tract infections Tuberculosis (e.g. glandular compression of airways) HIV disease (e.g. lymphocytic interstitial pneumonitis)
Congenital/perinatal problems	Tracheomalacia Cystic fibrosis Bronchopulmonary dysplasia Congenital malformation causing narrowing of the intrathoracic airways Primary ciliary dyskinesia syndrome Immune deficiency Congenital heart disease (e.g. left-to-right shunts)
Mechanical problems	Foreign body aspiration Gastro-oesophageal reflux

Treatment

- Avoid trigger factors.
- Avoid/reduce exposure to identified allergens and irritants.
- Control co-morbid conditions, e.g. allergic rhinitis, sinusitis and gastro-oesophageal reflux.

Medication

- *Relievers* (rapid-acting β_2 agonists): prescribe for all patients.
- *Controllers* (inhaled corticosteroids, leukotriene receptor antagonists and long acting β_2 agonists): all patients with persistent asthma should be on a controller.

Controllers:
- *Inhaled corticosteroids* (ICS) are the first-line controller therapy for persistent asthma. Most children will be controlled on low daily doses of ICS (Table 11.3). Some children require higher doses for control. ☆☆☆☆☆

> **Practice point:**
>
> Inhaled corticosteroids are the most effective controller therapy.

Table 11.3 The estimated equipotent daily dosage for inhaled glucocorticosteroids for children

Drug	Low daily dose (µg)	Medium daily dose (µg)	High daily dose (µg)
Beclomethasone dipropionate	100–200	200–400	> 400
Budesonide*	100–200	200–400	> 400
Ciclesonide *	80–160	160–320	> 320
Fluticasone	50–100	100–250	> 250

* Approved for once daily dosing in patients with mild asthma

As CFC preparations are withdrawn from the market, medication inserts for CFC-free preparations should be carefully reviewed for the equivalent correct dosage.

- *Leukotriene receptor antagonists (LTRAs)*:
  - LTRAs may be used as monotherapy for mild persistent asthma where ICS cannot be administered. ☆☆☆☺
  - LTRAs are recommended as add on therapy to ICS for mild to moderate persistent asthma. ☆☆☆☺
- *Long-acting β-agonists (LABAs)*:
  - Ineffective as monotherapy for control of asthma and associated with an increased risk of asthma mortality in children. ☆☆☆☺
  - Primarily indicated as add-on therapy in children > 4 years whose asthma is not controlled with moderate to high doses of ICS. ☆☆☆☆

> **Practice point:**
>
> Inhaled therapy, where possible, is preferred. Different age groups require different inhalers for administration of therapy (Table 11.4). In general inhaled therapy via a metered dose inhaler (MDI) with a small volume spacer is preferable to nebulised therapy (convenient, more effective lung deposition, fewer side effects and lower cost). For children older > 5 years of age, a dry powder device (DPI) or breath actuated MDI is also effective. ☆☆☆☆☆

Table 11.4 Choice of inhaler device for children

Age group	Preferred device
< 4 years	MDI *plus* dedicated spacer with face mask
4–6 years	MDI *plus* dedicated spacer with mouthpiece
> 6 years	DPI, *or* breath-actuated MDI, *or* MDI with spacer and mouthpiece

MDI = metred dose inhaler
DPI = dry powder inhaler

Asthma education

- Education should be staged over several visits.
- Discuss the nature of the disease and avoidance of triggers.
- Detailed written management/action plans should be drawn up.
- Teach self-management skills – improves outcomes.

Regular review

- Asthma control may be assessed at each visit using a simplified scheme for recognizing controlled and uncontrolled asthma in a given week (Table 11.5).
- Check adherence and inhaler technique at each visit.
- Monitor growth.
- Enquire about side effects of medication.

Table 11.5 Levels of asthma control*

Characteristic	Controlled *(All of the following)*	Uncontrolled *(3 or more features in any week)*
Daytime symptoms	≤ 2/week	≥ 2/week
Limitation of activities	None	Any
Nocturnal symptoms/awakening	None	Any
Need for reliever/rescue treatment	≤ 2/week	≥ 2/week
Lung function (PEF or FEV_1)	Normal	< 80% predicted /personal best (if known)

Adapted from GINA 2006 guideline http://www.ginasthma.com 2006

Adjusting therapy based on control

Therapy incorporates medication, patient education, environmental control measures and regular follow-up. Treatment should be given for an initial period of at least 3 months to establish effectiveness in gaining control.

- If asthma is well controlled for at least 3 months, then treatment should be reduced. Therapy reduction should be gradual and closely monitored. There are few studies to guide therapy reduction. Stepping down is done as follows:
  - First discontinue oral steroids
  - Next reduce the dosage of ICS (if on high doses)
  - And thereafter discontinue additional controller treatment.

  The child should be maintained on the lowest effective dose of ICS. Assess control on a regular basis.

- If asthma is uncontrolled, the child's inhaler technique is optimal and adherence is assured, treatment must be stepped up as follows:
  - For children younger than 5 years: doubling the initial dose of ICS is the preferred controller option. Alternatively, consider adding a LTRA or LABA (LABA approved only in children > 4 years old) to the ICS. If uncontrolled on medium-dose ICS and a LTRA (or LABA in children > 4 years old), refer to a specialist for further evaluation and management.
  - For children older than 5 years: options for stepping up treatment include increasing the dose of ICS (medium to high dose) or adding a LABA or LTRA or SR theophylline (if LABA or LTRA unavailable). If still uncontrolled, refer to a specialist. The need for additional treatment should be reviewed at each visit and be maintained for as short a period as possible.

> ***Practice point:***
>
> Patients with uncontrolled asthma should be assessed for:
> - Poor adherence (common problem is confusing relievers and inhalers)
> - Poor inhaler technique
> - Exposure to trigger factors
> - Co-morbid conditions, e.g. rhinitis and sinusitis
> - Other causes of wheezing (Tables 11.1 and 11.2)
>
> Before stepping up or changing treatment, these factors should be excluded.

Acute severe asthma (status asthmaticus)

Table 11.6 Initial assessment of acute asthma in children

Symptoms	Mild	Severe[a]
Altered consciousness	No	Agitated, confused or drowsy
Oximetry on presentation[b] (SaO_2)	≥ 94%	< 90%
Talks in[c]	Sentences	Words
Accessory muscles, and suprasternal retractions	Usually not	Usually
Pulse rate	< 100 bpm[d]	> 200 bpm (0–3 years) > 180 bpm (4–5 years) > 160 bpm (> 5 years)
Pulsus paradoxus	Absent < 10 mm Hg	Often present 20–40 mm Hg
Central cyanosis	Absent	Likely to be present
Wheeze intensity	Variable	May be quiet
PEF after initial bronchodilator: % predicted or % personal best	> 80 %	< 60 %

[a] Any of these features indicates uncontrolled asthma.
[b] Oximetry performed before treatment with oxygen or bronchodilator.
[c] The normal development capability of the child must be taken into account.
[d] bpm = beats per minute

Initial management :

- *Hospitalize*: Preferably admit to a high-care or intensive care unit (ICU).
- *Oxygen*: By facemask or nasal prongs. Use a low flow rate and maintain SaO_2 > 92%.
- *Hydration*: 5% dextrose water at 60 to 80 ml/kg/day. Do not overhydrate.
- *Corticosteroids*: Prednisone 2 mg/kg/day orally for 5 days. If patient is vomiting then hydrocortisone 100–200 mg or dexamethasone 0.15 mg/kg 4–6 hourly may be given IV.

- *Inhaled β_2-agonist*: nebulized salbutamol or fenoterol (dosage < 2 yrs 0.5 ml; > 2 yrs 1 ml) added to normal saline 2 ml every 20 minutes for 3 doses (or continuously) then every 1–4 hours as needed; β_2-agonist given by metered-dose inhaler with spacer to a cooperative patient is as effective as nebulized treatment (4–8 puffs every 20 minutes for 3 doses then every 1–4 hours as needed). ☆☆☆👍
- *Inhaled ipratropium bromide* (< 2 yrs: 0.5 ml; > 2 yrs: 1 ml) may be added – possibly has a synergistic effect but no significant effect on improving lung function. ☆😐

Further management if incomplete or poor response:

- M*agnesium sulphate* 25 to 75 mg/kg/dose IV (maximum 2 g) infused over 20 min every 4 to 6 hours up to 3 to 4 doses. ☆☆☆😐
- *IV β_2-agonist* e.g. salbutamol (loading dose, followed by continuous infusion – see package insert for dosage) or *IV aminophylline* (administer only in an ICU setting and if serum theophylline levels can be monitored).

Subsequent management:

- Identify factors for poorly controlled asthma and rectify/address: adherence, inhaler technique, trigger factors, co-morbid conditions.

Recommended reading

1 Busse W et al. Expert Panel Report 3 (EPR-3): Guidelines for the diagnosis and Management of Asthma – Summary Report 2007. *J of Allergy Clin Immunol.* 2007; 120(5) Suppl. S.94–S138. Website: http://www.nhlbi.nih.gov

2 O'Byrne PM et al. GINA 2006. Guideline Executive Summary Report. *Eur Respir J.* 2008; 31(1): 143–78. Website: www.ginasthma.org

3 Motala C, Green RJ, Manjra AI, Potter PC, Zar HJ. 2009. Guideline for the management of chronic asthma in children – 2009 update. *S Afr Med J* 2009; 99:898–912. Website: www.allergysa.org

Allergic disorders

Allergic rhinitis (AR)

This affects 30–40% of children. The condition has a significant impact on quality of life, including school performance, sleep patterns and dental malocclusions. It is traditionally classified into *seasonal* (hay-fever) or *perennial* (all-year round). The classification has been revised, based on frequency of symptoms (intermittent or persistent) as well as severity of symptoms (mild, moderate or severe). (Figure 11.1)

Figure 11.1 Classification of allergic rhinitis

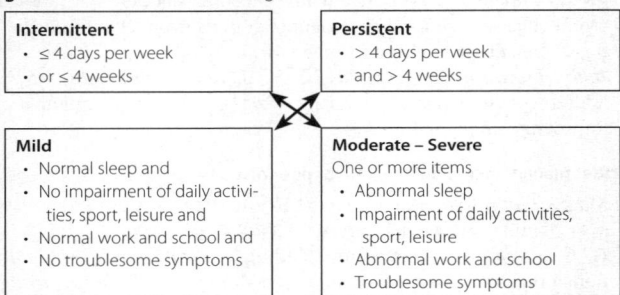

Diagnosis

- History:
  - *Symptoms*: (intermittent or persistent)
    - Nasal: congestion, rhinorrhea, pruritus, sneezing
    - Ocular: pruritus, tearing
    - Postnasal drip: sore throat, cough, pruritus.
  - *Patterns*:
    - Seasonal: depends on local allergens (grass or tree pollen)
    - Perennial: (house dust mite, grass pollen if exposure is long, moulds and pets)
    - Coexisting atopic diseases common (e.g. asthma – 40 to 80%, conjunctivitis – 50%).
- Physical examination:
  - 'Allergic facies' with shiners, mouth breathing, transverse nasal crease
  - Nasal mucosa may be normal to pink to pale gray
  - Injected sclera with or without clear discharge.
- Investigations
  - Nasal smear (Hansel's stain) for presence of eosinophils: quick, easy screen with good positive predictive value
  - Total immunoglobulin E (IgE): non-specific due to wide overlap between atopic and non-atopic subjects
  - Skin prick testing (SPT): gold standard for identifying allergen(s)
  - Radio allergosorbent testing (RAST): serum IgE to specific allergen(s) – alternative to SPT but more expensive
  - Nasal provocation test: research test only.

Differential diagnosis

This includes:

- *Vasomotor rhinitis*: Symptoms made worse by scents, alcohol, or changes in temperature or humidity
- *Adenoidal hypertrophy*
- *Rhinitis medicamentosa*: rebound rhinitis from prolonged use of nasal vasoconstrictors
- *Sinusitis*: acute or chronic
- *Non-allergic rhinitis with eosinophilia syndrome (NARES)*
- *Nasal polyps*.

Treatment

- Allergen avoidance:
  - Relies on identification of triggers.
  - Difficult to avoid ubiquitous airborne allergens.
- Medications
  - *Oral antihistamines:*
    - Effective for histamine-related symptoms such as itching, rhinorrhoea and sneezing but little effect on nasal blockage. ☆☆☆☺
    - Second-generation preparations (Table 11.7) non- or less-sedating; long-acting, preferable to older antihistamines (sedating and psychomotor adverse effects; required more frequently). ☆☆☆☆

Table 11.7: Recommended daily dosage of new generation antihistamines in children

	2–5 yrs	*6–11 yrs	≥12 yrs
Cetirizine*	2.5–5 mg	5–10 mg	10 mg
Fexofenadine			120 mg
Loratadine*	2.5 mg	5–10 mg	10 mg
Desloratadine	1.25 mg	2.5 mg	5 mg
Levocetirizine			5 mg

* *children < 30 kg: 5 mg; > 30 kg: 10 mg*

  - *Intranasal corticosteroids*:
    - Treatment of choice for persistent moderate-severe AR.
    - Most effective maintenance therapy for nasal congestion. ☆☆☆☆☆
    - Available preparations: beclomethasone, budesonide, fluticasone, mometasone, triamcinolone.

- Dosage: 1 puff/nostril daily (NB: beclomethasone ideally to be given twice/day)
- Adverse effects: nasal irritation, sneezing, bleeding. No proven adverse effect on long-term growth.
  - *Decongestants*:
    - May be effective in the short term (5–7 days).
    - Adverse effects (with prolonged use): anxiety, insomnia, rebound symptoms, tachycardia.
  - *Nasal rinsing*:
    - Hypertonic saline.
    - Well tolerated and inexpensive.
- *Immunotherapy* (injection or sublingual): effective in selected patients (e.g. monosensitive to grass pollen or house dust mite). Consider when pharmacotherapy is ineffective, unacceptable side effects of medication occur or triggering allergens are difficult to avoid. Not recommended in poorly compliant patients or those with uncontrolled asthma and children < 5 years. ☆☆☆☺

Food allergy

Definition

Immunologically mediated adverse reactions to food (IgE or non-IgE). IgE-mediated reactions occur less than 2 hours after food ingestion; non-IgE mediated reactions occur several hours or days later. Few foods commonly provoke symptoms: cow's milk, eggs, and peanuts in infants and young children; fish, shellfish, fruit, peanuts, tree nuts and spices in older children and adults.

Manifestations

- IgE-mediated allergic reactions to food: several organ systems may be involved, including the gastrointestinal (GI) tract, the skin, the cardiovascular system (anaphylaxis) and the respiratory tract (Table 11.8). The skin and the GI tract are the most commonly affected systems. It is unusual for respiratory symptoms to be the only manifestations of food allergy. Anaphylaxis is the most severe allergic reaction to food.
- Mixed IgE/Non-IgE mediated reactions: include atopic dermatitis and the eosinophilic enteropathies (oesophagitis, gastroenteritis, proctocolitis).
- Non-IgE mediated reactions: include food-induced enterocolitis and food-induced colitis in young children. Most commonly caused by allergy to cow's milk and soya proteins.

Table 11.8 IgE-mediated manifestations of food allergy

Gastrointestinal tract:	Oral allergy syndrome, infantile colic, vomiting, diarrhoea, abdominal pain
Skin:	Urticaria, angio-oedema, atopic dermatitis
Respiratory tract:	Rhinitis, asthma, laryngeal oedema
Cardiovascular system:	Anaphylaxis

Diagnosis

The accurate diagnosis of food allergy is critically dependent on a good history.

- History:
  - Identify suspected foods
  - Establish timing and nature of reactions; patients should keep a food diary.
- Physical examination: findings will depend on the manifestations of food allergy.
- Investigations – for IgE-mediated food allergy:
  - *Skin prick testing*:
    Has a modest positive predictive value (PPV), but very good negative predictive value. Fresh food extracts are more sensitive and specific than commercial allergen extracts. Ideally, should be performed in a setting where resuscitation facilities are readily available (because of small risk of anaphylaxis). Skin tests are interpreted by comparing the size of the wheal and flare responses to positive (histamine) or negative (diluent) controls. The tests may be scored using either qualitative (0–4+) or quantitative (diameter of wheal and flare in millimetres) measurements. In the case of inhalant and injectant allergens, a prick test producing a wheal at least 3 mm larger than the negative control usually indicates a clinically significant response. The cut-off values of positive or negative SPTs for food allergens are much higher. (Table 11.9).
  - *RAST immunoassay (specific IgE levels)*:
    specific IgE level > 0.35 ku/L has poor positive predicted value; < 0.35 ku/L has good negative predictive value. Levels above a certain threshold have increasing positive predictive value and vary for individual food allergens. (Table 11.9) ☆☆☆☺
  - *Oral challenge testing*:
    must be performed under medical supervision with intravenous (IV) access for giving emergency treatment if needed. Double-blind-placebo-controlled food challenge testing, using graded doses of disguised food, is the gold standard (performed in

specialized units only). Open challenges useful for refuting the diagnosis of food allergy.

Table 11.9 Diagnosis of food allergies with the use of 95% PPV for specific skin-prick tests and IgE

Food	95% PPV for skin-prick test wheal diameter * mm	95% PPV for specific IgE** kU/liter
Egg	7 (5+)	7 (2+)
Milk	8 (6+)	15 (5+)
Peanuts	8 (4+)	14
Fish	7	20
Tree nuts	8	15

+ cut-off value for infants < 2years
* Adapted from Sporik et al: Clin Exp Allergy 2000; 30:1540–1546
** Adapted from Sampson HA: J Allergy Clin Immunol 2001; 107:891–896

> ### Practice points:
>
> In patients with a strongly suggestive history of an IgE-mediated food allergic reaction, food challenges should be performed even if the food specific IgE level is below the cut-off values.
>
> No reliable diagnostic tests are currently available for non-IgE-mediated food allergy – diagnosis depends upon history, observation of the effect of exclusion diets and where necessary, blinded food challenges, endoscopy and biopsy.

Treatment

- Avoidance of the offending food(s) is the mainstay of treatment.
- Patients must be managed in collaboration with a dietician.
- Pharmacotherapy for the specific manifestations may be necessary, e.g. topical steroids and emollients for eczema.

Anaphylaxis

Definition

Anaphylaxis is the clinical syndrome of immediate hypersensitivity. It is characterized by cardiovascular collapse, respiratory compromise, cutaneous symptoms (e.g. urticaria) and gastrointestinal symptoms (e.g. vomiting).

It may be IgE-mediated (allergic anaphylaxis) or non-IgE mediated (anaphylactoid or non-allergic). Different *patterns* include uniphasic, biphasic (late phase 3–8 hours after initial reaction) or protracted (duration 3–21 days). *Causes* include foods (e.g. peanuts), antibiotics (e.g. penicillin) and stinging insects (e.g. bee).

Initial investigation

- *Serum tryptase*: most useful test for confirming occurrence of anaphylaxis. Tryptase level increased in anaphylaxis, peaks at 45–60 minutes and may remain elevated for several hours. Should be measured within an hour of the reaction and a second sample taken within 24 hours.

Initial management

- *ABCs*: establish *airway* if necessary. Assess *breathing*; supply with 100% O_2 with respiratory support as needed. Assess *circulation* and establish IV access. Place patient on cardiac monitor.
- *Adrenaline*: give 0.01 ml/kg (1:1000) intramuscularly (IM), maximum dose 0.5 ml. Repeat every 15 minutes as needed. The site of choice is the lateral aspect of the thigh due to its vascularity. ☆☆☆☆◈
- *ß₂-agonist*: give nebulised salbutamol 0.05–0.15 mg/kg in 3 ml normal saline solution (quick estimate: 2.5 mg for < 30 kg, 5 mg for > 30 kg) every 15 minutes as needed.
- *Antihistamine-1 receptor antagonist*: such as diphenhydramine, 1–2 mg/kg IM, IV, or oral (PO) route (maximum dose 50 mg); promethazine 0.25–0.5 mg/kg IM.
- *Corticosteroids*: help prevent the late phase of the allergic response. Administer methylprednisolone in a 2 mg/kg IV bolus, then 2 mg/kg per day IV or IM divided every 6 hours, or prednisone, 2 mg/kg PO in a bolus once daily. Observe for 6 to 24 hours for late-phase symptoms depending on clinical condition and stability.

Management of hypotension

- *Trendelenburg position*: put patient's head at 30-degree angle below feet.
- *Fluid*: administer 20 ml/kg IV normal saline or Ringer's lactate solution over 5 to 15 minutes. Repeat bolus as necessary.
- *Adrenaline*: Give 0.1 ml/kg (1:10 000) IV every 2–5 minutes while an adrenaline or dopamine infusion is being prepared.

Post-treatment steps

- Identify the offending allergen:
  - IgE-mediated reactions: RAST as a first step, SPT if RAST is negative. Challenge testing: if SPT and RAST negative: preferably performed in ICU setting (facilities available for prompt resuscitation).
  - Non-IgE mediated reactions: currently no reliable laboratory tests are available for detecting these reactions.
  - Strict avoidance of offending agent *(patient education)*.
- *Provide injectable adrenaline* (Epipen® or adrenaline vial plus syringe and needle). Training on correct use is essential.
- *Immunotherapy* in the case of bee venom sensitivity.

Urticaria and angio-oedema

Definition

Intensely itchy lesions vary from erythema with minimal oedema to massive wheals of the skin and mucosal surfaces with or without respiratory compromise.

Classification

Urticaria may be acute (< 6 weeks duration) or chronic (> 6 weeks duration). *Chronic urticaria* may be episodic (recurrent) or persistent. Approximately 50% of affected patients have both urticaria and angio-oedema, 40% urticaria alone, and 10% only angio-oedema.

Differential diagnosis (clinical evaluation)

The diagnosis of urticaria is primarily clinical. The duration of wheals, features of the rash and identification of the triggering factor (stimulus) may be helpful in arriving at an initial diagnosis.

- The wheals of *ordinary urticaria* last less than 24 hours. *Acute ordinary urticaria* is more likely to follow a mild viral infection than an allergy. *Episodic urticaria* may be due to drug or dietary exposures but often remains unexplained. *Chronic urticaria* frequently follows a remitting and relapsing course and is worse at night (30% have autoantibodies – this is autoimmune urticaria).
- *Urticarial vasculitis*: clinical clues include systemic symptoms (fever and arthralgia or arthritis) and lesions lasting for more than 24 hours, or associated with tenderness, petechiae, purpura or skin staining as the lesions fade.
- *Physical urticarias*: wheaIing occurs in response to a specific physical stimulus (mechanical trauma, temperature change, light and water).

Usually appear within 10 minutes of the physical stimulus and clear within an hour, except delayed pressure urticaria (develops 2–4 hours after exposure to pressure and lasts for 24–48 hours). *Cold urticaria* is commonest of physical urticarias, affects extremities and face, and may be induced by cold weather, handling cold objects, cold shower or skiing. Diagnosis is confirmed by application of an ice cube.
- *Angio-oedema* may accompany wheals in most patterns of urticaria but may, less commonly, occur without wheals, as in hereditary angio-oedema (C1 esterase inhibitor deficiency).
- *Contact urticaria*: wheals localized, develop within minutes of stimulus and usually short-lived, e.g. contact urticaria to allergens such as peanuts or latex.

Investigations

- These should be guided by the history and clinical presentation. In general laboratory tests are unnecessary for mild ordinary urticaria that responds to antihistamines.
- *Baseline investigations* for chronic ordinary urticaria should include FBC, ESR and urine dipsticks for underlying infection, systemic disease or urticarial vasculitis.

Treatment

- Avoidance of identified triggers is the first step.
- *Antihistamines* are the mainstay of treatment for acute and chronic urticaria. The new generation antihistamines are preferred to the older antihistamines. Combinations of antihistamines may improve symptom control, e.g. use of 2 different second-generation antihistamines; alternatively a second-generation antihistamine in the morning and short-term use of a first-generation antihistamine in the evening. ☆☆☆☆☆

> *Practice point:*
>
> Higher than recommended doses of antihistamine are frequently required for adequate control. Patients with difficult-to-control chronic urticaria should be referred to a specialist/tertiary centre.

Recommended reading

1. Donald YM, Leung Hugh A, Sampson Raif S, Geha Stanley, Szefler J *Pediatric Allergy – Principles and Practice*. Mosby 2003. St. Louis, Missouri
2. *The ALLSA Handbook of Practical Allergy*. Cape Town. Available from the Allergy Society of S.A. PO Box 88, Observatory, 7935. Website: www.allergysa.org
3. Useful website: www.foodallergy.org

Immunology

Immunodeficiency diseases

Definitions

Primary immunodeficiency diseases (PIDs): a rare group of genetic conditions that result in a spectrum of intrinsic immunological defects, affecting various aspects of immunological function. Broad groups include antibody deficiencies, T-cell disorders, combined T- and B-cell deficiencies, phagocyte disorders, and complement deficiencies. More than 50% of all patients with PIDs manifest as antibody deficiencies.

Secondary immunodeficiency diseases (SIDs): a group of acquired conditions in which exogenous factors impair immunological function, e.g. protein-energy malnutrition, protein losing states, infections such as HIV, CMV and measles, and immunosuppressive therapy.

Clinical features

Immunodeficiency diseases may present with a wide spectrum of clinical manifestations including bronchiectasis, chronic liver disease, autoimmune manifestations, adverse reactions to vaccines and delayed umbilical cord separation. Recurrent or atypical infection is common.

Table 11.10 Common manifestations of primary immunodeficiency

Eight or more ear infections per annum
Two or more serious sinus infections per annum
Two or more months of antibiotics with little effect
Two or more pneumonias within 1 year
Recurrent deep-seated or organ abscesses
Persistent thrush of mouth, nails or skin
Two or more deep-seated infections, e.g. osteomyelitis, meningitis, septicaemia
Infection caused by unusual organisms
Failure to thrive
Family history of primary immunodeficiency disease

Normal pre-school children may experience between 6 and 12 minor infections per annum. Children with more frequent, severe, persistent, or atypical infections should be investigated for underlying causes. In addition to the immunodeficiency diseases, several groups of conditions may cause or mimic recurrent infection:
- *Increased exposure to microorganisms:* overcrowding, poor environmental hygiene, poverty, and pre-school attendance increase the exposure of young children to microorganisms, especially during the winter months.
- *Anatomical abnormalities*: obstruction to drainage of secretions promotes microbial growth and chronicity. Examples include middle ear infection caused by Eustachian tube obstruction, chronic sinusitis and upper respiratory tract infection due to adenoidal hypertrophy, and persistent lung infection due to a bronchial foreign body or bronchial narrowing. Furthermore, urinary tract abnormalities, cerebrospinal leaks, and upper gastrointestinal disorders (e.g. gastro-oesophageal reflux or tracheo-oesophageal fistula) are associated with recurrent infection. A distinctive feature of anatomical abnormalities is that infection recurs at the same site.
- *Allergy:* allergic inflammation and mucosal swelling frequently mimics recurrent infection. Allergies may be associated with recurrent infection due to subtle PIDs.
- *Delayed maturation of the immune system:* at birth innate immunity (complement, neutrophils, and local barriers) is immature and specific immunity (B and T lymphocytes) is naïve, reducing the responsiveness of the immune system. Passively acquired maternal IgG (transplacentally) and IgA (breast milk) provides protection during the first 6 to 9 months of life. The immune system gradually develops, usually reaching a state of maturity during early childhood. IgG (particularly IgG_2 and IgG_4 subclasses) and IgA levels are slow to mature. Transient hypogammaglobulinaemia of infancy may occasionally persist until the age of 2 years or longer, causing increased infectious susceptibility during early childhood.

Diagnosis

Before investigating children for PIDs, SIDs, increased environmental exposure to infection, anatomical abnormalities, and allergy should be considered. HIV infection must be specifically excluded.

General immunological testing should follow a structured approach (Table 11.11, steps 1–3). Interpretation of the results and advanced testing (step 4) requires consultation with a specialist.

Table 11.11: Immunological testing

Step 1
History, physical examination, mass and height
Exclude HIV infection
Full blood count and differential count
Immunoglobulin levels (IgA, IgM, IgG, IgE)
Step 2
Specific antibody responses (tetanus, diphtheria)
Response to pneumococcal vaccine (pre- and post-titres)
IgG subclass analysis
Step 3
Lymphocyte subsets (CD3, CD4, CD8, CD19, CD16/56)
Complement screen (CH50)
Neutrophil oxidation burst
Step 4
Advanced testing

Adapted from the approach of the Jeffery Modell Foundation

Treatment of PIDs

Treatment depends on the type of PID. Many antibody deficiencies and combined deficiencies require immunoglobulin replacement therapy (IVIG), generally 300–600 mg per kg every 3 to 4 weeks. ☆☆☆☆☆

Life-long replacement is required for severe, genetically confirmed deficiencies. In conditions without a molecular genetic diagnosis, IVIG should initially be administered for 1 to 5 years followed by re-evaluation of serum immunoglobulin concentrations, since hypogammaglobulinaemia may be transient and resolve spontaneously. IVIG is not indicated for IgA deficiency.

Adverse reactions to IVIG: anaphylactic reactions are extremely rare but have been described in IgA-deficient patients with circulating anti-IgA antibodies. Infusions should be given under the same supervision as required for blood transfusions. Common side-effects (nausea, chills, headache, backache, malaise, fever, pruritis, and tingling) occur in ± 10% of infusions and are mainly related to the rate of infusion. Therefore the initial infusion rate should be 10 ml/hour and, if tolerated, gradually increased to 40 ml/hour. Recurring side-effects can be modified or prevented by administering aspirin (15 mg/kg/dose, PO) ibuprofen (5 mg/kg/dose, PO) or hydrocortisone (6 mg/kg/dose, IV, maximum 100 mg) 1 hour before infusion. There is no risk of HIV or hepatitis B transmission. Some immunoglobulin preparations have been associated with outbreaks of non-A, non-B hepatitis, including hepatitis C.

In children receiving long-term IVIG, alanine aminotransferase (ALT) levels should be monitored 6-monthly. IVIG is expensive. Local products (e.g. Polygam®, National Bioproducts Institute) have reduced cost.

In milder conditions (e.g. IgA deficiency and transient hypogammaglobulinaemia of infancy) recurrent infections may be controlled with prophylactic antibiotics, e.g. amoxicillin, 10–25 mg/kg/dose twice daily or azithromycin, 10 mg/kg/dose weekly. ☆☆☺

Bone marrow transplantation (BMT) is the treatment of choice of severe immunodeficiencies such as severe combined immunodeficiency (SCID) or T-cell deficiencies. ☆☆☆☆⚑

During the pre-BMT phase, children with SCID may benefit from broad-spectrum antimicrobial prophylaxis plus IVIG. Other therapies include cytokines such as interferon-γ for chronic granulomatous disease, myeloid haematopoietic growth factors for congenital and cyclical neutropaenia, and enzyme replacement for adenosine deaminase deficiency.

> *Practice point:*
>
> Blood products for patients with T-cell dysfunction should always be irradiated to prevent graft-versus-host disease.

12 Development

V. Ramanjam

An approach to developmental disabilities

Definitions

Development is the progressive acquiring of new skills over time and reflects the integrity of the CNS. It is assessed in the following areas:
- Gross motor
- Fine motor
- Language and communication
- Adaptive and social functioning.

Developmental delay is the failure to attain appropriate milestones for a child's corrected age in 1 or more areas of development (corrected until 2 years in premature infants). All children do not develop at the same rate, nor do they develop at the same rate in all areas of development. When milestones are below average they should be monitored and intervention recommended. Milestones reflected in a chart usually represent the average.

Impairment is an abnormality of body structure or function.

Disability is a failure of a function or skill, e.g. seeing, hearing, walking, writing, conceptualising, or any other function within the normal range for age.

Handicap is a disability with substantial or permanent effect on normal growth (WHO).

Prevalence of developmental disability

- Approximately 1 in 10 children are affected.
- Low morbidity, milder disorders occur more frequently and are more common, e.g. learning disability, attention deficit hyperactivity disorder (ADHD).
- High morbidity, more severe disorders are less common and tend to have an organic cause, e.g. cerebral palsy.

Developmental disorders: classification into global or focal

Global disorders

These include:
- Intellectual disability
- Pervasive developmental/autistic spectrum disorders
- Cultural or environmental deprivation.

Focal disorders

These include:
- Disorders of language and communication:
  - Hearing impairment
  - Speech impediments
  - Developmental language disorders.
- Gross motor disorders:
  - Cerebral palsy
  - Neuromuscular disorders
  - Orthopaedic problems
  - Chronic disease
  - Motor maturational delay.
- Fine motor disorders:
  - Developmental coordination disorder (DCD)
  - Visual-motor integration problems (VMI)
  - Sensory integration problems
  - Visual impairment secondary to gross motor problems.

An approach to intellectual disability

Definitions

Intellectual disability is defined as:
- Significant limitations in intellectual functioning and in adaptive behaviour including everyday social and practical skills, which originates before 18 years of age.
- Measured as > 2 standard deviations below the norm on a psycho-educational assessment (IQ) with 2 or more deficits in adaptive functioning:
  - Mild (IQ 50–74): can be included in mainstream education if the necessary support is provided. Unlikely to manage in mainstream without support.
  - Moderate (IQ 35–50): generally attend 'special needs schools', which cater to individual disabilities, most cannot live

independently as adults but may be able to participate in supervised tasks.
- Severe (IQ 20–34) and Profound (IQ < 20): individuals are fully dependant for daily needs, eligible for care dependency grants.

Prevalence

- 1–3% of the population.
- Mild intellectual disability is more common and may be secondary to chronic illness, malnutrition, prolonged poverty, and other social causes.
- Moderate to severe intellectual disability is more likely due to a specific or organic cause.

Global developmental delay

- Usually implies a younger child (< 5 years) who has a functional level 2 or more standard deviations below the population mean in 2 or more developmental areas, i.e. gross motor, fine motor, speech and language, personal and social.
- Global developmental delay may overlap with, but is not synonymous with, intellectual disability, e.g. a child with cerebral palsy with significant gross and fine motor delay, but cognition may be spared. Some of these children catch up with intervention.

Aetiology of developmental disabilities

This is illustrated in Table 12.1.

Table 12.1 The aetiology of developmental disorders

Time of Insult	Cause	Example
Prenatal	Genetic/chromosomal abnormality	Down's syndrome Fragile X syndrome
	Structural brain malformations	Schizencephaly Lissencephaly
	Intra-uterine insult	Antenatal bleed Trauma
	Toxins/drugs	Fetal alcohol syndrome Maternal tik use
	Intra-uterine infection	Rubella, toxoplasma, CMV, HIV
	Unknown	Multiple congenital abnormalities
Postnatal	Complications of prematurity	Intraventricular bleeds Hypoxia and/or infection – causing cerebral palsy

Time of Insult	Cause	Example
Postnatal	Complications of labour	Hypoxic ischaemia Encephalopathy Meconium aspiration Sepsis
	Sepsis	Meningitis HIV TB
	Head injury	Accidental/abuse
	Other	Severe dehydration Chronic illness Malnutrition
Idiopathic	No cause identified after full investigation	

Approach to a child with developmental delay

- Identify children at risk at every health care visit, e.g. neonatal unit, routine immunisation visits, when seen with acute illness.
- Children with environmental risk factors need regular surveillance, e.g. poverty, community and family deprivation/dysfunction, exposure to substance abuse, abuse, neglect, or mental health problems in parents.

Figure 12.1 An approach to a child with developmental delay (see next page)

Cerebral palsy

Definition

- An umbrella term for a group of non-progressive but changing motor impairment syndromes caused by an insult to the developing brain. While the lesion does not progress or resolve, the clinical presentation may change with time. Gross motor signs and symptoms predominate but all areas of development may be affected, and there may be many other associated complications, e.g. seizures, cognitive impairment etc.

Prevalence

- The most common motor disability in childhood
- In developed countries prevalence is approximately 2 per 1 000.
- Presumed to be higher in developing countries.

Figure 12.1 An approach to a child with developmental delay

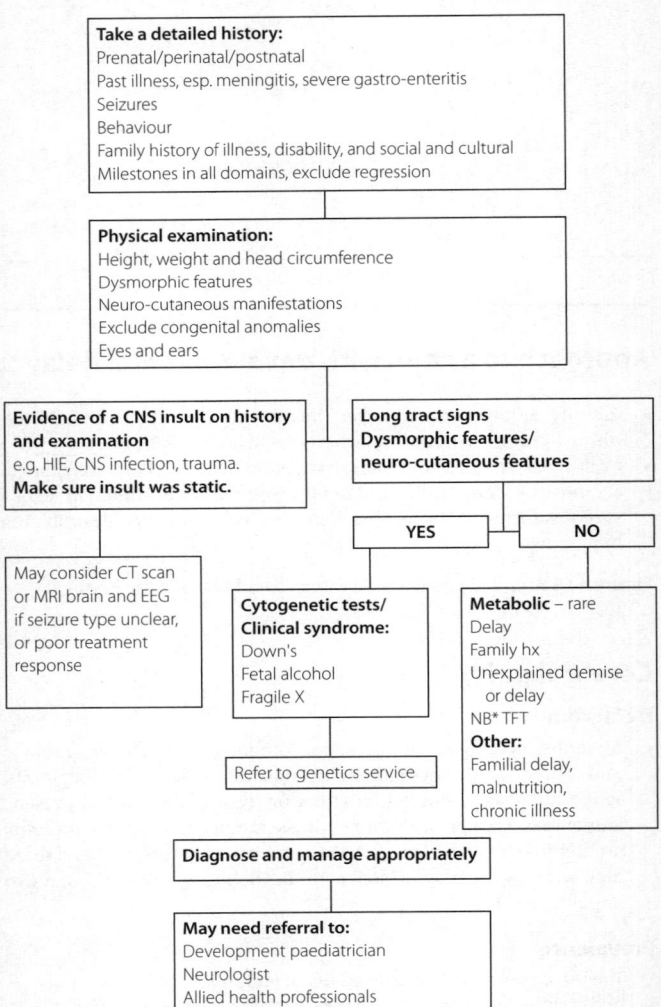

Classification
- Usually according to the physiological type and topography.
- Should also emphasize functional limitation.
- Gross motor function classification system – describes 5 groups based on functional ability.
- NB: Isolated hypotonia and intellectual disability is not cerebral palsy.

Types:
1. Spastic (most common): quadraplegic, hemiplegic, diplegic, triplegic.
2. Dyskinetic: Athetoid, choreo-athetoid, dystonic (variable tone).
3. Ataxic: often associated with hypotonia, need to exclude other causes of ataxia.
4. Mixed: all forms may co-exist.

Approach to management of a child with cerebral palsy

1. Detailed history to identify aetiology (NB: Follow up all high risk neonates)
2. Make sure insult was static and non-progressive
3. General, systemic and detailed CNS examination:
   - Exclude co-morbid conditions
   - Assess nutrition and growth
   - Ability to swallow/ feed/cough
   - Vision and hearing
   - Mobility
   - Secondary complications, e.g. contractures, scoliosis, constipation.
   - Assess functional ability
   - Developmental assessment.
4. Investigations:
   - CT scan or MRI if cause not clear or needs clarification
   - Vision and hearing
   - EEG if seizure type unclear
   - Others: exclude gastro-oesophageal reflux if symptoms suggest
   - X-ray: spine and hips if clinical scoliosis or dislocation of hips
5. REFER EARLY:
   - Physiotherapy

- Speech and feeding therapist
- Occupational therapy
- Dietician
- Developmental paediatrician/child neurology
- Social worker
- Orthopaedic surgeon
- Treat associated complications early, e.g. seizures, gastro-oesophageal reflux, painful dislocated hips.
- Early intervention maximizes the child's developmental potential.

The optimal management of a child with cerebral palsy/global delay involves a multidisciplinary team focusing on early intervention therapy.

Developmental milestones and warning signs

Areas to consider
- Gross motor
- Fine motor/vision
- Hearing and speech
- Personal/social
- Warning signs.

Expected skills	Warning signs
Newborn period	
• Almost complete head lag. Ventral suspension: head droops, hips flex, limbs hang downwards. Moro, palmar and plantar grasp reflexes present. • Hands closed. Closes eyes to sudden bright light. • Stills to sound. Startles to sudden loud sounds. • Alternates between drowsiness and alert wakefulness – findings during examination are dependent on these states. • Vigorous cry.	• Poor sucking. • Lack of arousal (stupor or coma). • High-pitched or weak cry. • Abnormal (incomplete or absent) Moro response • Opisthotonus. • Flaccidity or hypertonia. • Convulsions. • Tremulous limbs. • Failure of tonic deviation of eyes on passive movement of head or of head and body.

Expected skills	Warning signs
6 weeks	
• Some head control. Prone: head to side, buttocks moderately high. Ventral suspension: head is in line with body and hips well extended. • Moro reflex present. • Stares, eyes fixated on objects. Follows horizontally to 90°. Places hand in mouth. • Startle response. • Smiles at mother. Suckles vigorously. • Adopts tonic asymmetrical neck postures (tonic neck reflexes). • Support and stepping unelicitable • Vertical suspension—legs flex, head up. • Optokinetic nystagmus elicitable.	• No visual fixation or following. • Failure to smile. • No response to sound. • Absence of any or all of the normal functions. • Convulsions. • Hypotonia or hypertonia of neck and limbs.
3 months	
• Pull to sit: little/no head lag. • Prone: supports on forearms, lifts head, buttocks flat. Beginning to develop reflex standing when held, i.e. primary extension phase. Rolls over. Moro begins to disappear. • Follows through 180°. Hands loosely open. Holds rattle placed in hand. Watches own hand. Pulls at clothes. • Coos and chuckles. Quieting with familiar sounds. Turns head to sound. • Excited when fed. Reacts to familiar situations. • Adopts tonic asymmetrical neck postures (tonic neck reflexes) • Support and stepping unelicitable • Vertical suspension – legs flex, head up • Optokinetic nystagmus elicitable.	• As for previous weeks. Excessive startling to visual stimuli – does not hear well. • Absent vocalization.

Expected skills	Warning signs
5–6 months	
- Pull to sit: braces shoulders and pulls to sit. Sits with support. Prone: lifts up head and chest. Support on extended arms and hands. Reaches out with one hand while supported on the other. Supine: lifts leg and plays with feet; feet to mouth. - Reaches for objects with the centre of palm, grasps with all fingers. Radial approach to toy. Shadow reaction in opposite arm (have not usually started transferring). - Babbling begins at about 4 months, repetitive and vowel-like (sing-song). Turns to mother's voice across the room. Laughs aloud. - Takes everything to mouth. Responds to mirror image. Starts holding bottle. Shows likes and dislikes. - Discriminates between family and strangers. - Primitive reflexes disappear. - Tries to recover lost object. - Landau response (postural reflex) is present.	- Failure to use both hands. - Squint. - Failure to turn to sound. - Poor response to people. - Little vocalization. - Obligatory postures. - Cannot sit or roll over. - Hypo- or hypertonia. - Persistent primitive reflexes. - No Landau response.
9 months	
- Sits without support and can move body without losing balance. Rolls. Crawls forwards or backwards. Rocks on all fours. Pulls to stand. - Immediately reaches out. Holds a cube in each hand, with flexible finger approach. Picks up small toy with ends of fingers. Removes peg man or object from hole; cannot return it. Points.	- Unable to sit. Hand preference present. Fisting. Squint. Persistence of primitive reflexes. Monotonous vocalization. - Fails to attain these motor, verbal, and social milestones. - Persistent automatisms and tonic neck reflexes or hypo- or hypertonia.

Expected skills	Warning signs
9 months (continued)	
• Vocalizes deliberately. Babbles. Imitates sounds. Understands 'bye-bye' or 'no'. • Stranger anxiety. • Drinks from cup. • Sociable; plays 'pat-a-cake', seeks attention. • Landau response present. • Parachute response present.	
10 months	
• Pulls to stand. Lifts one foot. Walks with both hands held. May cruise around furniture. Sitting: beginning protective extension of arms backwards. • Picks up small objects between thumb and index finger. Voluntary release begins. • Shakes head for no. Waves bye-bye. Says one word with meaning. • Plays peek-a-boo/hide and seek.	• As for previous months.
12 months	
• Bear walks. Stands alone. Walks around furniture lifting one foot and stepping sideways. May walk alone with feet wide and arms in high-guard. • Pincer grasp. Releases object on request. Begins to throw objects to floor. Mouthing virtually stopped. Looks for toys when out of sight. • Knows own name. Jargons. Two to 3 words with meaning. Echoes sounds. Understands simple instructions. • Finger feeds. • Pushes arm into sleeve. • Plays games.	• Unable to sit or bear weight. Abnormal grasp. • Failure to respond to sound. No spontaneous vocalization. • Failure to attain 12-month milestones. • Persistence of automatisms.

Expected skills	Warning signs
15 months	
- Walks alone with uneven steps. Steps with arms out for balance. Collapses backward. Creeps upstairs, goes downstairs backwards. - Two-cube tower. Holds 2 cubes in one hand. - Jabbers with expression. Two to 6 words spoken. Points at objects on request. - Picks up, drinks from, and puts down cup. Attempts feeding with spoon and spills most. - Indicates wet nappy. - Scribbles with crayon. - Interest in sounds, music, pictures, and animal toys.	- Retardation in reaching milestones expected at this age. - Persistent abnormalities of tone and posture. - Sensory discriminations defective.
18 months	
- Walks well with arms down, and can stop and start. Cannot turn unless still. Pulls a toy. Throws a ball. Climbs onto a chair. Seats self on chair. - Three-cube tower. Scribbles. May show hand preference. - Uses 6 to 20+ recognizable words. Begins to put 2 words together. - Handles spoon and cup. Enjoys picture books. Takes off shoes, socks. Domestic mimicry. - Says at least 6 words. - Feeds self; uses spoon well. - May obey commands. - Runs stiffly; seats self in chair. - Hand dominance. - Throws ball. - Plays several nursery games. - Uses simple tools in imitation. - Removes shoes and stockings.	- Failure to walk. - No pincer grip. - Inability to understand simple commands. - No speech. - Mouthing. Drooling.

Expected skills	Warning signs
18 months (continued)	
• Points to 2 or 3 parts of body, common objects, and pictures in book.	
24 months	
• Up and down steps with 2 feet per steps. Runs. Can kick a ball. Squats, rises without hand support. Can plan movement (under/over).	• Unable to understand simple commands. • Tremor. • In-coordination. • Severe clumsiness.
• Six-cube tower. Train with cubes. Imitates vertical line. Scribbles	
• Hand preference usually obvious.	
• Short phrases. Uses 50+ words. Puts 2 or 3 words together. Asks for drink, toilet, food. Helps to undress	
• Listens to stories with pictures	
• Spoon feeds without spilling. Clean and dry by day.	
• Pretend play.	
30 months	
• Jumps on both feet; walks on tiptoes if asked.	
• Knows full name; asks questions	
• Refers to self as 'I'.	
• Helps put away toys and clothes.	
• Names animals in book, knows 1 to 3 colours.	
36 months	
• Rides a tricycle. Up steps 1 foot per step. Down steps 2 feet per step. Climbs. Walks on tiptoe. Throws and kicks ball. Stands on one foot momentarily.	• Ataxia. Using single words only.

Expected skills	Warning signs

36 months (continued)

- Nine-cube tower. Builds bridge with cubes. Copies circle. Cuts with scissors. Three-piece form-board; threads large beads.
- Knows name and sex. Uses pronouns. Talks incessantly. Large vocabulary, intelligible to strangers.
- Toilet trained. Dresses with supervision.
- Washes and dries hands.
- Plays simple games.
- Identifies 5 colours.

48 months

- Up and down stairs with 1 foot per step. Stands on 1 (preferred) foot for 3 to 5 seconds. Hops on preferred foot.
- Copies cross. Five-cube gate/bridge. Coloured form-board 5 out of 5.
- Cuts out pictures with scissors. Copies cross and circle. Draws a human figure with 2 to 4 parts other than head.
- Starting to count. Knows big and small.
- Full name and age. Recognizes colours.
- Speech is grammatically correct and intelligible.
- Eats with spoon and fork. Dresses and undresses. Make-believe play. Always asking questions.
- Goes to toilet alone.

Warning signs (48 months):
- Speech difficult to understand because of poor articulation or omission of consonants.
- Poor gross or fine motor skills.

Expected skills	Warning signs
60 months	
- Walks easily on narrow line. Can hop on each foot separately. - Six-cube steps. Copies square and triangle. Draws a man with all features. Can print a few letters, good pencil control. - Fluent speech. Full name, age, birthday, address. Uses complex sentences e.g. the use of conjunctions such as 'although' (if English speaking). Knows 3 opposites. - Uses knife and fork competently (if culturally appropriate). Undresses and dresses alone. Chooses own friends. - Names 4 colors; counts to 10.	- Emotional immaturity. - Clumsiness and poor fine motor skills.
72 months	
- Sits up without help of hands. Walks backwards along straight line (10 paces). - Ten-cube steps. Copies diamond but oddly shaped. - Learns irregular forms of nouns and verbs. Learns comparatives. - Cooperative play – leadership and division of labour.	- Clumsy. - Poor posture. - Poor pencil grip.

—Adapted from Kibel and Wagstaff. *Child Health for All*. 2nd ed. Cape Town. Oxford University Press. 1995.

Recommended reading

1. Roberts G, et al. A rational approach to the medical evaluation of a child with developmental delay. *Contemp Pediatr.* March 2004.
2. Shevell M, et al. Practice Parameter: Evaluation of the Child with global developmental delay. *Neurology* 2003;60:367–380
3. Bax M et al. Proposed Definition and Classification of Cerebral Palsy. *Dev Med Child Neurol* 2005, 47:571–576
4. Kibel, MA and Wagstaff, LA. (Eds) *Child Health for All* 2nd ed. Cape Town. Oxford University Press. 1995
5. Adams and Victor's Neurology. Normal Development and Deviations in Development of the Nervous System. *Access Medicine*. June. 2009. http://www.accessmedicine.com

13 Child psychiatry

A. Flisher, G. Riordan

Autistic-like conditions and autism

Definition

These fall within the group of pervasive development disorders (PDDs). They manifest in early childhood and are characterized by serious delays and deviations in development such as impairment in social interaction, communication and imagination (associated with repetitive and stereotyped patterns of behaviour, interests and activities).

Many children have mental handicap, but an increasing number with normal intelligence are now recognized (the PDD-NOS 'borderline' or 'atypical' child).

Although the outcome for severely affected children is poor, early detection and referral is crucial. Timely intervention provides an opportunity for social integration and may affect the developmental outcome, particularly in mild cases.

Clinical features

Clinical features can include:
- Poor eye contact
- Failure to show communicative intent, i.e. to use sounds/words for communication (not just repetitively)
- Inability to engage in 'pretend' games, e.g. peek-a-boo
- Failure to develop joint attention (e.g. failure to look at an object pointed out by the mother – the child looks at her finger, not at the object)
- Failure to point to objects of interest.

These signs indicate that the child is not developing a shared social language. In some cases a socially deviant pattern of interacting may be observed before 18 months.

Autistic children who are mildly affected present in the pre-school years as social 'misfits' or 'strange' with idiosyncratic preoccupations and abnormalities of speech/behaviour. This pattern is common.

Less common, but more typical, are those who appear to live in their own world, act 'as if deaf' and have various behavioural disturbances.

Diagnosis
- Obtain a careful medical and family history of the child's development, particularly the early interactions with the caregiver (e.g. 'Did your child point out things to you?' 'Could you engage him/her in a little game such as peek-a-boo?').
- Arrange comprehensive psychiatric, medical and developmental evaluations (including Griffith scale).
- Exclude associated medical conditions such as anatomical CNS pathology, genetic abnormalities, epilepsy, visual and hearing problems.

Treatment
- Refer for specialist evaluation and treatment as early as possible (a 'wait and see approach' loses valuable time). ☙☆☆☆
- Medication generally does not have a significant role and should be commenced only after specialist consultation. ☙☆☆☆
- In supporting the family, be realistic but encouraging - it is not helpful to have parents react to diagnoses with such despair that effective parent-child work becomes impossible. ☙

Attention deficit hyperactivity disorder

ADHD is the most commonly diagnosed neurobehavioural disorder in childhood, especially in boys. Girls with inattention may be underdiagnosed.

Definition and diagnosis
To make the diagnosis, the child must display 6 or more symptoms of either inattention or hyperactivity/impulsivity that have persisted for 6 months to a degree that is maladaptive and inconsistent with developmental level. The relevant symptoms are as follows.

Inattention:
- Poor attention to detail, careless errors
- Cannot sustain attention
- Does not listen
- Does not follow instructions or complete tasks
- Poor organization
- Avoids tasks requiring sustained attention

- Loses things
- Easily distracted
- Forgetful.

Hyperactivity:

- Fidgets
- Leaves seat recurrently
- Runs, climbs excessively
- Noisy
- 'On the go'
- Talks excessively.

Impulsivity:

- Blurts out answers
- Fails to wait turn
- Interrupts.

In addition, the symptoms need to be present before 7 years; be associated with impairment in 2 or more settings; produce clinically significant impairment in social, academic or occupational functioning; and not be attributable to pervasive developmental disorder, psychosis or other mental disorder.

Exclude other potential causes of the symptoms, such as:
- Upper airway obstruction/snoring
- Normal preschool activity
- Developmental delay or learning disability
- Iron deficiency
- Drugs – phenobarbitone, clonazepam, caffeine
- Emotional or mood disorder
- Traumatic brain injury
- Genetic syndromes – Fragile X, William's, fetal alcohol
- HIV
- Hyperthyroidism (rare).

Assess for the presence of common comorbidities, such as:
- Developmental and learning problems
- Mood disorder
- Oppositional defiant disorder, conduct disorder
- Pervasive developmental disorders
- Tourette syndrome
- Chronic illness – cardiac, renal, asthma, epilepsy.

Treatment

Psychosocial: (all 🖐☆☆☆)

- Provide education to caregivers, educators and other key figures.
- Ensure that the daily routine is as stable and predictable as possible.
- Organise the home space to minimize distractions.
- In class, arrange for the child to be seated such that s/he is close to the teacher and protected from distractions from peers.
- When communicating with the child, ensure that her/his attention has been secured, for example by using her/his first name.
- Provide concise, clear and direct instructions, and follow up to ascertain whether the instructions have been complied with.
- Supervise homework and other tasks, while avoiding being unnecessarily intrusive.
- Divide time-linked tasks into short intervals.
- If necessary, arrange learning support.
- Ensure sufficient sleep.
- Avoid inappropriate or excessive television or computer games.
- Encourage and facilitate physical play.
- Provide a diet that is balanced and nutritious, avoiding caffeine and non-nutritive foods.
- Focus on strengths to build self esteem.

Pharmacological:

Methylphenidate: 🖐☆☆☆☆

- History should include inquiry into sudden death/possible cardiac arrhythmias in the family.
- A full physical examination including BP, heart rate and cardiovascular examination is mandatory.
- ECG is recommended where available.
- Commence with 5 mg, (half a tablet) or 0.2 mg/kg, after breakfast, with a second dose 4 hours later. Increase to 10 mg, or higher, as necessary in 5 mg increments. Maximum single dose is 20 mg. Thrice daily dosing may be required but avoid using after 4 pm. Where long acting formulations are available, these may be substituted after a trial for efficacy, and the dose adjusted according to symptoms.
- Adverse effects include appetite suppression, headache, abdominal pain, anxiety, insomnia, increased heart rate, increased blood pressure (mild), lower seizure threshold and tics.
- Contraindications include hyperthyroidism and cardiac arrhythmias
- Rating scales can be used to monitor response (Connors, SNAP, NICHQ, Vanderbilt)

- Assess 2-4 weeks after initiating treatment
- Review quarterly BP, heart rate, weight, height, rating scales, scholastic progress on stable dose.

Atomoxetine ☾☆☆☆☆
- Useful where methylphenidate is contraindicated, significant anxiety or tics, no response to methylphenidate
- Expensive, currently not in EDL
- 0.5 mg/kg/day-1.2 mg/kg/day UP TO 70 kg, maximum 100 mg/day. May take several months to achieve a response.
- Suicidal ideation has been reported.

Conversion disorder

Definition
The symptoms of conversion disorder (CD) are psychological in origin and involve motor and sensory functions that are suggestive of an organic disease. They are not feigned or intentional and cause functional impairment or significant distress. They may warrant medical investigation.

Clinical features
The symptoms are biologically implausible and/or inconsistent. They may be acute or chronic, stable or fluctuating and single or multiple. The presentation may be obscure if the symptoms are associated with existing organic pathology.

Diagnosis
Exclude possibilities such as:
- Illness that can mimic CD: e.g. temporal lobe epilepsy, subacute sclerosing panencephalitis, Guillain-Barré syndrome; and
- Malingering (physical symptoms are intentional).

Identify associated psychological factors such as:
- Stressors (including physical and sexual abuse)
- Unresolved grief
- Concern about parental illness or depression
- Family conflict and/or communication difficulty
- Secondary gain, e.g. remaining at home with a parent who is the focus of the child's concern
- Inappropriate lack of concern on the part of the child.

Treatment

Once the diagnosis is suspected:
- Indicate to the child and family that the physical and psychological aspects will be evaluated.
- Interview the child alone and with the family.

Once there is firm evidence for the diagnosis: ☙☆☆☆
- Disclose it to the child and family in a supportive and non-judgemental manner.
- If appropriate, point out the association between the onset of the symptoms and the recent psycho-social stressors.
- Implement simple interventions to address these stressors.
- Offer reassurance that the symptoms will improve.
- Resist pressure to undertake additional unnecessary diagnostic procedures.
- Consider referral for physiotherapy if motor symptoms are present, especially if they are long-standing.

Consider referral for specialized psychiatric intervention if:
- The CD is not associated with a time-limited environmental source of stress
- The symptoms do not resolve with explanation and/or simple interventions
- The child has other psychiatric pathology, or
- There are serious family problems.

After referral maintain contact with the child and family, and continue to liaise with the colleague to whom the child was referred.

Delirium

Definition

This transient and usually reversible mental disturbance is manifested by a variety of neuro-psychiatric symptoms. Mild forms may be mistaken for regressive, provocative, manipulative, or uncooperative behaviour. Undetected delirium can lead to unsympathetic management, self-harm or hindrance of medical treatment.

Clinical features

The symptoms fluctuate and usually develop over hours or days, but can be abrupt, e.g. after head injury or an operation. Clinical features include the following:
- Fluctuating awareness and attention, e.g. perseveration in answer to a question, wandering off during a conversation
- Disturbed sleep-wake cycle, e.g. frequent daytime naps
- Restlessness, irritability, anxiety, emotional lability; alternatively, decreased psychomotor activity
- Disorientation, particularly for time
- Disorganized thinking, e.g. rambling or incoherent speech, constructional apraxia, dysnomia
- Memory impairment
- Hallucinations and other perceptual disturbances, e.g. perceiving a catheter to be a snake; these are often threatening and lead to unco-operative behaviour or attempts to run away.

Diagnosis

- Suspect delirium when the above disturbances fail to respond to comforting and the presence of familiar persons.
- Identify and treat any associated medical conditions such as:
  — Systemic infection (encephalitis, meningitis, AIDS) – thiamine deficiency
  — Toxins (pesticides and solvents) – post-operative or post-ictal states
  — Metabolic disorder – hypertensive encephalopathy/serum glucose disturbances
  — Fluid/electrolyte imbalance – burns
  — Hepatic or renal disease – sequelae of head trauma.
- Attend to predisposing factors such as pyrexia or medication (e.g. anticholinergics).
- Consider an EEG. This may show slowing or low-voltage fast activity.

Treatment (all ✎☆☆☆)

- Arrange close observation and ensure safety in a well-lit room.
- Encourage a familiar nursing attendant or relative to allay fears and to offer direction (e.g. 'It is lunchtime now').
- Reassure family members and encourage them to visit often and to bring familiar objects from home.
- Avoid excessive sedation. Consider haloperidol to reduce agitation.

Major depressive disorder

Definition

Children rarely present with depression. Major depressive disorder (MDD) is frequently detected when investigating secondary symptoms. The diagnosis can be made when at least 5 of the following symptoms have been present for the same 2-week period:
- Depressed or irritable mood
- Diminished interest or pleasure or loss of pleasure in almost all activities
- Sleep disturbance
- Weight change (or failure to achieve expected weight gain) or appetite disturbance
- Decreased concentration or indecisiveness
- Suicidal ideation or thoughts of death
- Psychomotor agitation or retardation
- Fatigue or loss of energy
- Feelings of worthlessness or inappropriate guilt.

At least 1 of the first 2 symptoms must be present. The symptoms must be sufficiently severe to cause significant distress or functional impairment. A substance or a medical condition should not have precipitated the features.

Diagnosis

- A child may complain of the above features but the following are more common:
  - Behavioural changes such as irritability, whining, aggression and antisocial behaviour
  - Deteriorating scholastic performance
  - Somatic complaints or anxiety
  - Withdrawal from social and other previously enjoyed activities, or
  - Alcohol or other substance misuse.
- Identify and manage medical mimics of MDD such as:
  - Infections (e.g. encephalitis, pneumonia, tuberculosis, HIV)
  - Neurologic disorders (e.g. epilepsy)
  - Endocrine disorders (e.g. diabetes mellitus, thyroid pathology)
  - Electrolyte abnormalities
  - Anaemia
  - Alcohol or other substance abuse/withdrawal.
- Exclude pharmacological causes of depression such as aminophylline, anticonvulsants, barbiturates, steroidal contraceptives and corticosteroids.

- Assess suicide risk and take preventive steps if indicated.
- Identify aetiological psycho-social factors such as family disharmony, academic difficulties, poor peer relationships, community stresses and recent losses.
- Identify co-morbid conditions such as anxiety disorders and substance abuse.

Treatment
- Counsel the child and family with a view to addressing these factors.
- If the response to counselling is inadequate, consider fluoxetine. ☙☆☆☆
- Consider referral for more specialized intervention if:
  - There are psychotic features such as persecutory delusions.
  - The depression is too severe to respond to the above measures.
  - There is a significant risk of suicide.
  - There is other psychiatric pathology.
  - The depression does not remit within a few weeks in response to the above measures.

Traumatic stress

Clinical features and diagnosis
Children who witness or experience an overwhelmingly frightening event may show signs of traumatic stress in how they think, feel and behave. Their various responses are sometimes delayed and are often overlooked or regarded as misbehaviour.

The following reactions commonly occur immediately after a traumatic event:
- Sleep disturbances, bad dreams, nightmares
- Clingy behaviour and anxiety about separating from parents
- Inattentiveness, poor concentration
- Regression, e.g. bed-wetting, thumb-sucking
- Withdrawal and preoccupation with the event
- Physical complaints, e.g. headaches, stomach-ache
- Other behavioural problems and irritability.

In many, these are temporary and can be regarded as 'normal'. However, they do reflect a disturbance of emotional equilibrium (insecurity, anxiety, and/or depression), which requires observation until recovery has occurred.

Reactions that persist for more than a few weeks and that affect the daily functioning of the child should be regarded as abnormal.

Distressing symptoms that appear within 3 months of the traumatic event may continue as an adjustment disorder. Serious reactions may persist as a post-traumatic stress disorder (PTSD). They reflect the child's helplessness and intense fear and horror of the traumatic event. Typical symptoms of PTSD include:

- Recurring 'flashbacks' of the event – the trauma is also re-experienced in bad dreams, repetitive compulsive play, etc.
- Deliberate efforts to avoid thoughts and feelings about the trauma.
- A persistent hyper-arousal state – jumpiness, disturbed sleep.

Continuing post-traumatic stress disorder interferes considerably with a child's functioning and development.

Treatment

- Attend primarily to factors that affect the child's sense of security.
- Encourage the family to speak about the trauma in a way that allows the child to reveal concerns about the event (e.g. 'Do you think Sandile is worried that something like that will happen again – and someone may be hurt/killed?'). The family should acknowledge the child's feelings and correct any misapprehensions about the event.
- Discuss the trauma with the parents in the child's presence. This sometimes serves to release bottled-up feelings for parents and child.
- Interview the child privately if possible. Previous undisclosed concerns may need to be clarified for the parents.
- Use medication symptomatically for sleep disturbance, anxiety or depression. Propranolol or fluoxetine may be indicted for post-traumatic anxiety. ☆ ☆ ☆
- Refer those with persistent and clear-cut post-traumatic or adjustment disorders for psychiatric evaluation and treatment.

Recommended reading

1. American Academy of Child and Adolescent Psychiatry. http://www.aacap.org
2. Flisher, AJ. Psychiatric problems. In: Kibel, M, Westwood, ATR, Saloojee Y, (Eds.). *Child Health for All* (4th ed). Cape Town. Oxford University Press. 2008.
3. Robertson, B. *Handbook of Child Psychiatry*. Cape Town. Oxford University Press. 1996.
4. Taylor, E, Döpfer, M, Sergeant, J. et al. European guidelines for hyperkinetic disorder – first update. *Eur Child Adolesc Psychiatry*. 2004; 13 (suppl. 1): 1-7.
5. http://www.ADHD.net/

14 Endocrinology

M. Carrihill, S.V. Delport, A. Spitaels

Diabetic emergencies

- Diabetic ketoacidosis (DKA)
- Hypoglycaemia in diabetics
- Sick day management

Diabetic ketoacidosis (DKA)

Definition

- Glycosuria and ketonuria
- Hyperglycaemia (blood glucose > 11 mmol/l)
- Acidaemia (pH < 7.3, bicarbonate < 15 mmol/l)
- Dehydration

> ***Practice points:***
>
> Diagnostic pitfalls in undiagnosed diabetics:
> - Inappropriate polyuria
> - Acute abdomen
> - Respiratory distress.

Management

- See algorithm (Figure 14.1)
- Evidence shows that outcomes are better when the same protocol is used throughout a unit. This algorithm may be adapted to suit a specific unit.

> ***Practice points:***
>
> Management pitfalls in DKA:
> - The patient may appear deceptively well despite gross metabolic imbalances.
> - Cerebral oedema occurs, and is potentially fatal.
> - DKA can occur without pronounced hyperglycaemia.
> - Too rapid rehydration is associated with cerebral oedema.
> - Consider infection as a precipitant.

Figure 14.1 Management of DKA

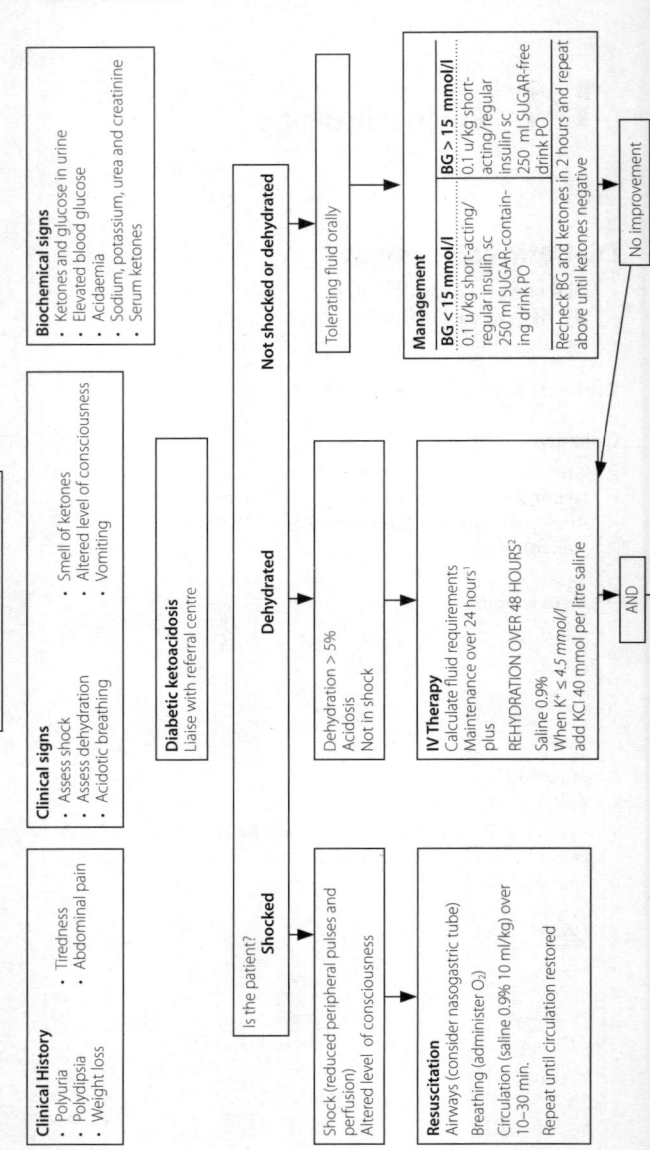

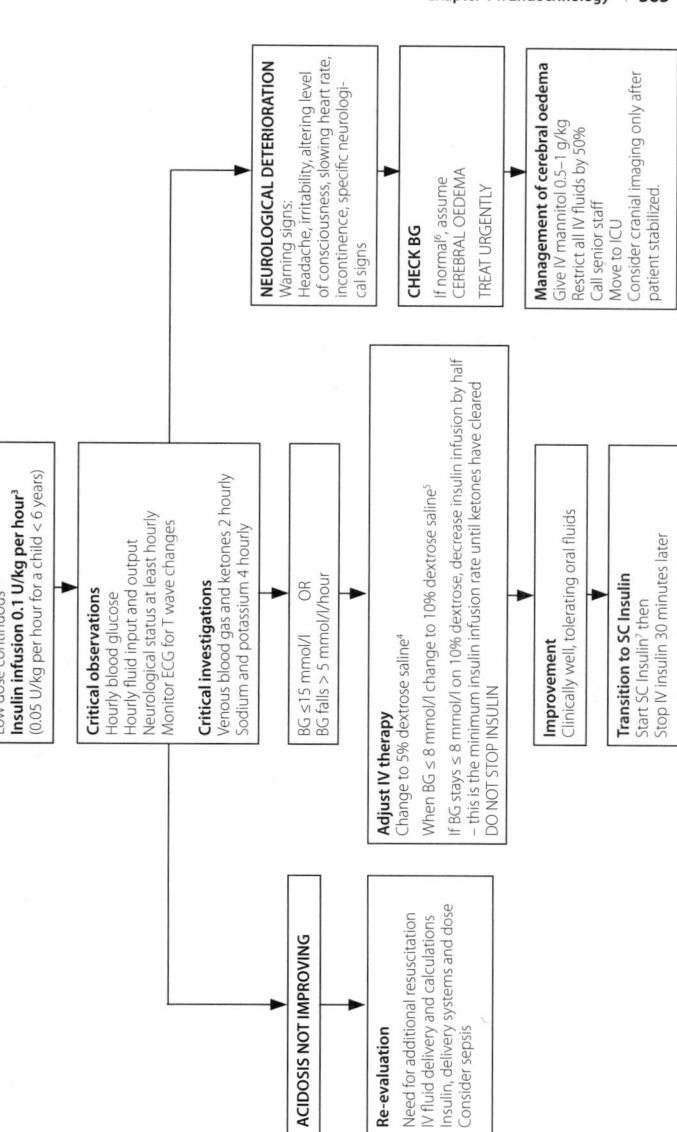

KEY TO FLOWCHART

1 Daily maintenance fluid volumes for different ages:

Age (years)	Weight (kg)	ml/kg per day
< 1	3–9	80
1–5	10–19	70
6–9	20–29	60
10–14	30–50	50
> 15	> 50	35

2 Rehydration:

Hydration state	Moderate (~ 5% dehydrated)	Severe (~10% dehydrated)
Volume over 48 hours	$\frac{50 \text{ ml/kg} \times \text{body weight in kg}}{48}$ = ml/hr	$\frac{100 \text{ ml/kg} \times \text{body weight in kg}}{48}$ = ml/hr

3 Insulin infusion:
   - Use only clear soluble regular insulin such as Actrapid HM (ge) or Humulin R.
   - Use only orange-coded (no dead-space) insulin syringes to draw up insulin.
   - Make up the insulin/saline mixture before priming the giving set. Run about 20 ml of the mixture through the set to prime the tubing and to saturate insulin binding sites. ENSURE CLEARLY LABELLED AS CONTAINING INSULIN.
   - To ensure safety, connect the insulin solution to the IV rehydration line by a 3-way tap or by 'piggy-back' (watch for leaks!) and control the flow with an adjustable-rate pressure pump.
   - During transport or transfer of the patient STOP AND DISCONNECT the insulin infusion.
   - If insulin infusion is not possible, or for prolonged transport, give hourly IV insulin stat injections (0.1 unit/kg/hr) into the rubber stopper of the IV rehydration set. Ensure accuracy of the intermittent doses. Since only U-100 insulins (100 units/ml) are available, use low-dose insulin syringes (0.3 or 0.5 ml) with widely spaced gradations.

For 0.1units/kg/hr

Patient weight < 25kg	Mix 25 units insulin solution in 100 ml saline run insulin solution at (0.4 x patient's mass in kg) ml/hr
Patient weight > 25kg	Mix 50 units insulin solution in 100 ml saline run insulin solution at (0.2 x patient's mass in kg) ml/hr

For 0.05units/kg/hr, halve the above rate.

4 5% dextrose saline = 900 ml normal saline + 100 ml 50% dextrose

5. 10% dextrose saline = 800 ml normal saline − 200 ml 50% dextrose

6. If blood sugar < 4 mmol/l, stop the insulin infusion. Treat the hypoglycaemia to a level of 8 mmol/l. Recommence the insulin infusion at half the rate.

7. Subcutaneous insulin:

Regimen 1: Short-acting and intermediate insulins, 3 daily doses
Total daily dose = 0.6 units/kg/24 hours (< 6 years = 0.4 units/kg/24 hours)

Breakfast	am = 2/3 of total daily dose	short-acting insulin (1/3 of am dose) + intermediate acting insulin (2/3 of am dose)
Supper	pm = 1/3 of total daily dose	short-acting insulin (1/3 of pm dose)
At night (± 21h00)		intermediate acting insulin (2/3 of pm dose)

Regimen 2: Short-acting and intermediate insulins, basal bolus doses
Total daily dose = 0.6 units/kg/24 hours (< 6 years = 0.4 units/kg/24 hours)

Breakfast	20% short-acting insulin
Lunch	20% short-acting insulin
Supper	20% short-acting insulin
At night (± 21h00)	40% intermediate acting insulin

Regimen 3: Premixed insulin, twice daily doses (least flexible, most likely to cause nocturnal hypoglycaemia)
Total daily dose = 0.6 units/kg/24 hours (< 6 years = 0.4 units/kg/24 hours)

Breakfast	am = 2/3 of total daily dose	Premixed insulin short-acting/intermediate 30/70
Supper	pm = 1/3 of total daily dose	Premixed insulin short-acting/intermediate 30/70

Regimen 4: Insulin analogues, multiple daily injections
Aspart/glulisine/lispro rapid acting analogue insulin
Detemir/glargine long-acting insulin analogue

Breakfast	Rapid-acting analogue Dose adjusted for blood sugar, carbohydrate load and insulin sensitivity
Lunch	
Supper	
Any carbohydrate snack	
Daily	Long-acting analogue Adjusted for basal requirement

Sodium bicarbonate

- There is no evidence that bicarbonate is necessary or safe in DKA and it should not be used at all. It may exacerbate cerebral acidosis, precipitate hypokalaemia and cause low ionised calcium, excessive osmolar load and tissue hypoxia.

Phosphate

- Severe hypophosphataemia in conjunction with unexplained weakness should be treated.

Sodium

- With hyperglycaemia plasma sodium readings are fictitiously low (< 130 mmol/l). Corrected sodium = plasma sodium + 2 × ([plasma glucose-5.6]/5.6) mmol/l.
- The measured sodium should increase with effective therapy.

Long term management

- Ideally the child and family should be managed by an expert multi-disciplinary team (Figure 14.2).

Figure 14.2 Principals of holistic management of diabetes

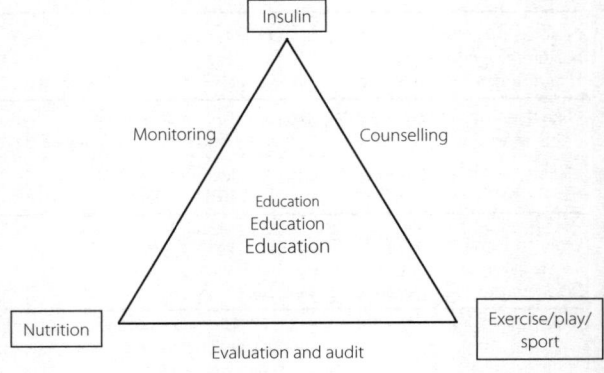

Hypoglycaemia in diabetics

Hypoglycaemia is a frequent acute complication in type 1 diabetes with the potential to cause permanent brain damage.

Definition
- Blood glucose < 4 mmol/l
- Normally physiological counter-regulation commences when blood glucose falls below 4 mmol/l. This physiological response becomes abnormal when on exogenous insulin.

Clinical features

Table 14.1 Symptoms and signs of hypoglycaemia in children with type 1 diabetes mellitus

Neuroglycopaenic and autonomic	Behavioural
Reported by children:	Headache
Weakness	Argumentative
Trembling	Aggressive
Dizziness	Irritability
Poor concentration	Naughty
Hunger	
Sweating	
Confusion	
Blurred vision	
Slurred speech	
Double vision	
Observed by parents:	
As above plus	Nausea
Pallor	Nightmares
Sleepiness	
Convulsions	

Management

Table 14.2 Management of hypoglycaemia in the diabetic child and adolescent

Severity	Definition	Management
Mild	Aware of, responds to and self treats the hypoglycaemia (Children < 6 years should not be classified as mild because they are unable to help themselves)	Immediate oral rapidly absorbed simple carbohydrate 5–15 g glucose or sucrose OR 100 ml sweet drink Repeat as required
Moderate	Cannot respond to hypoglycaemia, and requires help. Oral treatment is successful	Follow with complex carbohydrate snack/meal
Severe	Altered level of consciousness ± convulsions. Requires parenteral intervention	Glucagon IMI < 12 years 0.5 mg > 12 years 1 mg If glucagon is unavailable/recovery inadequate: glucose 10% IVI 2–5 ml/kg stat. Follow with carbohydrate snack/glucose 10% infusion

Retest after 15 min and repeat therapy as needed. Continue to monitor BG every 15 min until BG ≥ 6 mmol/l

Never use glucose 50% IVI.

Sick day management

(See Tables 14.3 and 14.4.)
- Children with well controlled diabetes do not get more illnesses or infections than other children.
- Mild illnesses such as sore throats and colds may only reduce appetite and make a child feel miserable without much effect on diabetes.
- More severe children's illnesses such as 'flu', tonsillitis and chest infections often cause a raised temperature and tend to increase the blood glucose because stress hormones like adrenaline, growth hormone and cortisol make the liver release extra glucose to help resist the infection.
- Illnesses with diarrhoea and vomiting (gastroenteritis) often decrease the blood glucose because less food is digested and absorbed from the stomach.

NB: Never stop the insulin.

Table 14.3 High blood glucose

	Mild illness with loss of appetite but no vomiting	More severe illness with fever, blood glucose more than 15 mmol/l, but no vomiting	High blood glucose (above 15 mmol/l) with 1 or 2 vomits	High blood glucose (more than 15 mmol/l) with persistent vomiting (and ketones may be present)
Insulin	Normal dose, plus extra if BG > 15 mmol/l	Increase all doses by 20%, plus extra if BG > 15 mmol/l	Increase all doses by 20%, plus extra if BG > 15 mmol/l	Treat as DKA (see Fig. 14.1)
Food/fluid	Replace usual food with small frequent amounts of easily digestible carbohydrate food or drinks	Replace usual food with small frequent amounts of easily digestible carbohydrate food or drinks	Stop the usual solid meals; give small frequent amounts of easily digestible carbohydrate food or drinks	
Blood test	Every 2-4 hours	Every 2 hours	Every 2 hours	

Table 14.4 Normal or low blood glucose

	Normal or low BG, feeling sick and beginning to vomit ± diarrhoea	Normal or low BG, not tolerating oral fluids
	Treat hypoglycaemia	Treat hypoglycaemia
Insulin	Decrease all doses by 20%	Admit for 10% dextrose IVI and insulin infusion 0.05 U/kg/hr
Food/fluid	Stop solid food. Small frequent amounts of sugary drinks	NPO
Blood test	Every 2-4 hours	Every hour

Endocrine emergencies

- Hypoglycaemia
- Acute adrenal insufficiency
- Ambiguous genitalia.

Hypoglycaemia

NB: Measure blood glucose in every sick child. Hypoglycaemia causes brain damage.

Definition
Blood glucose < 2.6 mmol/l at all ages

Clinical features

Table 14.5 Clinical features of hypoglycaemia

Autonomic	Neuroglycopaenic	Non-specific malaise
Sweating	Confusion	Hunger
Palpitations	Drowsiness	Abdominal pain
Shaking	Odd behaviour	Headache
Hunger	Speech difficulty	
Pallor	In-coordination	
Anxiety	Convulsions	
	Coma	

Management
- Confirm diagnosis.
- Insert IV cannula. Do laboratory blood glucose; if there is no overt cause (Table 14.6) for the hypoglycaemia, take further samples (Table 14.7).
- Give glucose 10% IVI 2-5ml/kg stat.
- Continue glucose 10% maintenance infusion.
- Measure BG every 15 min until ≥ 6 mmol/l.
- If still hypoglycaemic, give hydrocortisone IV stat:
    < 3 years 50 mg   > 3 years 100 mg
- Treat the cause.

NB: Never use glucose 50% IVI.

Table 14.6 Overt causes of hypoglycaemia

Drugs	Poisons – plants/chemicals
Include: oral hypoglycaemic agents, insulin, alcohol, salicylates, propranolol, valproic acid, pentamidine, quinine, trimethoprim/sulfamethoxazole	Sepsis
	Liver failure
	Malnutrition
	Severe systemic illness
	Malaria

Table 14.7 Investigations for hypoglycaemia

	First line	**Second line**	
Blood	Venous gas Cortisol Insulin Growth hormone (Save tube of serum)	C-peptide if insulin detectable Ammonia Free fatty acids Lactate and pyruvate	Alanine Amino acids Carnitine profile β-hydroxybutyrate and acetoacetate
Urine	Ketones	Organic acids Carnitine profile Reducing substances	

Acute adrenal insufficiency

Definition
- An emergency caused by inadequate cortisol.

Clinical features

Table 14.6 The clinical features of adrenal insufficiency

Symptoms	Signs	Investigations
Vomiting Abdominal pain Lethargy Anorexia Fever Loss of weight Seizures Dizziness	Lethargy Hypotension Shock Increased skin pigmentation	Hypoglycaemia Hyponatraemia Hyperkalaemia Metabolic acidosis

- Symptoms and signs are non-specific and can vary depending on the cause.
- Crisis may be precipitated by any acute illness, trauma, surgery and exposure to excess heat.

Management
- Treat shock
- Treat hypoglycaemia
- Give hydrocortisone IVI stat
  < 1 year 25 mg   1-3 years 50 mg   > 3 years 100 mg
  Hydrocortisone is the only glucocorticoid with mineralocorticoid effects
- Continue hydrocortisone at 2 mg/kg/dose 6 hourly IVI for 48 hours
- Start oral replacement hydrocortisone with fludrocortisone
- Refer.

Ambiguous genitalia

Definition
- Anomalous development of the external genitalia
- This is an emergency because it may be congenital adrenal hyperplasia (CAH) with acute adrenal insufficiency
- Disorders of sex development (DSDs) may present with ambiguous genitalia, but include other conditions with an unambiguous phenotype. DSDs develop due to abnormalities in the pathways in Figure 14.3.

Figure 14.3 Sexual determination and differentiation in the foetus

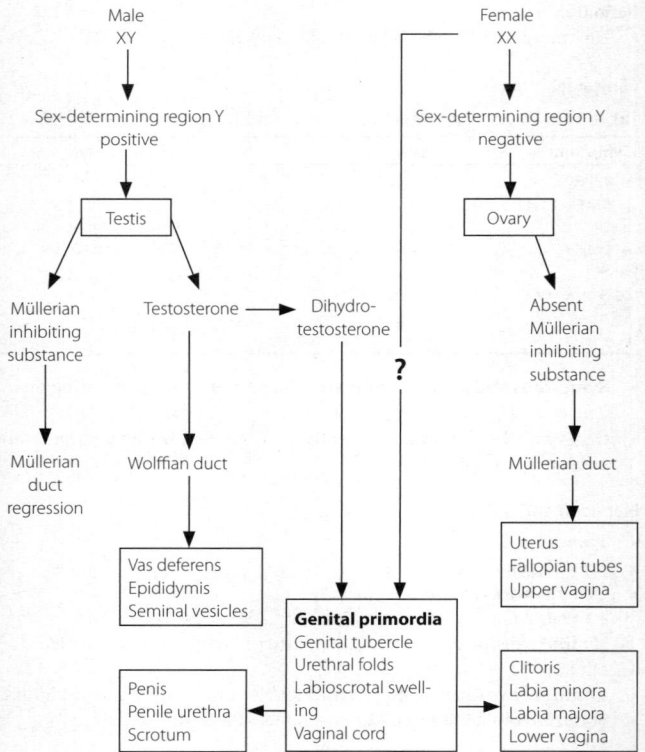

Management

- Presume CAH: monitor blood glucose, sodium and potassium daily
- Send blood for karyotype and 17-hydroxyprogesterone
- Refer to a paediatric endocrinologist.

Table 14.7 Dos and don'ts of indeterminate genitalia

DOs	DON'Ts
• Refer!	• Panic!
• Assure parents that you will seek expert advice	• Assign gender
• Assure parents a gender will be assigned after careful evaluation	• Avoid the parents
• Talk about 'your baby/child'	• Call the baby 'he, she or it'
• Delay registration and formal naming of the baby	• Lie to parents
• Celebrate the birth of the baby!	

Growth and development

- Short stature
- Tall stature
- Obesity
- Abnormal puberty.

Short stature

Definition

- A height < −2SD for age, OR
- A height < 3rd centile for age, OR
- A height < target height (see below).

Table 14.8 Target height in boys and girls

Mid-parental height	
For boys:	MPH = [father's height + (mother's height +13)] / 2 cm
	Target height = MPH ±7.5 cm
For girls:	MPH = [(father's height -13) + mother's height] / 2 cm
	Target height = MPH ±6 cm

—Hintz RL. Management of disorders of size. In: Brook C.G.D, Hindmarsh P.C, editors. *Clinical pediatric endocrinology* 4th edition. Oxford: Blackwell Science Limited. 2001. p127.

Differential diagnosis

An algorithm for the diagnosis of a short child is shown in Figure 14.4 on p. 377.

Management

Refer for assessment if the child meets the definition of short stature, or if the growth velocity is less than expected for age.

Tall stature

Definition

- A height > +2SD for age
- A height > 97th centile for age
- A height > target height (see above)

Differential diagnosis

An algorithm for the diagnosis of tall stature is shown in Figure 14.5 on p. 378.

Management

Refer for assessment if the child meets the definition of tall stature, or if the growth velocity exceeds that expected for age.

Obesity

Definition

- > 120% expected weight for height
- > 95 centile for BMI, where BMI = wt (kg)/[height(m^2)]

(http://www.cdc.gov/GrowthCharts/ and http://www.who.int/childgrowth/standards)

Conditions presenting with obesity

Table 14.9 Causes of obesity

Common causes
Nutritional (exogenous obesity)
Psychosocial *
*(Listed separately from nutritional to ensure that psychosocial causes are not missed as a primary issue.)
Rare causes
Syndromes – for example, Prader-Willi, Bardet-Biedl
Endocrine
Hypothyroidism
Cushing's
Hypothalamic lesions
Single gene defects

Arch Dis Child Educ Pract Ed 2004; 89: 57–62.

Figure 14.4 Algorithm for the diagnosis of short stature

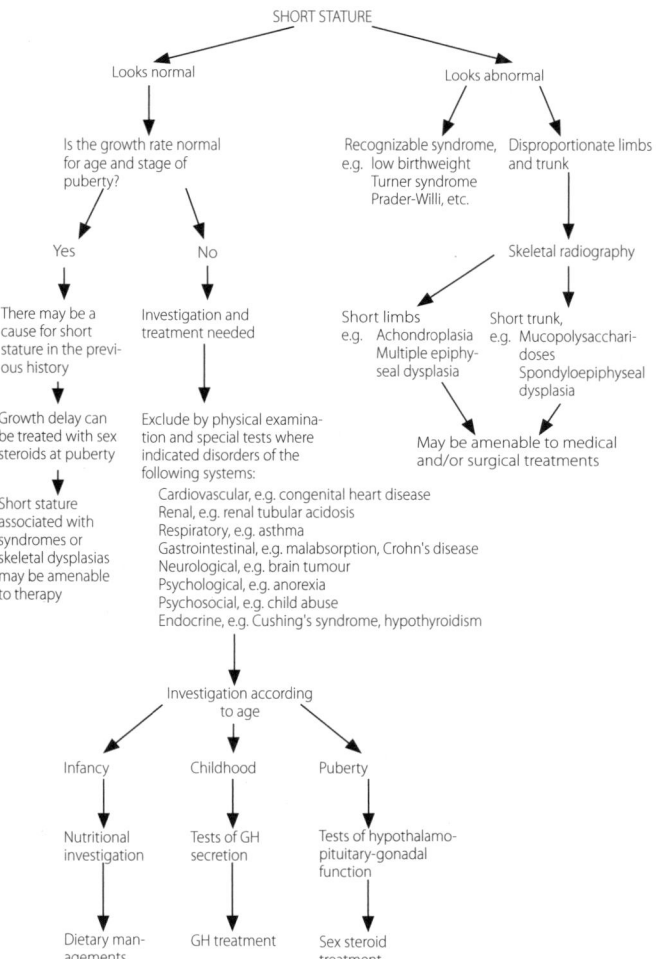

From *Guide to the Practice of Paediatric Endocrinology,* Ed. C. Brook. Cambridge University Press. 1993.

Figure 14.5 Algorithm for the diagnosis of tall stature

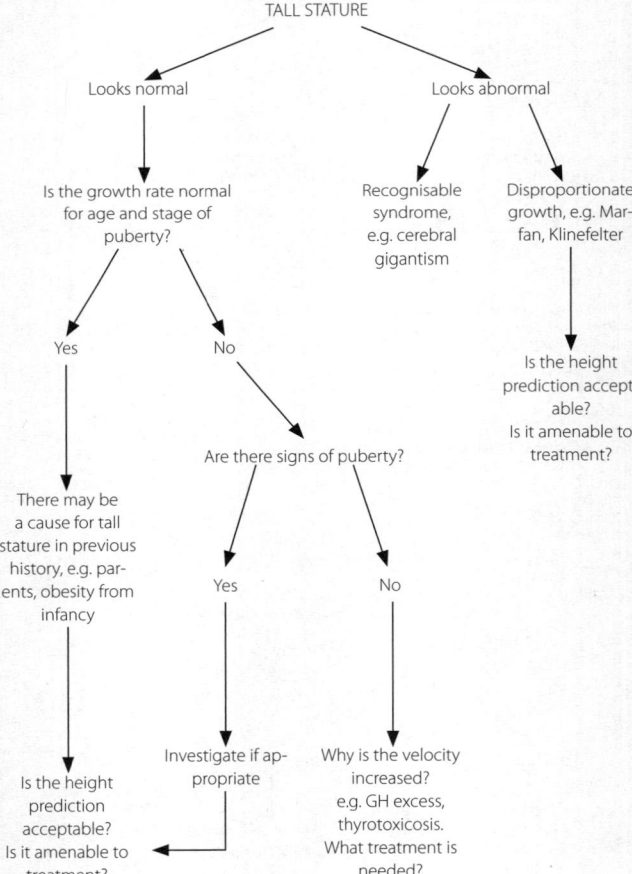

From *Guide to the Practice of Paediatric Endocrinology*, Ed. C. Brook. Cambridge University Press. 1993.

Management

- Identification of a medical cause
- Identification of any consequences of obesity
- Promotion of weight loss/control
- Management of medical problems
- An obese child who is short or has a slow growth velocity for age must be referred.

Table 14.10 Clinical features suggesting a genetic syndrome associated with obesity

Short stature
Severe unremitting obesity
Onset of obesity before the age of 2 years
Dysmorphic features
Microcephaly
Learning disability
Hypotonia
Hypogonadism
Eye abnormalities
Skeletal abnormalities
Sensorineural deafness
Renal abnormalities
Cardiac abnormalities

—*Arch Dis Child Educ Pract Ed* 2004; 89: 57–62.

Table 14.11 Consequences for the obese child

Overt	Occult
Emotional and behavioural	Impaired glucose tolerance
Orthopaedic	Hypertension
Blounts's disease	Dyslipidaemia
Slipped capital femoral epiphyses	Steatohepatitis
Asthma	
Sleep apnoea	
Pseudotumour cerebri	
Polycystic ovary syndrome	

—*Arch Dis Child Educ Pract Ed* 2004; 89: 57–62.

Puberty

Physical changes

The stages of puberty for boys and girls are shown in Figures 14.6 and 14.7.

Figure 14.6 Stages of puberty for males

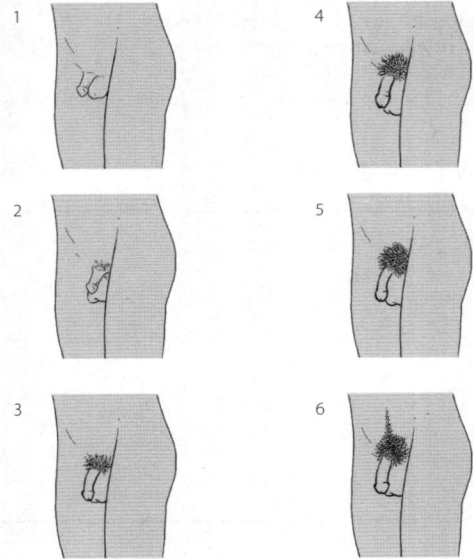

Genitalia	Stage	Pubic hair
Preadolescent testes, scrotum, and penis are about the same size and proportion as in early childhood	1	Preadolescent: the vellus over the pubes is not developed more than that over the abdominal wall (i.e. no pubic hair)
Enlargement of the scrotum and testes. Skin of scrotum reddens and changes in texture. Little or no enlargement of penis.	2	Sparse, long, slightly pigmented downy hair, straight or slightly curly, chiefly at the base of the penis.
Length of penis increases. Further growth of testes and scrotum.	3	Considerably darker, coarser, and more curled. The sparse hair extends over the pubic junction.
Breadth of penis increases and glans develops. Testes and scrotum enlarge; scrotal skin darkens	4	Now adult in type, but still sparse. None on the medial thigh
Genitalia adult size and shape	5	Adult in quantity and type with a horizontal ('feminine') pattern.
	6	Spread to the medial thigh. Spread up linea alba.

Figure 14.7 Stages of puberty for females

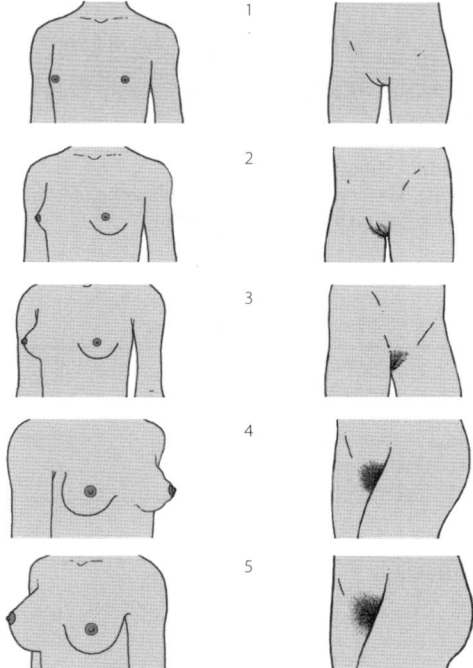

Stage	Breast size
1	Preadolescent elevation of papilla only.
2	Breast bud stage: elevation of breast and papilla as small mount. Enlargement of areola diameter.
3	Further enlargement and elevation of breast and areola with no separaton of their contours.
4	Projection of areola and papilla to form a secondary mound above the level of the breast.
5	Mature stage projection of papilla only, due to recession of the areola to the great contour of the breast.

Pubic hair stages 1–5 for females.

Abnormal puberty

Definition:

- Precocious: signs of puberty before the age of 8 years in a girl and 9 years in a boy
- Delayed: no signs of puberty by 13 years in a girl and 14 years in a boy
- Non-consonant:
  - abnormal order of puberty stages
  - abnormal timing of puberty stages
  - > 5 years between thelarche and adrenarche in a girl
- > 5 years for genital development in a boy

See figures 14.8 and 14.9

Table 14.12 Classification of precocious puberty

Gonadotrophin-dependent precocious puberty
Gonadotrophin-independent precocious puberty

Variants of the normal pubertal development:
     Isolated precocious thelarche
     Isolated precocious pubarche
     Isolated precocious menarche

Table 14.13 Aetiology of gonadotrophin-dependent precocious puberty

No CNS abnormalities	CNS abnormalities
Idiopathic	Hypothalamic hamartoma
Genetic causes	Tumours
Secondary to previous chronic exposure to sex steroids	Congenital malformations
After exposure to endocrine disrupters	Acquired diseases: infections and inflammatory processes of the CNS

Table 14.14 Aetiology of gonadotrophin-independent precocious puberty.

Exogenous use of sex steroids
Tumours
Autonomous ovarian cysts
Severe long-term untreated primary hypothyroidism
Genetic causes, e.g.   McCune-Albright syndrome   Testotoxicosis

—Adapted from *Arq Bras Endrocrinol Metab* 2008;52/1

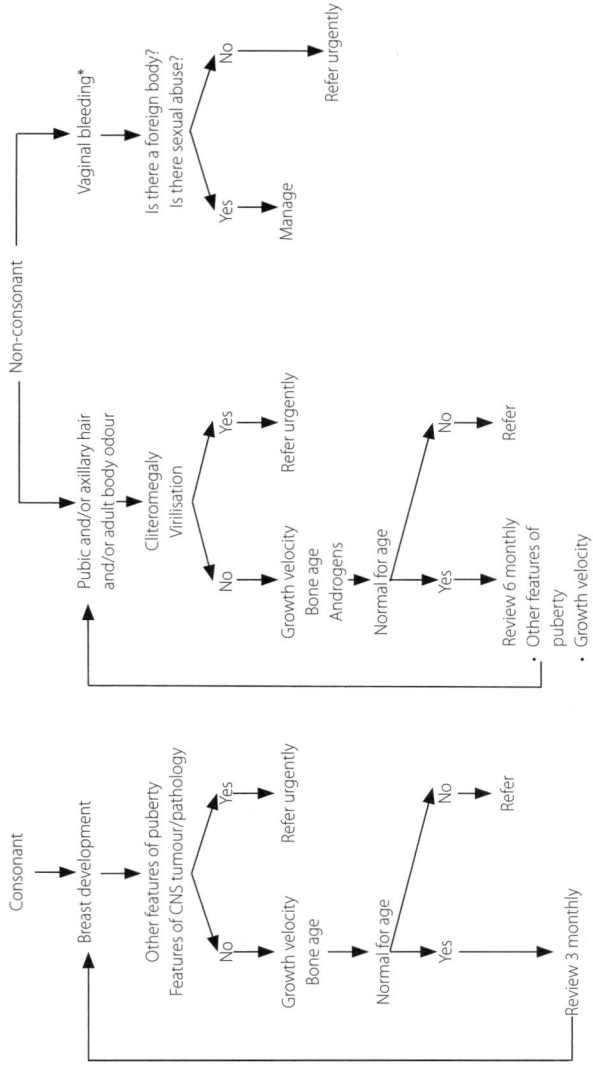

Figure 14.8 Approach to precocious puberty in girls

*Neonates can have a normal withdrawal bleed

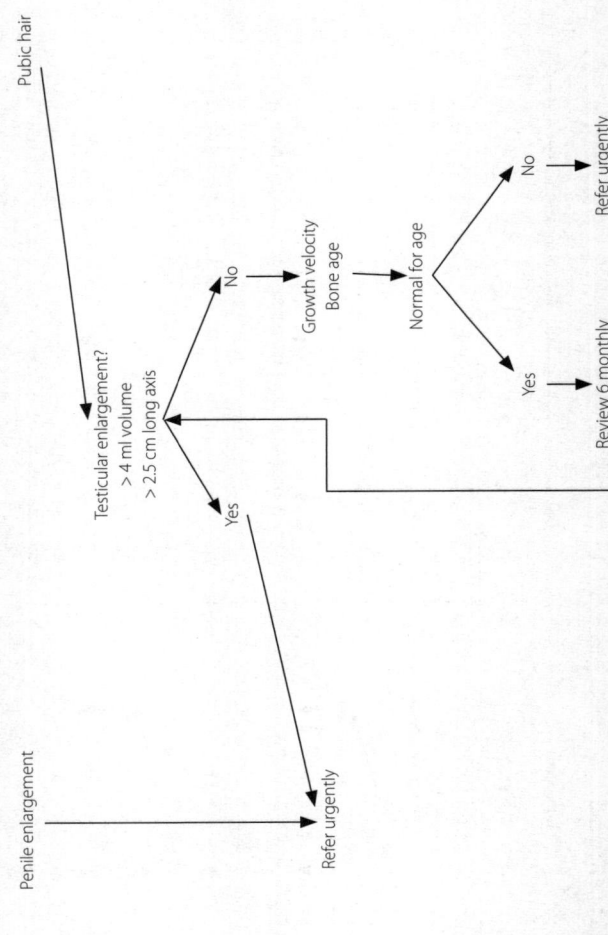

Figure 14.9 Approach to precocious puberty in boys

Delayed puberty

- The most common cause of late puberty is a constitutional delay of growth and puberty. It occurs more often in boys than in girls. Pathological causes are more common in girls because of the high incidence of Turner's syndrome.
- Children with no signs of puberty by 13.5 years may simply have delayed maturation but could permanently lack the ability to develop in puberty and should be referred for investigation. Assessment includes a careful physical examination and calculation of height velocity.

Table 14.15 A simple classification of delayed puberty

Constitutional
Chronic disease
Hypogonadotrophic hypogonadism • Idiopathic • Genetic, e.g. Kallman syndrome • Hypothalamic-pituitary pathology
Hypergonadotrophic hypogonadism • Primary gonadal failure, e.g. Turner's syndrome, Klinefelter's syndrome • Secondary gonadal failure, e.g chemotherapy

Disorders of the thyroid gland

Table 14.16 Laboratory values in thyroid disorders

Disorder	TSH	Free T4
Primary hyperthyroidism	Low	High normal/high
Primary hypothyroidism	High	Low
Secondary/tertiary (Pituitary/hypothalamic) hypothyroidism	Low/normal/ slightly high	Low
Non-thyroidal illness or euthyroid sick syndrome	Low/normal/ slightly high	Low/low normal
Subclinical hypothyroidism	High	Normal

Hypothyroidism

Causes

Table 14.17 Causes of hypothyroidism

Congenital disorders
primary (thyroid)
dysgenetic gland, dyshormonogenesis
secondary (pituitary)
thyroid-stimulating hormone (TSH) deficiency (isolated or multiple hormone defect)
Transient disorders
Acquired disorders
primary disease (thyroid)
iodine deficiency, goitrogens, autoimmune thyroiditis, post-irradiation, chemotherapy
secondary disease (pituitary)
TSH deficiency (isolated or multiple hormone defect)
tertiary disease (hypothalamic)
thyroid-releasing hormone (TRH) deficiency

Congenital hypothyroidism

Detection based on symptoms and signs is usually delayed, leading to intellectual impairment. This argues strongly for neonatal screening programmes. A high index of suspicion is needed to make the diagnosis on clinical grounds; and should be maintained even where screening programmes exist, as coverage is not 100%.

Early diagnosis and treatment improves intellectual outcome.

Clinical features

Table 14.18 Do a TSH in a child with any of these features.

Early	Late
Asymptomatic	
Umbilical hernia	Persists
Pallor and hypothermia	Persists
Large tongue	Increases
Hoarse cry	Persists
Constipation and feeding problems	Persist
Prolonged jaundice	Decreases
Large fontanelles	Delayed closure
Hypotonia	Worsens
Rough dry skin	Persists

Early	Late
Unexpected respiratory difficulties	
Mild post-maturity	
Birth weight > 3.5 kg	
	Facial puffiness
	Growth delay
	Developmental delay
	Myxoedema

—Adapted from: *Abnormal laboratory values.* In *Colour atlas of pediatric endocrinology and growth.* by Wales J.K.H., Rogel A.D., Wit J.M. London: Mosby-Wolfe. p. 125. © Elsevier, 1996.

Management

- If special investigations are not immediately available, start treatment.
- Thyroxine 100 µg/m^2 (single daily dose).
  - Measure TSH and T4 concentrations (monthly for 6 months and then 3 monthly) to adjust the dose of thyroxine and check adherence.
  - Maintain the free T4 in the upper range of normal for age. Note that the TSH may take some time to return to normal.
  - Monitor growth and neurodevelopment.
- NB: *Never* use thyroxine liquid formulation as dosing is extremely unreliable.

Determining the cause of congenital hypothyroidism:

- Thyroid technetium uptake scan (nuclear medicine):
  - Determines if and where thyroid tissue is present
- Thyroid ultrasound:
  - Determines whether or not a normal thyroid is present (in experienced hands)
- Maternal thyroid function and thyroid antibodies.

Acquired hypothyroidism

- It is easy to miss this diagnosis because the onset is gradual and may occur at any age. Consider this diagnosis in any child with growth delay, excessive weight gain *without tall stature*, abnormal pubertal development, and anaemia which does not respond to standard treatment.

Treatment:
- Thyroxine 100 µg/m^2 (single daily dose). Measure TSH and T4 concentrations (monthly until free T4 is in the higher range of

normal, then 6 monthly) to adjust the dose of thyroxine and check adherence. Monitor growth and pubertal development.
- NB: *Never* use thyroxine liquid formulation as dosing is extremely unreliable.

> ***Practice point:***
>
> **Warning:** In secondary and tertiary hypothyroidism, always check cortisol before commencing thyroxine therapy, as an Addisonian crisis can be precipitated if hypoadrenalism is not treated first.

Hyperthyroidism

This results from excessive circulating thyroid hormone. When thyrotoxicosis is associated with eye manifestations, the term 'Graves disease' is used.

Causes

Table 14.19 Causes of hyperthyroidism

Diffuse toxic goitre (Graves)
Thyroiditis with hyperthyroidism subacute thyroiditis chronic lymphocytic thyroiditis
TSH-induced hyperthyroidism TSH-producing tumour inappropriate secretion of TSH
Transient neonatal thyrotoxicosis

Clinical manifestations

Early findings are subtle. They include changes in behaviour and sleep pattern. Later more specific symptoms appear, including weight loss, sweating, palpitations, tremor and muscle weakness. The biochemical hallmarks are a raised T4 with a TSH suppressed below the normal range.

Treatment

- Carbimazole 0.5 to 1 mg/kg/day in 3 equal doses. The maximum dose should not exceed 30 mg/day. Propranolol may be required in the acute situation.
- Radioactive iodine should be considered if there is failure to remit after 12–18 months.

Rickets

Definition
A failure to mineralize bones in the growing child.

Clinical features

Table 14.20 Clinical features of rickets

Abnormal bone mineralization	Hypocalcaemia (if present)
Skull – delayed closure fontanelles, bossing Ribs and chest cage – prominent rib ends, Harrison's sulcus Wrists and ankles – widened Weight-bearing long bones - bowed Short stature Pain	Hypotonia Delayed motor milestones Seizures

Causes of rickets

Table 14.21 Causes of rickets

Calciopenic	
Calcium deficiency	Dietary Malabsorption
Vitamin D deficiency	Dietary Malabsorption No sunlight Liver disease Associated with anticonvulsant medication
Biosynthetic defect of vitamin D	Liver disease Renal disease 1 α-hydroxylase deficiency
Defective action of vitamin D	
Phosphopaenic	
Renal tubular loss of phosphate	Isolated defect X-linked hypophosphataemic rickets Autosomal recessive and dominant forms Mixed tubular disorders (e.g. Fanconi's, RTA)
Decreased phosphate intake / absorption	Prematurity Aluminium hydroxide
Abnormal bones	
Hypophosphatasia	
Renal osteodystrophy	

Approach and treatment

Figure 14.10 An approach to managing rickets

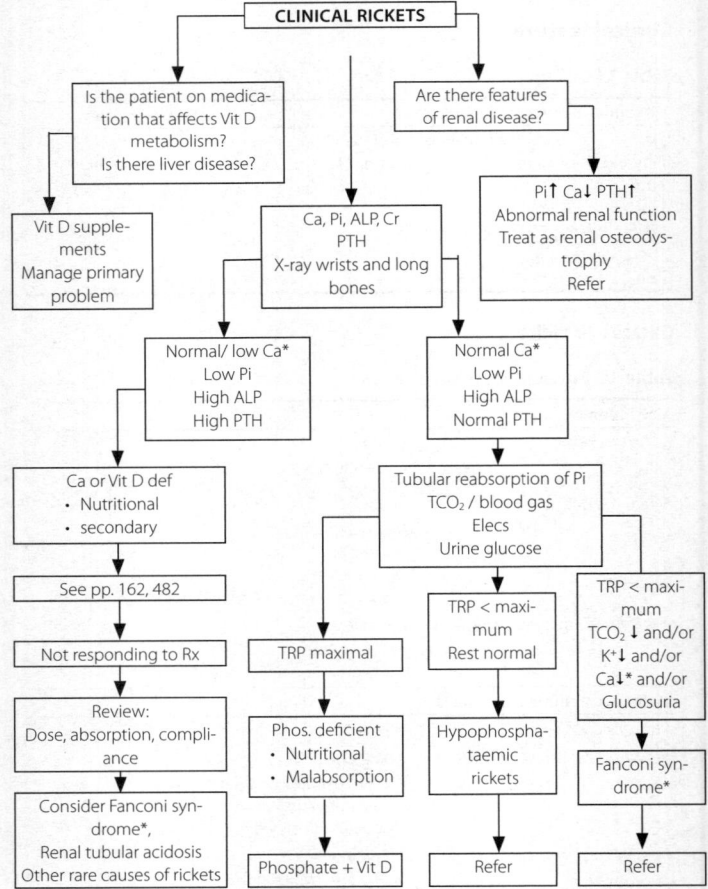

*Fanconi syndrome may start with only one abnormality and develop several over time

Problems with calcium and parathyroid hormone

A simple approach to management

Table 14. 22 The management of calcium and parathyroid hormone disorders

Low Ca*		
High PTH		Low or inappropriately normal PTH
Pi		HYPOPARATHYROIDISM
Normal or high	Low	Start treatment
PSEUDO-HYPOPARATHY-ROIDISM	Rickets**	Refer
Start treatment		
Refer		

High Ca***		
High or inappropriately normal PTH High urine Ca	Low PTH High urine Ca	Low or normal PTH Low urine Ca
HYPERPARATHYROIDISM	VIT D excess Ca excess Malignancy Immobilization Thiazide diuretics Subcutaneous fat necrosis Williams syndrome Granulomatous disease Hyperthyroidism Milk-alkali syndrome Bartter syndrome	Hypocalciuric hypercalcaemia
Manage hypercalcaemia***	Manage hypercalcaemia***	
Refer	Manage underlying condition/refer	

* Refer p. 482
** Refer p. 163, An approach to rickets
*** Refer Hypercalcaemia below

Table 14.23 The treatment of hypoparathyroidism and pseudohypoparathyroidism

Alfacalcidol	< 20 kg 0.05 mcg/kg/d PO	> 20 kg 1 mcg/d PO
Or calcitriol	0.01-0.04 mcg/kg/d PO	
Calcium elemental	30 mg/kg/d PO (1 calcium carbonate tablet = 168 mg elemental calcium)	
Do not use ergocalciferol – it is ineffective in these conditions		

Hypercalcaemia

Definition

Blood calcium above upper limit of normal for age.

Table 14.24 Normal laboratory values

Age	Total serum calcium (mmol/l)	Ionised calcium (mmol/l)
Premature infants	> 2.3	1.5
Full term infants	> 2.6	1.3
Children and adolescents	> 2.7	1.3

* Hypercalcaemic crisis: calcium > 3.5 mmol/l

Clinical features

Table 14.25 Clinical features of hypercalcaemia

Intestinal symptoms	Anorexia
	Nausea
	Vomiting
	Abdominal pain – peptic ulceration or acute pancreatitis
	Constipation
Urinary symptoms	Polydipsia
	Polyuria
	Nocturia
	Renal colic
Skeletal symptoms	Bone pain
Nervous system symptoms	Headache
	Muscular weakness
	Impaired concentration
	Increased sleep requirement
	Altered level of consciousness
	Convulsions
	Depression in an adolescent

Cardiovascular signs	Dehydration
	Hypertension
	Shortened QT interval

Emergency management

- Normal saline at 2-3 times maintenance rate (add maintenance potassium)
- Furosemide
- Severe or persistently elevated calcium – discuss dialysis, steroids, bisphosphonates or calcitonin use with specialist.

Recommended reading

1. *ISPAD Clinical Practice Consensus Guidelines 2006-2008.* Available under: Resources on http://www.ispad.org
2. *Practical endocrinology and diabetes in children* (2nd Ed.). Raine, JE. Blackwell. 2006.

15 Haematology and oncology

F. Desai, M. Hendricks

Haematology

The haemoglobin concentration and mean corpuscular volume vary according to age. Normal values are shown below.

Table 15.1. Average haemoglobin and mean corpuscular volume according to age.

Age	Hb g/dl	MCV fl
0–2 weeks	14.0	> 100
6 weeks	9.5	80 – 96
3 months	10.0	72 – 96
6– 8 months	11.0	70 – 96
18–48 months	11.5	75 – 96
4–12 years	11.5	76 – 95
> 12 years	Girls 12 Boys 14	78 – 96

Anaemia

Anaemia is the most common haematological abnormality in childhood.

Diagnosis of anaemia

- Take a thorough history (birth weight, diet, pica, recurrent jaundice, ethnicity, drug exposure or infections, family history of splenectomy or cholecystectomy, travel history).
- Examine the patient (dysmorphology, pallor, jaundice, signs of cardiac failure, hepatosplenomegaly, purpura and lymphadenopathy).
- Identify that the haemoglobin value is low for age.
- Establish whether the anaemia is simple (low Hb with a normal WCC and platelet count) or complex (low Hb with low or abnormal WCC and/or platelets).
- Complex anaemias warrant consultation with a specialist paediatrician or haematologist for further appropriate investigation or referral (e.g. bone marrow biopsy).

- In the case of simple anaemia establish the type based on the mean corpuscular volume: microcytic, macrocytic or normocytic.
- Tailor investigations according to the morphology.

Figure 15.1 Management of simple anaemia

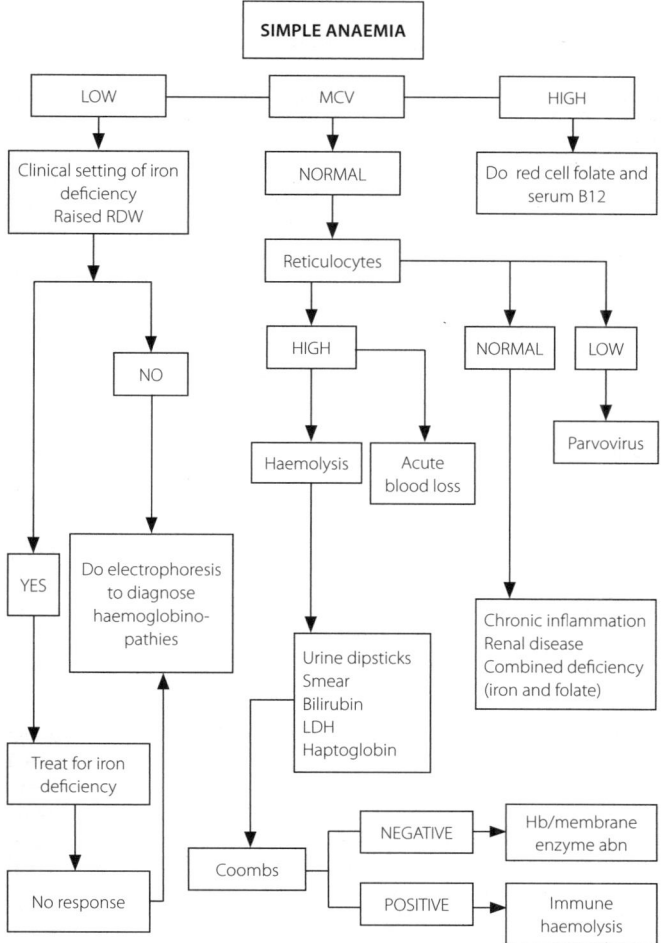

Iron deficiency

This is the most common cause of anaemia worldwide. The peak incidence occurs between 6 months and 2 years of age and is primarily dietary. Blood loss is a common cause in older children.

Prophylaxis

Give oral iron to artificially fed infants from 1 month of age and to breastfed infants from 3 months of age. Use iron-enriched milk powders or an oral elemental iron supplement: term infants 1 mg/kg/day; preterm infants 2 mg/kg/day.

Treatment

- Treat empirically with elemental iron 3–6 mg/kg/day as ferrous sulphate in 2 divided doses along with oral vitamin C to enhance gut absorption. Check the haemoglobin after 4 weeks.
- If no improvement, consider: poor compliance, continued blood loss or infection interfering with iron utilization. If iron studies do not confirm the diagnosis of iron deficiency another cause for the anaemia must be sought, for example thalassaemia. Effective iron therapy should correct anaemia within 1 to 2 months. Continue iron therapy for a further 2 months to replenish body iron stores.

Folate deficiency

- Risk factors:
  - Preterm infants
  - Goat's milk diet
  - Intestinal malabsorption
  - Anticonvulsants.
- In children with macrocytic anaemia, measure red cell folate and serum B12 levels.
- Treatment: folic acid PO 2.5 mg–5 mg daily.

Haemolytic anaemia

Congenital haemolytic anaemia arises as a result of intrinsic red cell abnormalities (membrane, haemoglobin or enzyme defects). Acquired haemolytic anaemia can be immune or non-immune and is secondary to infections, toxins, malignancies and microangiopathy of varying causes. In auto-immune haemolysis warm antibodies (IgG) are associated with brisk haemolysis whereas cold antibodies (IgM) are associated with more indolent haemolysis.

Figure 15.2 Congenital red cell abnormalities

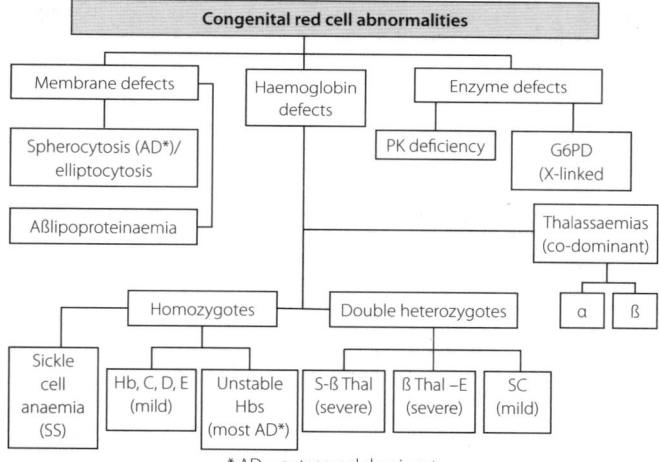

* AD = autosomal dominant

Figure 15.3 Red cell microenvironment abnormalities

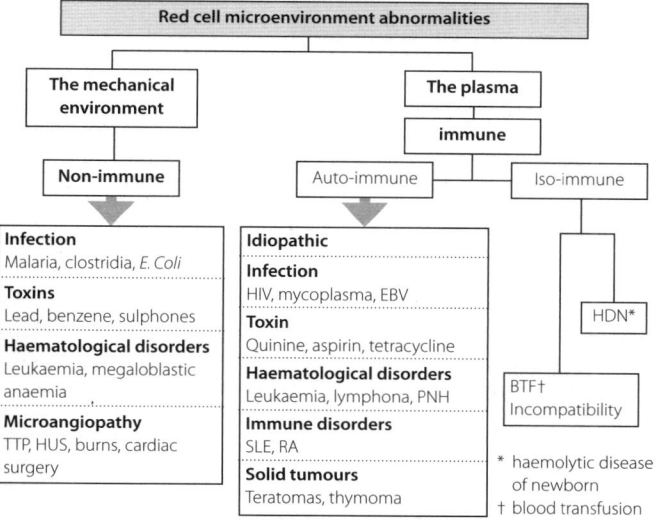

Diagnosis

Establish if the anaemia is haemolytic, where the site of destruction is and what the cause is.

Table 15.2 Investigation of haemolysis

Characteristics of haemolyisis	Appropriate initial investigations
• Pallor • Jaundice (unconjugated hyperbilirubinaemia) • Raised LDH • Urobilinogenuria • Decreased haptoglobin (heme scavenger)	• FBC, retics and Coombs. Cross match if blood transfusion is required • Total and conjugated bilirubin, ALT, LDH • Urine dipstix • Serum haptoglobin (if available)
• Macrocytosis, polychromasia and fragments	• Blood smear
• Sickle cells, spherocytes, bite and blister cells (G6PD)	• Blood smear
• Radiological changes reflecting chronic erythroid hyperplasia	• Skull X-ray

Congenital haemolytic anaemias

Sickle cell anaemia

This is the most important congenital haemolytic anaemia in children of Central African and South and Middle East Asian descent.

This disorder is most severe in children with homozygous sickle cell disease, of intermediate severity in double heterozygotes (e.g. haemoglobin SC) and mild in those with a sickle cell trait.

Four classic crises are described:
1. Vaso-occlusive crisis
2. Haemolytic crisis
3. Aplastic crisis
4. Splenic sequestration.

Recurrent infections also complicate this condition because of functional asplenia. The commonest cause of death under 2 years of age is infection due to encapsulated organisms (*Pneumococcus* and *Haemophilus* species). The recent addition of conjugate pneumococcal vaccine to the national vaccination schedule, in addition to the already available Hib vaccine, will, over time, alter this profile for South African born children.

Diagnosis

- History:
  - Family history
  - Ethnic origin
  - Previous dactylitis
  - Recurrent episodes of jaundice, anaemia and infection.
- Investigations:
  - Basic investigations for haemolytic anaemia
  - Sickle preparation
  - Haemoglobin electrophoresis for definitive diagnosis.
  - Screening of siblings.

Management

- Prevention of infection:
  - Penicillin prophylaxis from diagnosis, Penicillin VK PO 125 mg bd under 3 years of age, and 250 mg bd thereafter.
- Routine immunisation:
  - Hib and HepB
  - Pneumovac at age 2 and every 5 years thereafter
  - Less than 2 years give pneumococcal conjugate vaccine
  - Influenza vaccine yearly.
- Treatment of acute infections:
  - Prompt administration of broad spectrum antibiotics is mandatory following the relevant cultures:
    - Ambulatory patients: oral co-amoxiclav PO 25 mg/kg tds according to weight
    - Patients requiring IV antibiotics: ceftriaxone IV 50 mg/kg/day. Tailor antibiotic choice according to culture positivity and sensitivity.
- Treatment of vaso-occlusive crises:
  - Hydrate with maintenance IV fluids.
  - Cover empirically with broad spectrum antibiotics.
  - Provide adequate analgesia: start with oral paracetamol/codeine combination regularly every 6 hours and progress to IV opiates if necessary.
  - Most children will respond to adequate hydration and oral analgesia.
  - If pain persists or worsens try IV methylprednisolone 15 mg/kg/day for 2 days. Watch for rebound pain. ☆☆☆☺
  - Children with recurrent severe crises should be considered for hydroxyurea therapy: 15 mg/kg/day. ☆☆☆☆☢ Monitor Hb F levels. Aim for 10%. Must be done in consultation with a haematologist.

Table 15.3 Indications for transfusion and for referral

Indications for blood transfusion	Indications for referral
Acute splenic sequestration (resuscitation with blood and discussion with a paediatric haematologist is *mandatory* before referral)	
	Stroke
Acute chest syndrome (chest pain, dyspnoea, pallor, respiratory distress, hypoxaemia, abnormal CXR)	
Aplastic crisis (low reticulocyte count, parvovirus IgM)	
Brisk haemolysis (high reticulocyte count, pallor and jaundice)	
Preparation for anaesthetic or surgery	
Priapism	

Bleeding disorders

Haemostatic defects result from a deficiency of platelets or clotting factors or both. All children with a significant bleeding history or abnormal haemostatic screening tests should be discussed with a haematologist for possible referral to a tertiary paediatric centre.

History

Is the child a bleeder?
- Bruises at abnormal sites
- Any spontaneous bleeding
- Bleeding following dental extraction or surgery
- Bleeding disproportionate to the degree of trauma.

What type of bleeding?
- Thrombocytopenia:
  - Mucosal bleeding (epistaxis, GIT bleeding, menorrhagia)
  - Petechiae and small bruises.
- Coagulation defects:
  - Deep seated haematomas
  - Haemarthroses
  - Haematuria.

How severe is it?
Is it inherited?

Investigations

- Platelet count
- INR
- PTT: if the PTT is prolonged, a mix with normal plasma must be performed. If the PTT corrects to within 6 seconds of the control then there is a clotting factor deficiency in the test sample, most commonly FVIII or FIX deficiency. If the PTT does not fully correct consider an inhibitor, like heparin.
- Bleeding time: perform this only if platelet count and coagulation screen are normal and there is a history of superficial bleeding.

Clotting abnormalities

Figure 15.4 Clotting screen

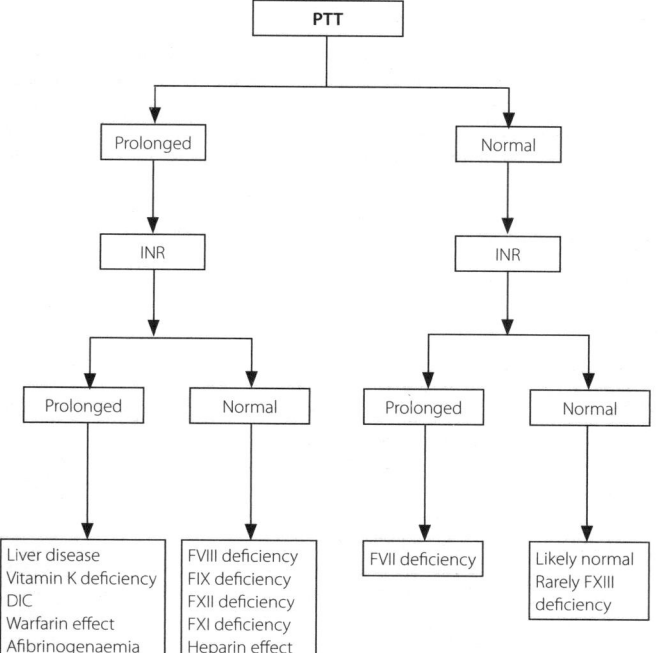

Acquired bleeding disorders

Disseminated intravascular coagulation (DIC)

- Consumption of platelets and clotting factors and fibrinogen is followed by fibrinolysis with the production of fibrin-split products. Consider DIC in suspected Gram-negative infection, severe systemic illness, purpura fulminans and burns.
- In neonates, DIC can follow septicaemia, birth asphyxia, acidosis, hypothermia and respiratory distress syndrome.
- Correct the underlying cause. In a bleeding patient, transfuse with blood and platelets. Use fresh frozen plasma (FFP) 15–20 ml/kg to correct the PTT. Wet cryoprecipitate 10 units/kg may be given for severe hypofibrinogenaemia.

Thrombocytopenia

- Isolated thrombocytopenia with a sudden onset of bruising, petechiael rash or epistaxis in an otherwise well child is usually immune in origin (immune thrombocytopenic purpura (ITP)). This is usually idiopathic or may be secondary to immunizations, viral infections, like HIV, or less commonly collagen vascular disease especially in the older child.
- Other causes include drugs, hypersplenism, DIC, infections or marrow infiltration.

Management of ITP

- Restrict activity.

> **Practice point**
>
> Platelet transfusion is not routinely indicated as they are consumed.
> In the bleeding patient give prednisone PO 4 mg/kg/day for 4 days.
> ☆☆☆☆◊

- Prednisone should only be given if there is certainty about the diagnosis of ITP, i.e. no features to suggest leukaemia, e.g. blasts on the differential count or unexplained anaemia or neutropaenia, a raised LDH and the presence of significant adenopathy and/or hepatosplenomegaly.

- A bone marrow biopsy *must* be done before starting steroids if there is *any* doubt about the diagnosis of ITP.
- In the event of brisk or life threatening haemorrhage give IVIG 1g/kg/day for 2 days. ☆☆☆☆☆ Also consider concomitant high dose methyl prednisolone at 30 mg/kg/day for 3 days.
- All children with chronic ITP should have a bone marrow biopsy and auto-immune screen performed.
- Splenectomy is rarely indicated in chronic ITP.

Inherited bleeding disorders

Von Willebrand disease (vWD)

- This is the most common congenital bleeding disorder and affects up to 1% of the population. Bleeding is superficial and usually mild or moderate. Investigations: bleeding time, factor VIII and von Willebrand factor assays.
- Most patients (excluding the rare autosomal recessive Type III) will respond to desmopressin acetate (DDAVP) 0.3 µg/kg per dose IV. A DDAVP response test should be done prior to considering this treatment. DDAVP may also be given prior to minor surgery, e.g. tonsillectomy. Factor-VIII concentrate 20 U/kg IV is treatment of choice for severe bleeding.

Haemophilia A

Treatment

Give Factor VIII 15–20 U/kg for the average joint bleed; repeat it daily until the swelling subsides. Use 40 U/kg for suspected intracranial bleeding, following a head injury and prior to surgery. Phone a comprehensive haemophilia centre for advice once the first 40 U/kg have been given. If surgery is contemplated for a serious injury, phone a tertiary centre for advice once the first 40 U/kg dose has been given. ☆☆☆☆☆

Haemophilia B

Treatment:

Give Factor IX 25–30 U/kg or more for serious bleeding. Repeat every 24 hours. ☆☆☆☆☆

> ***Practice point***
>
> - *Do not* give IM injections or aspirin-containing compounds to patients with haemophilia or other bleeding disorders.
> - NEVER take blood from the jugular or femoral veins or perform arterial punctures.

Indications for transfusion of clotting factor:

- Pain or swelling in joint or muscle
- External bleeding not controlled by pressure
- Pre-operative
- Head trauma or headache should be treated urgently. Do not delay by waiting for imaging.

Oncology

Childhood cancer is uncommon (110–130 per million children per year in Western countries). Striking advances in management and prognosis have occurred in the last few decades and approximately 70% of paediatric cancers are curable. This has been achieved through clinical trials evaluating the most effective combinations of multi-agent chemotherapy, radiotherapy and surgery.

Leukaemia and brain tumours are the most common malignancies. The solid tumors are comprised mainly of embryonal malignancies (e.g. nephroblastoma, neuroblastoma) and sarcomas, rather than carcinomas.

> ***Practice point***
>
> Early diagnosis of all malignancies improves outcome.
>
> In addition children have a survival advantage if managed at a paediatric cancer centre and should be referred to paediatric oncologists for definitive care.

Warning signs in childhood cancer

- Pallor plus bleeding such as purpura, unexplained bruises or persistent oozing from the nose or mouth.
- Fever, apathy or weight loss that is persistent or unexplained, after excluding tuberculosis or HIV infection.

- Bone pain, often poorly localized and which may wake the child at night. It may present as a limp in the older child or a refusal to walk in a toddler. Persistent backache is sinister and may denote a spinal tumour. Backache is *always* abnormal in children and should be fully investigated.
- Localized lymphadenopathy that is persistent and unexplained. Discreet non-tender nodes (> 2 cm in diameter) that do not respond within 2 weeks to antibiotic therapy and all supraclavicular nodes should be biopsied.
- Unexplained mass (abdomen, testes, head and neck and limbs); an abdominal mass in a child under 5 is likely to be malignant.
- Unexplained neurological signs like longstanding or early morning headaches (> 2 weeks), early morning vomiting, ataxia or cranial nerve palsies.
- Eye signs: leucocoria (white spot in the eye or white light reflex), recent onset squint, proptosis and loss of vision.

Approach to a suspected malignancy in children

- All children with a suspected malignancy must be discussed promptly with a paediatric oncologist.
- Avoid unnecessary investigations that may delay diagnosis and referral.
- A few basic investigations are helpful and include a chest X-ray, HIV test, full blood count with a differential count, coagulation screen, ESR, urea, creatinine and electrolytes, ALT, LDH and serum urate.
- For suspected germ cell tumors or hepatoblastoma an α-fetoprotein and/or serum ß-chorionic gonadotrophin (ßHCG) is helpful.

Approach to febrile neutropaenia

Febrile neutropaenia is a common and potentially life threatening complication following intensive chemotherapy. Any child on chemotherapy who presents with a fever should have a full blood count and differential count done immediately to establish whether they are neutropaenic ($< 1 \times 10^9$/l or $< 1\,000$/mm^3).

- All children with leukaemia and non-Hodgkin's lymphoma should receive prophylactic oral trimethoprim-sulphoxazole twice daily 3 times a week to prevent *Pneumocystis jirovecii* pneumonia. ☆☆☆☆☆
- Culture blood, urine and any infected lesions and obtain a chest X-ray.

- Start broad spectrum empiric antibiotic therapy immediately, keeping in mind the local bacterial resistance patterns in your institution.
- Pathogens include *Staphylococcus aureus, Streptococcus viridans, Escherichia coli, Klebsiella* sp, and *Pseudomonas aeruginosa*. *Staphylococcus epidermidis* is a common pathogen in children with central venous access devices. Our first line therapy for febrile neutropaenia is:
  - Piperacillin tazobactam 90 mg/kg/dose 6 hourly IVI and
  - Amikacin 25 mg/kg/day IVI up to a maximum of 600 mg/day in children < 12 years and up to 900 mg/day in children > 12 years.
  ☆☆☆☆☆
- In children with central venous access devices consider changing IV amikacin to IV vancomycin 10 mg/kg 6 hourly, if there is no response to first line therapy after 48 hours.
- In those with prolonged neutropaenia consider a systemic fungal infection if fever persists despite broad spectrum antibiotic therapy. Treat empirically with amphotericin B.
- Varicella and now, much less commonly, measles, may be hazardous in immunosuppressed children:
  - Give varicella contacts zoster immune globulin 0.15 ml/kg IM.
  - To be effective, prophylaxis must be given within 72 hours of exposure.
  - Varicella: treat urgently with acyclovir 10 mg/kg IV 8-hourly for 10 days.
  - Oral herpes simplex: acyclovir 5–10 mg/kg orally 5 times daily.

Blood product transfusion

> *Practice point*
>
> All blood must be fully cross matched prior to administration except in the case of emergency resuscitation with O negative blood. Prior to administration of any blood product, the patient name and folder number, unit number, blood group and expiry date must be checked.

- Obtain written consent from the parent or guardian prior to transfusion.
- Transfuse packed red cells 15 ml/kg over 4 hours. Administer IV furosemide 1 mg/kg half way through. In neonates, very young infants, or children with recurrent transfusion requirements use lymphocyte

depleted or filtered red cells. Half hourly observations of pulse rate and temperature should be performed for the duration of the transfusion.
- Transfuse platelets 15–20 ml/kg IV fast in the child with thrombocytopenia and bleeding. Use a special blood transfusion filter and do not run the platelets through an IVAC. Premedicate patients with known reactions to platelet transfusions with IV promethazine 0.5 mg/kg. If apheresed platelets are used, 1 paediatric unit (50 ml) will suffice in younger patients, or 1 adult unit in older patients.

Recommended reading

1 Booth, IW, Aukett, MA. Iron deficiency in infancy and early childhood. *Arch Dis Child* 1997;76:549–554
2 Nojliana, B, Norman, R, Dhansay, MA, *et al.* Estimating the burden of disease attributable to iron deficiency anaemia in South Africa in 2000. *South Afr Med J* 2007;97:741–746
3 Beck, CE, Nathan, PC, Parkin, PC, *et al.* Corticosteroids versus intravenous immunoglobulin for the treatment of acute immune thrombocytopaenic purpura in children: A systematic review and meta-analysis of randomized control trials. *J Pediatr* 2005;147:521–527
4 Berntrop, E, Astermark, J, Bjorken, S *et al.* Consensus perspectives on prophylaxis therapy for haemophilia. *Haemophilia* 2003;9 (suppl 1):1–4
5 Wing-Yen Wong. Prevention and management of infection in children with sickle cell anaemia. *Pediatr Drugs* 2001;3(11):793–801

16 Dermatology

G. Todd

This chapter concentrates on the problems that are most common in a primary care setting. For any condition that is atypical in presentation or response to appropriate and adequate treatment, it is advised to seek a dermatology opinion.

Acne

See Figures 16.1 and 16.2 Acne.

Acne is an inflammatory reaction of the pilosebaceous unit. It is not an infection but is caused by the complex interplay between sex hormones, follicle hyperkeratosis, sebum secretion and follicular commensals. It occurs at puberty but can be seen in neonates. Drugs (steroids, contraceptives), chemicals (oils, greases and tars), cosmetics and occlusion can all aggravate acne.

The diagnostic lesion is the comedone. The open comedone (black head) is a dilated follicular pore packed with discoloured debris. The closed comedone (white head) is a skin coloured papule. Inflammation of the primary comedones leads to erythematous papules, nodules, pustules and cysts. The face, neck, back, chest, upper arms and buttock may all be affected.

> *Practice point*
>
> Acne causes significant psychological effects and heals with scarring and thus warrants treatment.
>
> Response to treatment is not immediate and it may be needed for months to years.

Treatment

Topical agents for mild to moderate acne include:
- Retinoids (adapalene, isotretinoin, tazarotene, tretinoin) used for the prevention and treatment of comedones. They are irritant, causing dryness and peeling. 💧★☆☆☆
- Benzoyl peroxide used for inflammatory acne. It is irritant, causing dryness and peeling. 💧★☆☆☆

- Topical antibiotic lotions (clindamycin, erythromycin) used for inflammatory acne ☝☆☆☆☆
- Topical cleansers may control mild acne. ☝☆☆☆☆

Systemic agents are reserved for the recalcitrant, more severe and extensive forms of acne, often in combination with topical agents. These include:

- Antibiotics (tetracyclines, doxycycline, minocycline, co-trimoxazole, erythromycin) are given for inflammatory acne in short courses of up to 4 months. ☝☆☆☆☆
- Hormonal manipulation combines oestrogens with progesterones of low androgenicity or the anti-androgens, cyproterone acetate or drosperinone, and is suitable for those requiring contraception who have moderate to severe acne. ☝☆☆☆☆
- Retinoids (isotretinoin) are extremely effective used over 6 months for severe or scarring acne. They are teratogenic and can only be used with extreme caution in women of child-bearing age who must use adequate contraception. ☝☆☆☆☆

General measures

- Maintain normal skin hygiene. Acne is not due to poor hygiene.
- Remove excess skin oiliness with topical degreasing preparations.
- Cosmetics should be water-based of low comedogenicity.
- Avoid squeezing lesions as this aggravates scarring.
- Maintain a healthy diet. Diet plays a minor role in acne.

Birthmarks

Pigmented (melanocytic) naevi

Refer all congenital naevi.

Refer naevi for an expert opinion if they develop:

- A change in size and colour
- Irregular borders or nodules
- Bleeding or ulceration
- Symptoms of itch or pain in the lesions.

Vascular naevi and malformations

Refer these for an expert opinion if they:

- Are very large or involve multiple sites
- Grow rapidly or ulcerate
- Are near an eye or are on the 'beard' area of the face
- Are on the tongue or oral mucosa
- Are in the genital area.

Eczema (or dermatitis)

See Figure 16.2 Acute eczema and Figure 16.3 Chronic eczema.

Eczema is the most common condition encountered in a paediatric dermatology clinic. It includes atopic, seborrheic, contact (irritant and allergic), napkin and nummular eczema/dermatitis.

Eczema may present acutely with the diagnostic features of vesicles, weeping, crusting and peeling on a background of erythema and possible swelling. In chronic eczema thickened, scaly, variably pigmented plaques with increased skin markings (lichenification) are seen, which suggest chronic scratching due to itching. Secondary infection with bacteria (*Staphylococcus aureus*, *Streptococcus pyogenes*), fungi (*Candida albicans*) or viruses (herpes simplex) may complicate eczema.

Atopic eczema

Atopic eczema occurs in infants at about 3 months of age when it commonly involves the face. Older children have lesions predominantly in flexures but in some cases only the extensor surfaces are involved. In severe cases the eczema is generalized. The skin is often very dry. There may be associated asthma, hay fever or other allergies. Contact dermatitis and urticaria may contribute to unresponsive atopic eczema. The role of food is controversial but may be considered in cases where a particular food has been associated with a well documented flare of the eczema in young children or when eczema is associated with other allergic disease.

Contact eczema

Contact eczema can be due to skin irritation or an allergic reaction to substances in contact with the skin. It often complicates other types of eczema. Irritant eczema is common and can occur after a single or repetitive exposure to irritant substances such as detergent, alkalis, acids, solvents or simply water or dry environmental conditions. Allergic contact dermatitis is less common but a wide range of allergens have been identified, which are included as standard allergens in patch testing series used for diagnostic testing. These include metals (nickel, chrome and mercury) perfumes and fragrances, rubber components, and anti-microbial and preservative components in water-based products. The body site involved is a good clue to the potential cause.

Napkin eczema

Eczema of the napkin area is a form of irritant contact dermatitis due to prolonged occlusive exposure of the skin to urine and faeces. It may complicate seborrhoeic and atopic eczema. It may be complicated by secondary infection with *Candida*. Use zinc-containing barrier creams applied to clean skin after every nappy change. As the differential for napkin eczema is broad, recalcitrant and unusual cases must be referred to a dermatologist.

Nummular eczema

Nummular eczema manifests as intensely itchy, round patches, often on the legs and may be associated with atopic dermatitis. It is often difficult to control, requiring potent topical steroids.

Pityriasis alba

See Figure 16.4.

This common condition is regarded as low grade eczema. Typically this consists of pale, scaly patches on the face. Central hyperpigmentation may occur.

Pityriasis alba is often mistaken for the fungal infection, pityriasis versicolor.

Seborrhoeic dermatitis

Seborrhoeic eczema occurs in the body folds, and on the scalp (cradle cap), face and napkin area in infants up to 3 months of age. It may be mildly itchy or asymptomatic and has a characteristic greasy scale. The cause is unknown. In the napkin region it may be complicated by *Candida* infection and irritant dermatitis.

Treatment of eczema

- Use topical steroids to rapidly control eczema and then wean to the lowest strength (this may be a simple moisturiser) needed to maintain control of the eczema. For mild cases, especially of the face and body folds, use hydrocortisone 1%. For more severe presentations, a more potent product, such as betamethasone, will be necessary. Do not apply potent steroids to the face and limit use in folds and flexures. ✎☆☆☆☆
- The fingertip method (Table 16.1) is a guide to applying topical steroid.
- When prescribing topical steroids, specify the amount required to last until the next visit.
- The efficacy of topical steroid can be increased by occluding the skin with wet or dry dressings. When there are signs of infection do not occlude the skin with wet wraps. ☺☆☆☆☆

- The non-steroid, cytokine inhibitors, tacrolimus and pimecrolimus, may be useful, but costly, alternates to topical steroids for selected patients and body areas. Lack of long term safety data limits their use. ☺︎☆☆☆☆
- For infected eczema, gently remove crusts and accretions with wet compresses and soaking and apply an antimicrobial (povidone-iodine, silver sulphadiazine, fusidic acid or mupirocin). In addition give a course of oral antibiotic such as erythromycin or flucloxacillin if widespread, severe or associated with systemic symptoms. ✋☆☆☆☆
- For suspected or proven contact eczema, identify and remove the cause.

General measures

- Skin hygiene is the cornerstone of good eczema care. Apply an emollient (aqueous cream) all over then soak the child in warm water and gently remove all crusts and old ointment.
- Avoid skin irritation. Triggers include soap, detergents, heat, certain clothing and scratching. Advise the use of an emollient as a soap substitute. Explain the itch-scratch cycle.
- Liberal use of moisturisers is recommended. Personal preference should direct the choice of the product which may be oil (grease/ointment) or water (cream/lotion) based. ✋☆☆☆☆
- Give an antihistamine for sleep disruption (sedating) or if urticaria (non-sedating) is present. ✋☆☆☆☆☆
- Topical salicylic acid 2%, precipitated sulphur 2% in aqueous cream is useful for the removal of scalp crusts and scale. ☺︎☆☆
- Any child not responsive to adequate topical care should be referred to a dermatologist for assessment.

Table 16.1 Finger tip unit (FTU) application of topical corticosteroids

FTU: amount of cream squeezed onto index finger from tip to first crease = 0.5g						
Age	face/neck FTU (g)	arm/hand FTU (g)	leg/foot FTU (g)	trunk-front FTU (g)	trunk-back FTU (g)	Full body FTU (g)
3–6 mths	1 (0.5 g)	1 (0.5 g)	1.5 (0.75 g)	1 (0.5 g)	1.5 (0.75 g)	4.25 g
1–2 yr	1.5 (0.75 g)	1.5 (0.75 g)	2 (1 g)	2 (1 g)	3 (1.5 g)	6.75 g
3–5 yr	1.5 (0.75 g)	2 (1 g)	3 (1.5 g)	3 (1.5 g)	3.5 (1.75 g)	9.0 g
6–10 yr	2 (1 g)	2.5 (1.25 g)	4.5 (2.25 g)	3.5 (1.75 g)	5 (2.5 g)	12.25 g
> 10 yr	2.5 (1.25g)	arm 3 (1.5 g) hand 1 (0.5 g)	leg 6 (3.0 g) foot 2 (1.0 g)	7 (3.5 g)	7 (3.5 g)	20.25 g

Drug reactions

See Figure 16.5 Blistering eruptions and Figure 16.6 Drug hypersensitivity syndrome.

Skin rashes are common side effects associated with medication. Most of these are morbilliform (measles-like) or urticarial and resolve spontaneously without sequelae, often despite ongoing use of the offending drug.

Some reactions are life-threatening and need urgent recognition. These include blistering eruptions (Stevens-Johnson syndrome, toxic epidermal necrolysis, erythema multiforme), systemic drug reactions (drug hypersensitivity syndrome) and angio-oedema.

The following clinical features should be looked for (see Figures 16.5a and 16.5b):

- Purple (necrotic skin) lesions
- Blisters
- Mucosal lesions
- Fever
- Systemic features (hepatitis, nephritis, pneumonitis, bone marrow suppression etc.)
- Facial, hand and foot oedema
- Problems with breathing.

All suspect medication should be discontinued and the patient stabilized pending immediate referral to a dermatologist or centre of expertise.

Fungal infections of the skin

Candida infection (thrush)

See Figure 16.7 Candida infection.

On the skin this causes white patches or a beefy-red scalded appearance with satellite pustules. Moist areas are particularly susceptible such as the buttocks, genitalia, axilla, neck and web spaces. On the oral mucosa it is recognized by white plaques, which are easily removed to reveal underlying erythema. It can also present with a red smooth tongue. Dysphagia may occur if the oesophagus is involved.

It is often associated with antibiotic use and if severe, extensive and recalcitrant to treatment could be a marker of immunosuppression.

Treatment

- Oral mucosa:
  - Oral nystatin 👆☆☆☆☆
  - Azole gel 👆☆☆☆☆
  - Consider oral azole for oesophageal involvement or if severe. 👆☆☆☆☆
- Skin folds (intertrigo):
  - Keep skin clean and dry and treat predisposing conditions.
  - Apply topical azole (clotrimazole, miconazole, ketoconazole or econazole) or nystatin cream twice daily until settles. 👆☆☆☆☆
  - Combined topical antifungals and steroids may be necessary to control associated dermatitis especially of the napkin area. 👆☆☆
  - Oral nystatin for bowel sterilization. 👆☆☆

Pityriasis versicolor

See Figure 16.8 Pityriasis versicolor.

This very common superficial fungal infection is caused by *Malassezia furfur*, a yeast commensal of the hair follicles of the skin. Pale or pigmented scaly patches are found, particularly on the trunk. The lesions are usually asymptomatic but can be itchy. The presence of scale indicates active disease. Post inflammatory hypopigmentation may persist for several weeks after eradication of the pathogenic form of the yeast.

Treatment

- Apply selenium sulphide, zinc pyrithione or an azole (ketoconazole) shampoo to all hair-bearing areas including the scalp. Wash off after 12 hours. Apply on 3 consecutive evenings or once a week for 3 weeks. 👆☆☆☆☆
- If extensive or recalcitrant consider using oral azoles. 👆☆☆☆☆
- The condition tends to be recurrent and may be controlled with the regular (twice weekly) use of selenium sulphide, zinc pyrithione or sulphur and salicylic acid containing soaps (Sastid®, Acne-Aid®). 🙂☆☆

Tinea (dermatophyte) infections

Dermatophyte fungi infect keratin. If infections are severe, recalcitrant and extensive, involving several body areas, underlying lowered immunity should be considered.

Fungal hyphae (skin) or spores (hair) can be seen with a microscope. The dermatophyte can be cultured from the scales or affected hairs taken from a lesion.

Tinea capitis (see Figure 16.9 a, b and c) is an infection of the scalp and hair and is commonly seen in prepubertal children. It presents as round scaly patches of variable hair loss in which broken-off hairs are seen as 'black dots' Less common presentations include diffuse scale with little hair loss or inflammatory forms with scalp pustules and vesicles or focal 'boggy' erythematous inflammatory swellings (kerions).

Tinea corporis (body) and faciei (face) are characterized by asymmetric annular (ring-like) lesions (see Figure 16.10), which have central clearing and an active edge of erythematous papules, vesicles or pustules and scale. Tinea faciei may be mistaken for eczema and lupus and inappropriately treated with topical steroids, which may mask the classic clinical features.

Tinea cruris is an infection of groin and natal cleft. The classic active edge is seen with inflammation or scale, which is usually symmetrically distributed. Occlusion and humidity promote recurrences

Tinea pedis and manuum are infections of the foot and hand respectively. They are uncommon in prepubertal children. Usually only one foot/hand is involved with variable erythema and scale, an active edge may be present. With inflammatory presentations vesicles and pustules may be present, especially of the instep. The webspaces of the feet usually show macerated hyperkeratosis and scale. If the nails are affected recurrences are the norm.

Tinea unguium (onychomycosis) is an infection of the nail plate. The infection can invade superficially, causing superficial white onychomycosis or it invades from the edge of the nail plate causing discoloured (yellow/brown), crumbly and deformed nails. Nail infections often act as reservoirs for repeated infections.

Tinea versicolor (see pityriasis versicolor).

Treatment

Skin:
- Topical agents are effective applied twice a day until all signs of infection have disappeared and remained away for 2 weeks. Any of the following can be used:
  - Whitfield's ointment (salicylic acid:benzoic acid 1:2 ointment). ☺☆☆
  - Topical over-the-counter preparations (undecanoic acid, tolnaftate) ☺☆☆☆☆
  - Topical azole preparations (clotrimazole, miconazole, ketoconazole or econazole) or allylamine preparations (terbinafine) ☽☆☆☆☆

- Systemic agents can be considered for extensive or recalcitrant lesions. 💧☆☆☆☆ Any of the following can be used:
  - Griseofulvin for 4-6 weeks
  - Ketoconazole for 1 week
  - Itraconazole for 1 week
  - Fluconazole once weekly for 2-4 weeks
  - Terbinafine for 2-6 weeks.

Scalp:
- Topical therapy is of no value used alone.
- Povidone-iodine shampoo is sporocidal. ☺☆☆☆
- Oral griseofulvin 10-20 mg/kg/day for 6 weeks. The tablets must be taken with food or milk. 💧☆☆☆☆
- If griseofulvin is contraindicated or not tolerated, consider any of the other oral antifungal agents listed above. 💧☆☆☆☆

Nails:
- Best results combine topical nail avulsion methods with topical (limited number of nails) or systemic antifungals. 💧☆☆☆
- Nail avulsion:
  - Chemical avulsion: urea 40% applied under occlusion for 24 hours, after which loosened, dystrophic nail is scraped away. Wash well and repeat daily until abnormal nail has been removed.
  - Physical avulsion: chiropodist.
- Antifungals:
  - Topical nail paints (limited nail involvement); amorolfine, tioconazole 💧☆☆☆
  - Systemic antifungals:
    - Griseofulvin for 3-6 months (finger nails) or 6-12 months (toe nails) ☺☆☆☆☆
    - Itraconazole for 1 week/month for 2 consecutive months (finger nails) or 3 consecutive months (toe nails) 💧☆☆☆☆
    - Terbinafine for 3 months 💧☆☆☆☆
    - Fluconazole weekly for 6-12 months. ☺☆☆☆☆

General measures:
- Prevent spread to others by advising patient not to share nail clippers, clothing or towels, walk barefoot, or contaminate shared ablutions.
- Consider predisposing causes (diabetes, steroid use, immunocompromise) if the infection is recalcitrant, severe, extensive or recurs.

- For unexplained recurrences consider untreated close contacts or contaminated communal environments
- If treatment fails, consider culture of skin scales or hair as not all organisms have the same antifungal sensitivity spectrum.
- If treatment fails, consider eczema and psoriasis.

Ichthyosis

See Figure 16.11.

This is characterized by dry skin with scaling. Ichthyosis is often seen in atopic eczema patients. Inheritance influences the type of ichthyosis, which may be part of a specific syndrome. Refer severe types for further investigation and specialized management.

Topical therapy includes emollients, with or without the addition of specific humectants such as urea and lactic acid.

Molluscum contagiosum

See Figure 16.12.

This is caused by a pox virus and consists of multiple flesh-coloured, dome-shaped umbilicated papules. Lesions resolve spontaneously without sequelae unless secondarily infected. In the immunocompromised child they may become severe, large, extensive and recalcitrant to treatment and need referral. Troublesome lesions involving the eyelids need referral to ophthalmology.

Treatment

- Allow the infection to resolve spontaneously.
- For cosmetically disturbing lesions consider the following destructive treatments, but they may be complicated by postinflammatory pigmentary change or scars:
  - Apply benzoyl peroxide, tretinoin cream or wart paint carefully to individual lesions. ☺☆☆
  - In a willing child, following local anaesthesia (Emla® cream), liquid nitrogen cryotherapy can be used for limited lesions. ☺☆☆
  - Imiquimod (immunotherapy) applied to individual lesions on alternate days may help recalcitrant lesions. ☺☆☆
- For severe or resistant cases consider physical removal (curettage) under anaesthesia. ☺☆☆

Papular urticaria

See Figure 16.13.

This is very common. It is due to an insect-bite allergy that causes recurrent itchy eruptions. These are polymorphous and include the initial urticarial papules with a central punctum, vesicles, and large bullae. Lesions may be grouped or linear and occur in crops. Older lesions are hyperpigmented or hypopigmented with variable scarring. The excoriated lesions may become impetigenized. Fleas are the most common insect implicated and the body areas affected are commonly the limbs and waist line.

Treatment

- Topical steroids relieve the itch during the active period of insect bites. ☝︎☆☆
- Antihistamines may be helpful for the itch (non-sedating) and sleep (sedating).
- Try to eliminate the offending insects (usually fleas, ticks or mosquitoes).
- Garlic in the diet, oral thiamine and the use of topical tar preparations at night may act as insect deterrents. ☺︎☆☆
- Inform the mother that the eruption may recur for years until the child develops tolerance to insect bites.
- Do not spray children's bedding with insecticides as this is not safe. Permethrin impregnated nets may be useful. ☝︎☆☆

Pediculosis

Lice can cause pruritus and crusted excoriations. These occur mostly on the scalp where nits are attached to the hairs.

Treatment

- Treat all affected people in the household.
- Repeat the treatment after 7 to 10 days to prevent re-infections from hatching nits that are still viable.
- Use any of the following:
  - Gamma-benzenehexachloride (1%) shampoo. Apply to scalp and hair and lather with a little water. Rinse off well after 5 minutes. ☺︎☆☆
  - Benzyl benzoate (25%; 12.5% toddlers; 6% infants) lotion. Apply to the scalp and hair, and leave on overnight then shampoo. ☺︎☆☆
  - Permethrin (1%) cream rinse. Apply to towel dried, clean hair and scalp for 10 minutes. Rinse off well. ☝︎☆☆☆☆

(continued on page 419, after colour section)

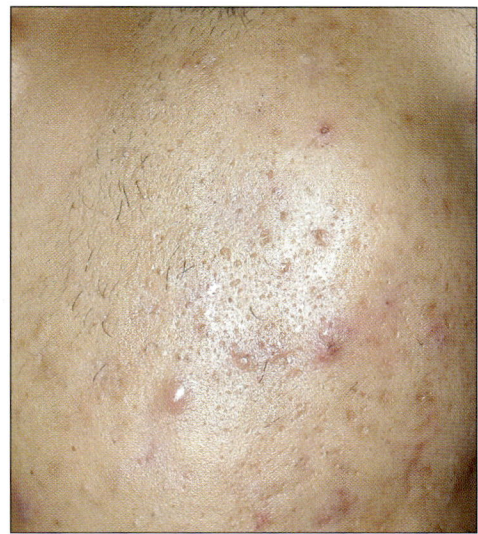

Figure 16.1
Acne: open comedones (dilated follicular pores packed with discoloured debris), closed comedones (skin coloured papules) with inflammatory erythematous papules and pustules and ice-pick scars

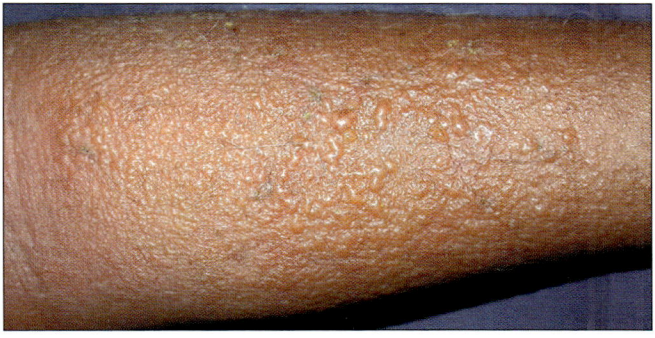

Figure 16.2
Acute eczema: vesicles, weeping, crusting and peeling on a background of erythema and swelling

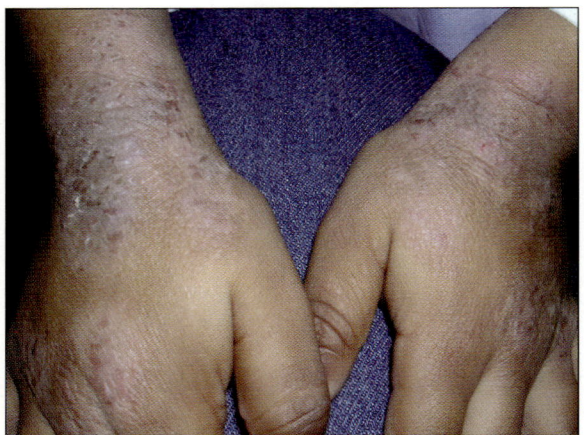

Figure 16.3
Chronic eczema: thickened, scaly, variably pigmented plaques with increased skin markings (lichenification)

Figure 16.4   Pityriasis alba:

Figure 16.4a
Pale, scaly macules

Figure 16.4 Pityriasis alba (continued)**:**

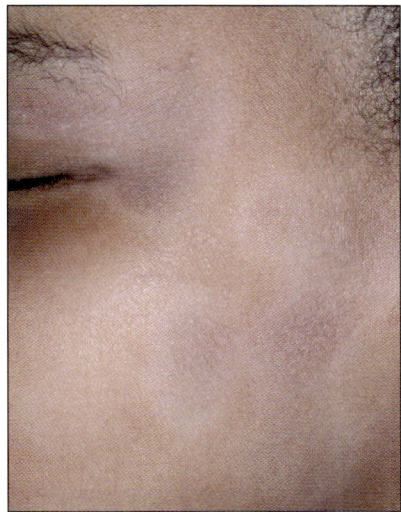

Figure 16.4b
Pale, scaly macules with central hyperpigmenation

Figure 16.5 Blistering eruptions

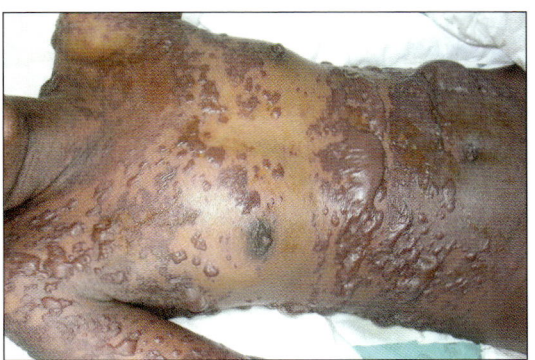

Figure 16.5a
Purple (necrotic skin) lesions with blisters

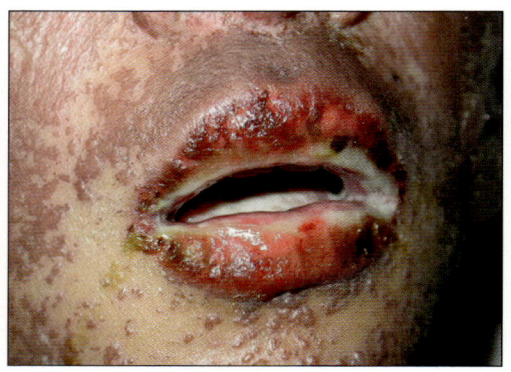

Figure 16.5b
Purple blistering lesions with haemorraghic chelitis

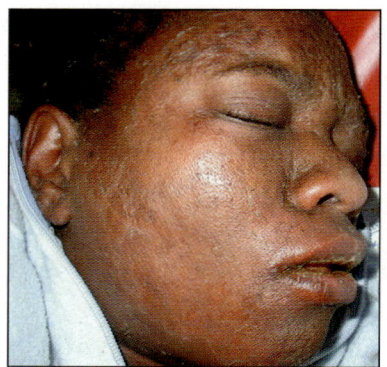

Figure 16.6
Drug hypersensitivity syndrome: swollen face with erythema and crusts

Figure 16.7 Candidiasis:

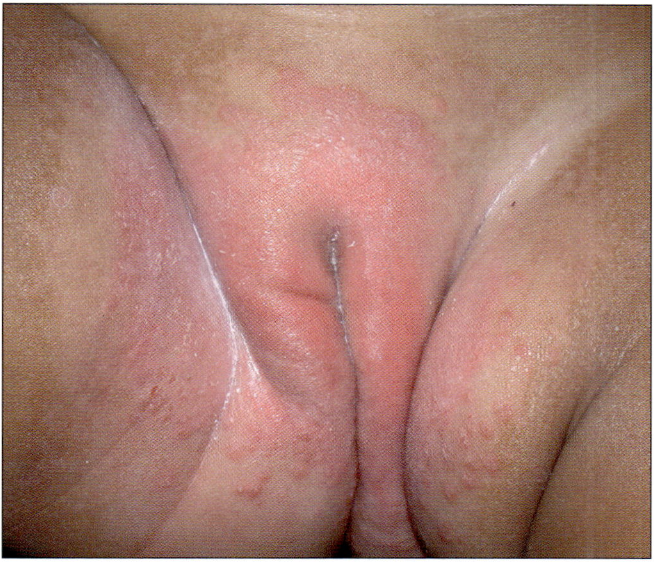

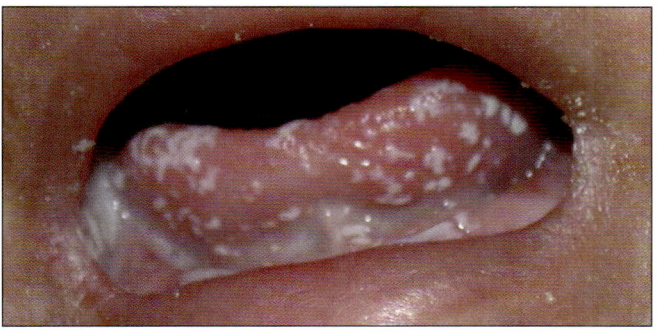

Figure 16.7a
Bright-red skin with satellite pustules

Figure 16.7b
White cheesy plaques with underlying erythema

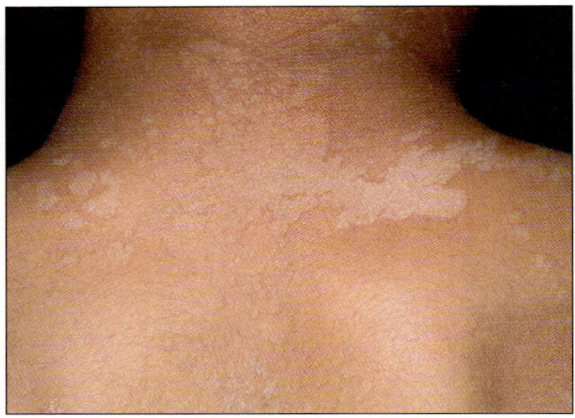

Figure 16.8
Pityriasis versicolor: pale macules with scale accentuated by stretching the skin

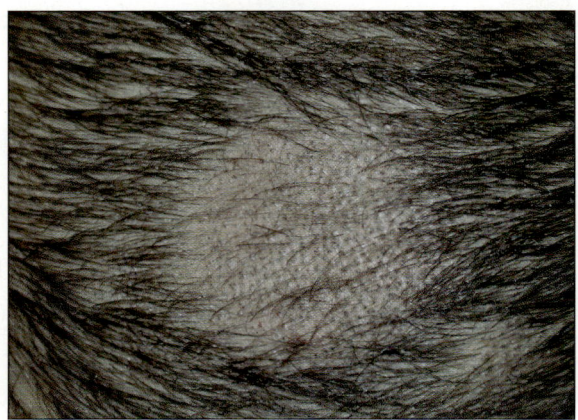

Figure 16.9a
Tinea capitus: scaly patches in which broken-off hairs are seen as "black dots"

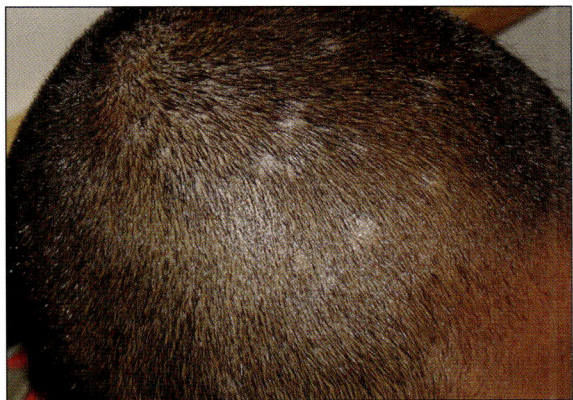

Figure 16.9b
Tinea capitus: diffuse patchy scale with little hair loss

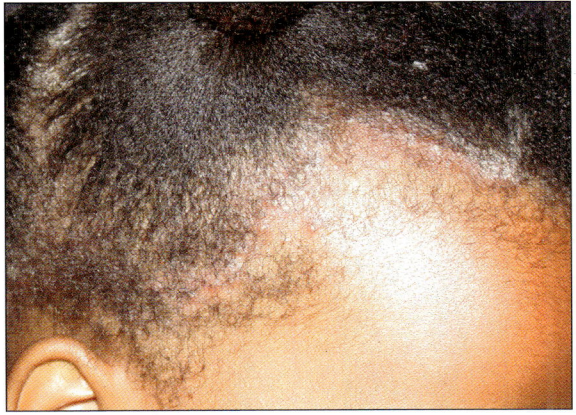

Figure 16.9c
Tinea capitus: inflammatory scalp scale, pustules and vesicles with variable hair loss

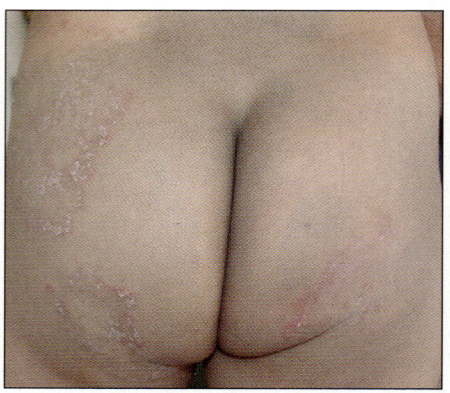

Figure 16.10
Tinea corporis: asymmetric annular (ring-like) lesions with central clearing and an active edge of erythematous papulo-vesicles and scale

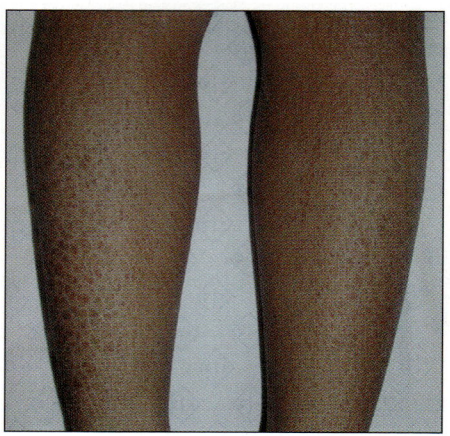

Figure 16.11
Ichthyosis: dry scaly skin with "crazy paving" appearance

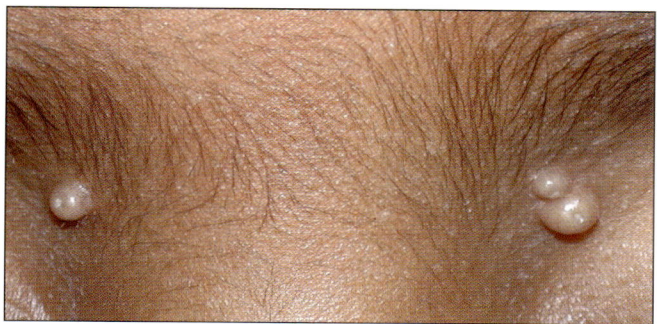

Figure 16.12
Molluscum contagiosum: flesh-coloured, dome-shaped umbilicated papules

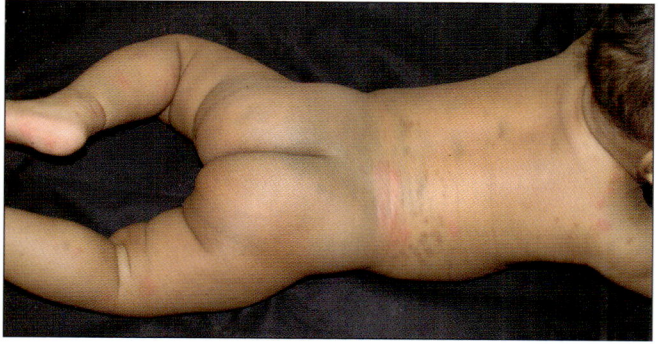

Figure 16.13
Papular urticaria: crops of polymorphous lesions include the initial grouped and linear urticarial papules with a central punctum and older hyperpigmented or hypopigmented macule with variable scarring

Figure 16.14 Psoriasis:

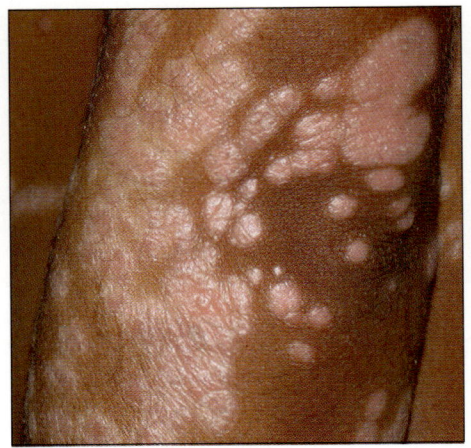

Figure 16.14a
Erythematous plaques with silvery scale on extensors

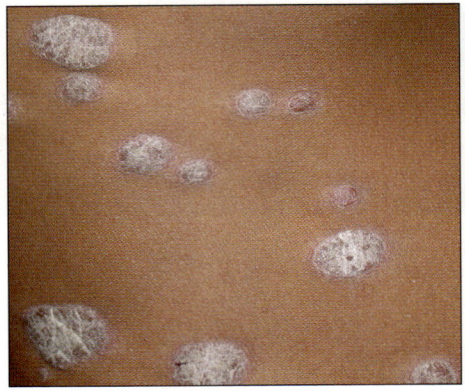

Figure 16.14b
Erythematous plaques with profuse silvery scales

Figure 16.15   Scabies:

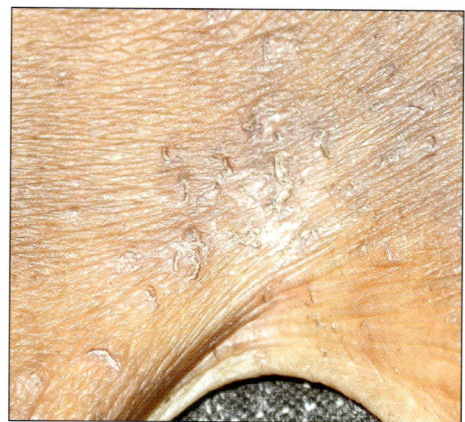

Figure 16.15a
Vesico-papules with diagnostic burrows of web spaces

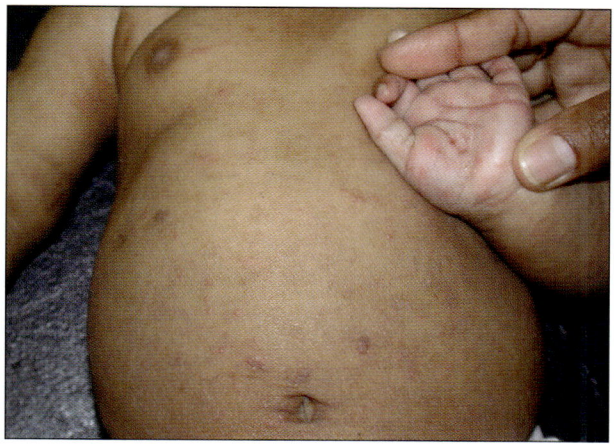

Figure 16.15b
Generalised discrete vesico-papules with diagnostic burrows

Figure 16.16   Impetigo

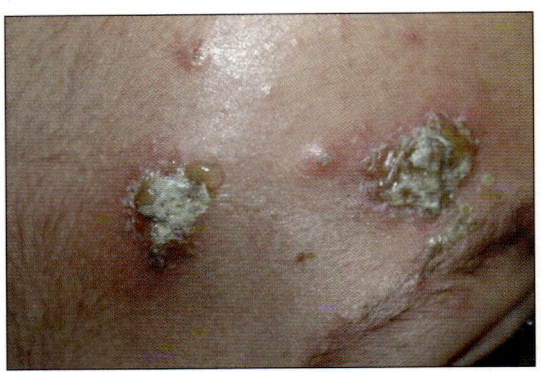

Figure 16.16a
Superficial pustules erosions and crusts

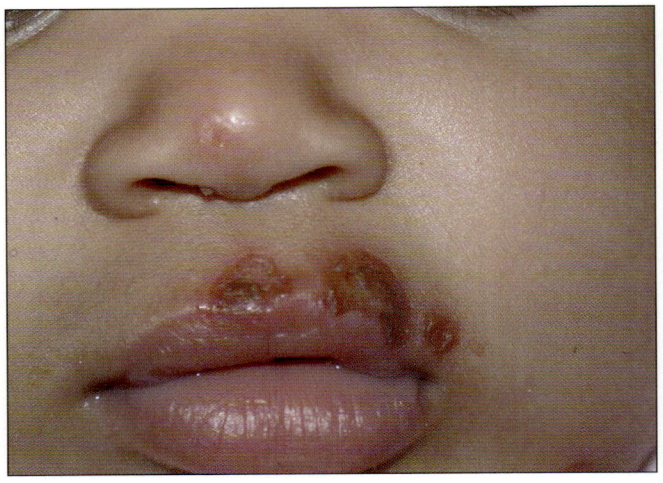

Figure 16.16b
Erosions and yellow (honey-coloured) crusts

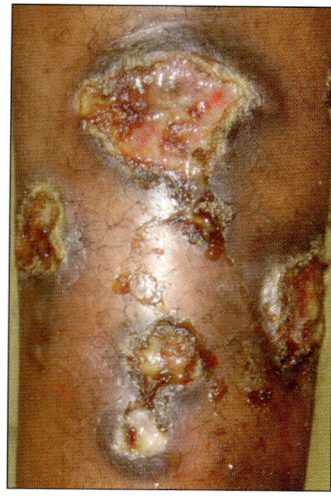

Figure 16.17
Ecthyma: deep crusted erosions and ulcers

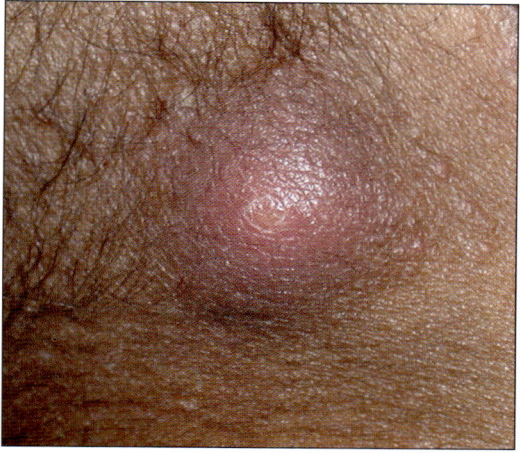

Figure 16.18
Furuncle: acute painful red swelling discharging pus

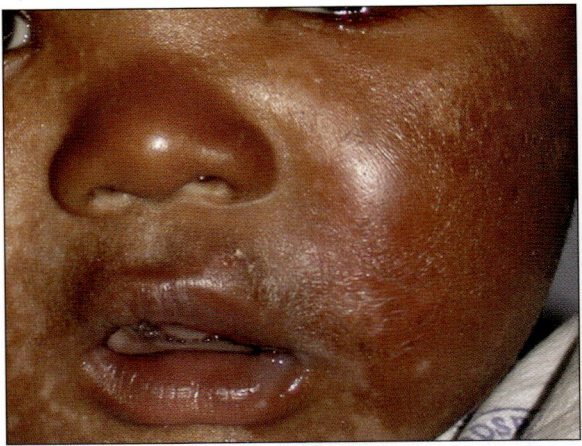

Figure 16.19
Cellulitis: erythematous, swollen, tender plaque of the left cheek deforming the mouth. Note the background rash and lesion on the left upper lip, the entry site for infection

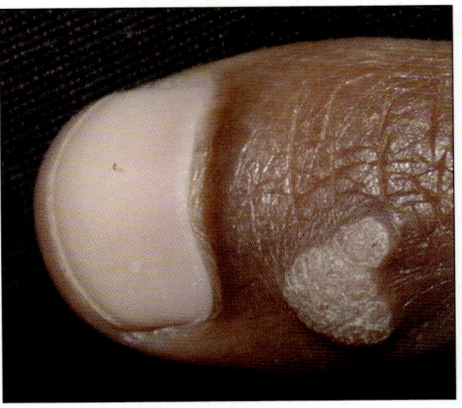

Figure 16.20
Common warts: skin-coloured papules with a rough, digitate surface

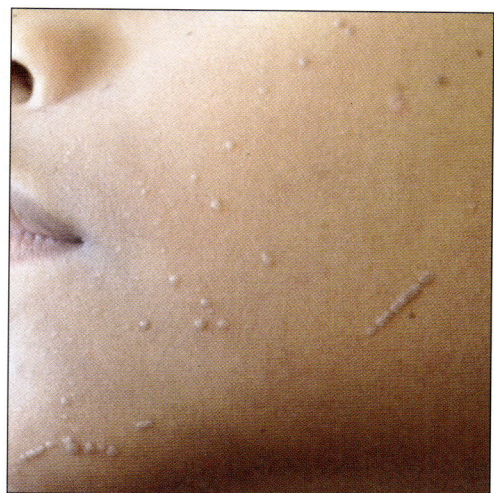

Figure 16.21
Plane warts: smooth surfaced skin-coloured or pigmented monomorphous papules showing Koebnerisation (linear lesions) into scratch marks

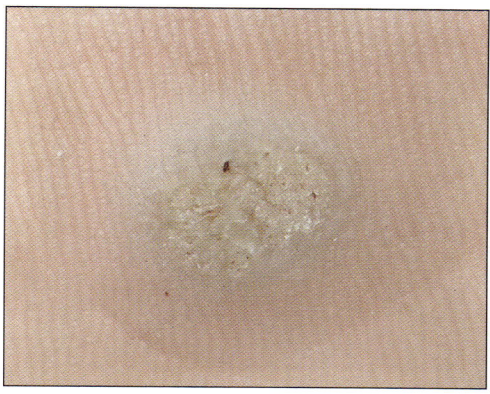

Figure 16.22
Plantar warts: Hyperkeratotic callus around the skin-coloured papules with a rough, digitate surface giving the appearance of a volcano

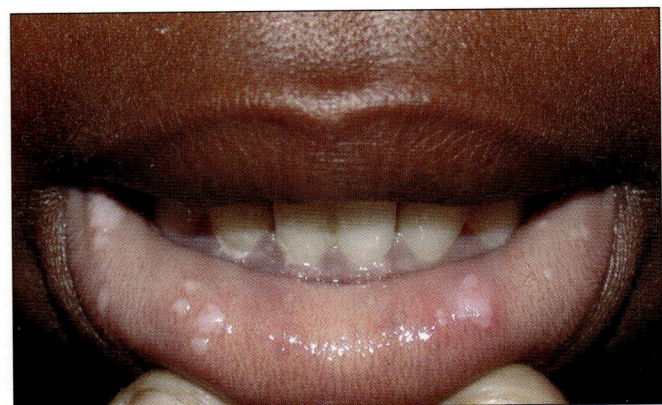

Figure 16.23
Mucosal warts: white papules

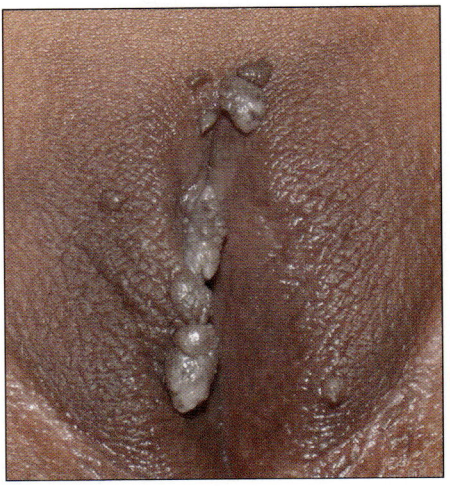

Figure 16.24
Condylomata accuminata: Exophytic, skin-coloured or pigmented papules with a rough, digitate surface. White lesions represent macerated hyperkeratoses

- Malathione (0.25%) or combination spray. Apply to the base of the hair and scalp till hair wet. Leave on for 10 minutes maximum then wash well. 👍☆☆☆
- Remove nits: comb the nits from the hair with a fine-tooth comb dipped in vinegar. 👍☆☆☆ Alternatively comb hair treated with hair conditioner (dimeticone) or essential oils (coconut, anise, ylang ylang) or shave the area. Apply petroleum jelly to the eyelashes twice daily. 👍☆☆

Pityriasis rosea

Widespread oval plaques with a collaret of scales appear on the trunk a few days after a herald patch. It is thought to be a viral exanthum.

- Reassure parents that the condition is self-limiting. It lasts about 6 weeks.
- Topical steroids ☺☆☆ or oral antihistamines ☺☆☆ may help symptomatically.
- Daily exposure to sunlight may hasten resolution. ☺☆☆

Pitfalls

The herald patch is often mistaken for tinea corporis. If there is no evidence of a herald patch remember the possibility of secondary syphilis. Check VDRL.

Psoriasis

See Figure 16.14 a and b.

This occurs at all ages and consists of erythematous lesions with silvery scales. There is often a family history of psoriasis. Arthritis may be present. Drugs (chloroquine, ß-blockers, lithium and steroid withdrawal), intercurrent infections and stress may all cause psoriasis to flare.

Treatment

Skin:

- Apply LPC (tar) 5% ointment twice daily. Continue applications until the lesions have cleared. 👍☆☆☆
- Use salicylic acid 2% to remove scale when necessary. 👍☆☆☆☆
- Topical steroids are effective acutely for psoriasis but need to be used with care as rebound flares are precipitated if the steroid is discontinued abruptly prior to stabilization on an alternate maintenance therapy. ☺☆☆☆☆

- Encourage daily exposure to sun to promote healing. 🖐☆☆☆☆
- Expensive, but more cosmetically acceptable alternatives include a 🖐☆☆☆☆ vitamin D preparation, calcipotriol and a ☺☆☆☆☆ topical retinoid, tazarotene.
- For extensive and recalcitrant psoriasis refer the child to a dermatologist for more specific management with dithranol, phototherapy or systemic agents.

Scalp:
- Wash regularly with a tar shampoo. 🖐☆☆☆
- If the response is poor add a topical steroid gel or a scalp preparation after washing. 🖐☆☆☆☆
- Apply salicylic acid 2% overnight to remove scale when necessary. 🖐☆☆☆☆
- Expensive, but more cosmetically acceptable alternatives include calcipotriol scalp lotion.

Scabies

See Figure 16.15 a and b.

The diagnosis is confirmed by finding the burrow and the mite. Look for burrows on the hands, between the fingers and on the genital area. In young boys check the scrotum and penile shaft. In infants, itchy vesico-papules are common on the trunk, palms and soles and in the axillae. Occasionally they may occur on the face.

Treatment
- Treat everyone in the household simultaneously and ensure that they have been given adequate instructions on what to do.
- Benzyl benzoate 🖐☆☆:

  Under 6 months of age: benzyl benzoate 6% lotion

  Over 6 months to 2 years: benzyl benzoate 12.5% lotion.

  Over 2 years of age: benzyl benzoate 25% lotion:
  - Apply the lotion to the body from the neck down. Keep it away from the eyes and mucous membranes.
  - Do not soak the child in a hot bath prior to treatment as the application may be absorbed.
  - Reapply preparation if the child's hands need to be washed.
  - Leave the lotion on for 12 to 24 hours and then wash it off thoroughly.
  - A second application after 1 week is necessary to kill any nymphs that may have hatched after the first treatment or if there is resistant scabies, re-infestation, or failure to comply.

- Sulphur compounds: 👍☆☆
  - Pregnant and nursing mothers: sulphur precipitate 10%. Apply daily for three days
  - Under 6 months of age: sulphur precipitate 5%. Apply daily for 3 days.
- Tetmosol® soap is used in institutions in addition to the above treatments as a prophylactic measure. It has little value for individual patients and their immediate contacts. ☺☆☆

Streptococcal and staphylococcal infections

Impetigo (Figure 16.16 a and b) is a superficial infection of the skin. It presents as blisters or yellow crusts and is highly contagious

Ecthyma (Figure 16.17) represents the infection of deeper layers of the skin. It presents as crusted erosions and ulcers that heal with scarring.

Folliculitis is a superficial infection of the hair follicles. It presents as individual pustules on a background of erythema. There are a number of causes for this presentation, not all of which are streptococcal or staphylococcal.

Furuncles (boils) (Figure 16.18) are deep necrotic infections of the hair follicle. They present as acute, painful red swellings, which develop pustular, necrotic centres which spontaneously discharge pus. They heal with scarring.

Erysipelas and cellulitis (Figure 16.19) are infections of the dermis and subcutaneous tissue and are usually associated with systemic features. An acute, red, swollen, tender, hot plaque is present, which may be accompanied by blistering and erosions. Lesions may heal with post inflammatory desquamation. Post infection complications may include abscess formation, lymphoedema or recurrent bouts of erysipelas/cellulitis.

These streptococcal and staphylococcal infections may be primary or may be superimposed on other dermatoses, e.g. eczema, scabies or insect bites.

Treatment

- All crusts should be gently removed with wet compresses and soaking. 👍☆☆
- An antimicrobial lotion or cream can be applied topically. Examples include: gentian violet, mercurochrome, povidone-iodine, silver sulphadiazine, fusidic acid or mupirocin. 👍☆☆☆☆

- Prevent spread and recurrences. Change soiled bedding, clothes and towels daily until infection resolved. Treat underlying predisposing conditions and dermatoses and eradicate carrier states.
- If widespread, severe or associated with systemic symptoms give oral flucloxacillin or erythromycin. ✋☆☆☆☆

> ### Practice point
>
> For acute erysipelas and cellulitis give parenteral antibiotics. Penicillin G and cloxacillin together are the first line choice. If there is clinical improvement after a few days, consider changing to co-amoxyclav. For milder infections consider oral co-amoxyclav, erythromycin or flucloxacillin. For recurrent attacks give Benzathine penicillin monthly and treat predisposing conditions. ✋☆☆☆☆

Carrier state eradication

- Wash hair, nails and body regularly (twice weekly) with an antiseptic such as povidone-iodine. ✋☆☆
- Keep nails short and clean.
- Apply antimicrobial nasal cream twice daily to nares (mupirocin, chlorhexidine) for 2 weeks. ✋☆☆

Warts

Warts represent an infection of the skin by human papilloma virus (HPV). The clinical presentation is varied and depends on the body area involved. They are usually asymptomatic and are spread by inoculation or direct contact. In the normal person warts last for months to years, but in the immunocompromised person they are often florid, extensive and recalcitrant to treatment. Wart virus has been associated with malignant transformation in women, and immunocompromised patients.

Common warts (Figure 16.20) are skin-coloured papules with a rough or digitate surface. They vary in diameter from 3 to 10 mm and are often found in clusters on the hands and fingers.

Plane warts (Figure 16.21) are smooth-surfaced, skin-coloured or pigmented monomorphous papules often seen on the face. Koebnerisation (linear lesions) into scratch marks is commonly seen. They are very difficult to treat.

Plantar warts (Figure 16.22) are found on the palms and soles and are often painful. Hyperkeratotic callus forms around the wart, which has an endophytic growth pattern giving the appearance of a volcano.

Mosaic warts form sheets of hyperkeratosis appearing as a mosaic pattern on the soles. They are very difficult to treat.

Mucosal warts (Figure 16.23) of the oral cavity appear as pink/white keratotic papules, which may extend to the vocal cords. Treatment is difficult.

Condylomata accuminata (Figure 16.24) are exophytic moist keratotic papules of the genital mucosa. They can be very exuberant

Treatment of common warts

- Allow them to resolve spontaneously.
- Alternatively use one of the following:
  - Wart paint: 👍☆☆☆☆
    - Apply a wart paint directly to the wart surface (salicylic acid 1 part, lactic acid 1 part, collodion 3 parts) and allow to dry (lesion turns white)
    - Cover the areas with waterproof plaster when the paint has dried and spillover onto normal skin has been removed.
    - Using fine sandpaper gently abrade the treated wart surface over paper to remove loosened scale after the daily bath. Remember the removed scale may contain infective material so dispose of the used sandpaper and paper immediately.
    - Wash well and dry the skin.
    - Repeat the above steps daily until the warts have disappeared.
- Occlude with duct tape or waterproof plaster. 👍☆☆☆
- Freezing with liquid nitrogen is a painful option, best done after debulking with wart paint. It is not feasible where there are many warts. 👍☆☆☆☆
- Imiquimod can be tried for recalcitrant cases. ☺☆☆
- In expert hands laser therapy is effective, especially for mucosal and some skin lesions. ☺☆☆

Treatment of genital warts

Children under 5 years:
- Assume that these have been caused by perinatal transmission unless proven otherwise.
- If the warts are not bothersome allow them to resolve spontaneously.
- Otherwise, apply topical 👍☆☆ trichloracetic acid (85% saturated solution in water) with a cotton-tipped applicator. The solution need not be washed off. Repeat once a week up to 6 weeks.
- Imiquimod applied to individual lesions on alternate days may help recalcitrant lesions. ☺☆☆

Children over 5 years:
- Consider sexual transmission and probe the likelihood of non-accidental injury.
- Do a VDRL test and consider testing for HIV.
- Apply ✦☆☆☆ podophyllin 25% in tinct. benzoin compound directly to the wart surface and dust with talc powder to fix. Wash it off well with soap and water after 4 hours. Repeat weekly as needed.
- Alternatively topical ✦☆☆ trichloracetic acid or ☺☆☆ imiquimod may be used.

Treatment of plantar warts
- Treatment with wart paint is effective in well motivated patients or families. ✦☆☆☆☆
- Alternately ✦☆☆☆☆ podophyllin resin 20%, salicylic acid 25% can be used topically 2-3 times a week.
- Physical paring by a chiropodist after ✦☆☆ silver nitrate stick or wart paint applications.

Recommended reading
1 *Handbook of Dermatology for Primary Care. A Practical Guide to Diagnosis.* Saxe, N, Jessop, S, Todd, G. 2nd Ed. Oxford University Press. Cape Town. 2007.
2 *Pediatric Dermatology.* Schachner, LA, Hansen, RC. (Eds). 3rd Ed. Mosby Elsevier. 2003.
3 *Hurwitz Clinical Pediatric Dermatology. A Textbook of Skin Disorders of Childhood and Adolescence.* Paller, A, Mancini, A. 3rd Ed. Elsevier. 2005.
4 *Textbook of Pediatric Dermatology.* Harper, J, Oranje, A, Prose, N. (Eds). 2nd Ed. Wiley Blackwell. 2006.

17 Bone and joint problems

T. Hoffman, P. Roux

Strong links between the orthopaedic surgeon, paediatric rheumatologist and physiotherapist are essential for optimal care of the child with bone and joint disease. This chapter demonstrates such a partnership.

An approach to a child with arthritis

Definition

Arthritis is inflammation of the synovial tissue in a joint space, with pain, swelling and limitation of movement. *Joint symptoms* and musculoskeletal pain also occur in non-inflammatory disorders. Juvenile rheumatoid (JRA), or juvenile chronic arthritis (JCA), is now termed juvenile idiopathic arthritis (JIA).

Diagnosis

Arthritis in 1 or more joints, present for at least 6 weeks in children less than 16 years old. This form of the disease is categorized according to the pattern of arthritis during the first 6 months of illness.

Classification

Table 17.1 Inflammatory causes of arthritis

Juvenile idiopathic arthritis (JIA - ILAR classification)	Other connective tissue disease	Infection-associated
• Systemic • Oligoarticular < 4 joints • Polyarticular 4 joints, RF (–) or • Polyarticular RF (+) • Psoriatic • Enthesitis-related • Undifferentiated – fitting no or more than 1 category	SLE Juvenile dermatomyositis Mixed connective tissue disease Scleroderma Vasculitides • Kawasaki disease • Polyarteritis • Henoch-Schönlein syndrome • Takayasu's arteritis	Infectious • Bacterial including mycobacterial • Viral • Spirochaetal Reactive • Rheumatic fever • Post-infectious

Table 17.2 Non-inflammatory causes of musculoskeletal pain

Benign hyper-mobility Pain amplification syndromes: • Fibromyalgia, reflex sympathetic dystrophy, diffuse or localized idiopathic pain Overuse syndromes: • Shin splints, stress fractures, chondromalacia patellae Trauma Spondylopathies Skeletal dysplasias Osteochondroses	Heritable connective tissue disorders: • Osteogenesis imperfecta • Ehlers-Danlos Storage diseases Metabolic disorders: • Rickets, osteoporosis, gout Systemic diseases: • Haemophilia, malignancies, haemoglobinopathies Benign nocturnal pains of childhood (growing pains)

Clinical assessment

History

The wide differential diagnosis for joint symptoms requires a thorough family history and a history of travel, trauma, sport and exposure to infection.

Table 17.3 Critical elements of the history

The pain	Other symptoms
Character (intermittent/persistent) Age-related expression of pain Stiffness of joints after resting, and morning stiffness Social, emotional and school-related features Sleep disturbance	Fever Weight loss School days or activity loss Change in behaviour or depression Gastrointestinal symptoms Muscle weakness Skin rashes

Examination

- General examination, at every visit note:
  - Any rash on body, limbs, hands, feet or face, including desquamation
  - Lymphadenopathy
  - Nail changes
  - Fever
  - Conjunctivitis or visual impairment.
- The musculoskeletal system (child in T-shirt and shorts)
  - Gait

- Examine each joint for signs of inflammation (swelling, heat, tenderness, limitation of movement), effusion, contracture and deformity
- Palpate muscle insertions and pressure points (tenderness and enthesitis)
- Assess muscle strength, atrophy and limb shortening. Record findings on a diagram.
• Slit-lamp examination of the eye by an ophthalmologist for iridocyclitis.

Table 17.4 Differential diagnosis: mono-arthritis, acute onset

Condition	Supportive evidence
Septic arthritis	Joint aspiration may yield pus for bacterial culture
Malignancy	Pain is adjacent to joint (but child may also have arthritis)
Trauma	History
Non-accidental injury	Story and findings do not match
Haemophilia	Boy, evidence of bleeding disorder
Slipped upper femoral epiphysis	Adolescent, obese, acute onset with no trauma
Reactive arthritis	Prior infection
Oligoarticular juvenile idiopathic arthritis (JIA)	Retrospective diagnosis – 6 weeks persistent signs and symptoms
Enthesitis-related arthritis	Enthesitis and inflammatory spinal pain
Osteochondritis	Radiographic features
Osteonecrosis (including Perthes')	Radiographic features
Idiopathic osteolysis of the hip	Radiographic features

Table 17.5 Differential diagnosis: mono-arthritis, gradual onset

Condition	Supportive evidence
Oligoarticular JIA	Most commonly pre-school girl (white race), develops further
Enthesitis-related arthritis	Back or buttock pain and/or tendonitis
Tuberculosis	Associated weight loss, cough, TB contact
Other conditions	Biopsy and culture diagnosis

Table 17.6 Differential diagnosis: polyarthritis

Condition	Supportive evidence
Polyarticular JIA	Five or more joints, symmetrical
Acute rheumatic fever	Modified Jones criteria, 'flitting' arthritis seldom involves small joints
Reactive arthritis	Often asymmetrical, large and small joints, non-erosive
Enthesitis-related arthritis	Back pain and enthesitis
Systemic lupus erythematosus	Skin changes, renal involvement, non-erosive arthritis
Osteochondritis/osteonecrosis	Better after rest, worse with exercise
Slipped upper femoral epiphyses	Adolescent, obese, acute onset, no trauma
Other conditions	Biopsy for diagnosis

Investigations for arthritis

- *Blood count* (normocytic anaemia, thrombocytosis)
- *ESR* or *CRP* (evidence of inflammatory disease)
- *Blood culture* (rule out septic arthritis – in monoarthritis).
- *ASOT/anti-DNAse B.* (rheumatic fever, post-streptococcal reactive arthritis)
- *TB skin testing (or quantiferon gold)* and *synovial biopsy* (tuberculous arthritis)
- *Rheumatoid factor* mostly negative in JIA, suggestive of a poorer prognosis when positive, (especially in conjunction with positive anti-citrullinated peptide)
- *Antinuclear antibodies, renal function tests* (SLE is suspected)
- *HLA B27* (for juvenile ankylosing spondylitis)
- *Radiographs of affected joints* (baseline at diagnosis and at annual intervals).

Prognosis in JIA

- *Oligoarticular* (60% of JIA): a 20% risk of uveitis, more frequently girls (5:1); good prognosis in RF seronegative children; peak incidence under age 2.
- *Rheumatoid factor-negative polyarthritis* (20% of JIA): peaks in preschoolers; more frequently girls (3:1); good long-term prognosis.
- *Rheumatoid factor-positive polyarthritis* (5–10% of JIA): adolescent girls; relatively poor prognosis. Outcome similar to adult RA.
- *Systemic onset JIA* (10% of all JIA): prolonged quotidian fever, rash, lymphadenopathy, hepatosplenomegaly and serositis; no gender preference; occurs in young children; poor joint prognosis. Macrophage activation syndrome is a fatal complication.
- *Enthesitis-related or psoriatic arthritis* usually chronic arthritis.

Outcome is assessed over years. The best prognosis comes from seronegative oligoarthritis (other than with uveitis). The worst prognosis with seropositive polyarticular arthritis and psoriatic arthritis. Most polyarticular disease will be in remission in 2 years. Overall remission: 55% after 14 years. Surgery is needed in 59% of patients and joint replacement in 22%. Children with persistent polyarticular JIA often have growth failure, osteoporosis and delayed sexual development. Delayed diagnosis and referral of arthritis affects outcome very negatively.

Management of JIA

Management includes:
- Education: parents, family and teachers must be well-informed members of the team. The South African Arthritis Foundation provides educational pamphlets.
- Physiotherapy and occupational therapy, orthopaedic surgeons.

Drug therapeutic guidelines for South Africa

Step 1: non-steroidal anti-inflammatory and drugs for pain relief: Paracetamol with ibuprofen, naprosyn, or indomethacin 25 mg bd, diclofenac 25 mg bd (tailor dosage to weight)

Arthritis non-responsive to NSAIDS and with unexplained findings such as persistent fever or unclear diagnosis should be referred to paediatric rheumatology.

Step 2: intra-articular injection (IAI) of steroids in *pauci-articular disease:* preferably triamcinolone hexacetonide – given with lidocaine under rheumatology or orthopaedic supervision.

Step 3: oral methotrexate (MTX) weekly, starting with 5 mg per dose, increasing to 20 mg weekly over 3 to 6 months, followed by folic acid 24 hours later ✋☆☆☆. Monitor blood count, reduce dose if absolute neutrophil count below 2 000/ml^3. Monitor liver function with ALT level guidelines. Use subcutaneous methotrexate in non-responders or with unacceptable side-effects.

Step 4: oral steroid with MTX in systemic onset disease and moderate to severe polyarticular disease. Maintenance dose is prednisone 5–10 mg daily. Titrate to the smallest effective dose against signs and laboratory indicators (platelet count, ESR, CRP) of inflammation.

Step 5: other disease modifying drugs (sulfasalazine – 40–60 mg/kg/day in divided doses ✋☆☆☆ may be tried for enthesitis-related arthritis instead of methotrexate). Chloroquine phosphate 250 mg daily for 3 days a week may be added in poorly responsive polyarticular disease or for patients with HIV-related arthritis.

Pulsed steroid: intravenous methylprednisolone 30 mg/kg daily for 3 days in systemic onset disease – only to be given in specialized units with monitoring facilities. Oral prednisone 1–2 mg/kg for relapse given for 1 week and reduced by 25% per week over the following 3 weeks.

Newer therapy

- Tumour necrosis factor a inhibitors: Etanercept 0.4 mg/kg subcutaneously twice weekly ☆☆☆☆. Expensive, not freely available
- Leflumomide: may be useful alternative to MTX responders who become intolerant
- Bone marrow transplant: experimental and hazardous.

Surgery

Joint replacement and reconstructive surgery are generally performed after the cessation of bone growth.

Table 17.7 An approach to the child with a limp

	Clinical	Special investigation
Acute		
• Fracture	Trauma, toddler (1 – 4 years)	X-ray: spiral fracture

• Pyogenic infection
  Bone
  Joint
	Temperature > 38.5 °C
	Metaphyseal tenderness
	Effusion, ↓ all movements
		FBC and diff: WCC > 12 000;
		ESR > 40
		Isotope bone scan: pelvis, hip

• Transient synovitis Hip	Temperature < 38.5 °C ↓ abduction, internal rotation	WCC < 12 000; ESR < 40
• Rheumatic fever	Flitting arthralgia, arthritis	
Insidious		
Diagnostic calendar • 0–5 years: DDH • 5–10 years: Perthes • 10–15 years: SUFE	Painless Trendelenburg Painful Trendelenburg Painful Trendelenburg	X-ray: AP pelvis, frog lateral hips
• Tuberculosis	Effusion + synovitis	ESR ↑, Mantoux, CXR + e 50%, synovial biopsy Can also do quantiferon gold
• JIA	Monarthritis, polyarthritis Effusion + synovitis	RF factor + e < 5%, ANA in 20%, synovial biopsy if in doubt
• Leukaemia	Bone pain ± effusion Hepatosplenomegaly Lymphadenopathy	X-ray: Bony changes 50% FBC and diff., uric acid, LDH Isotope bone scan Bone marrow biopsy

Acute haematogenous osteomyelitis (AHO) and septic arthritis (SA)

Pathology

Acute haematogenous osteomyelitis

- There is infection of the metaphysis.
- Neonate and infant: growth plate is not a barrier to infection and the patient presents with features of a septic arthritis. With delayed treatment the epiphysis is destroyed, with crippling consequences, especially in the hip.
- In the older child (mean age 7 years) pus decompresses subperiosteally. Delayed treatment results in sequestrum formation with a sinus (chronic osteomyelitis).

Septic arthritis

Haematogenous synovial infection or decompression of an intra-articular metaphyseal infection, e.g. the hip. Delayed treatment results in chondrolysis and/or avascular necrosis in the hip.

Bacteriology

Acute haematogenous osteomyelitis

- Neonatal: 75% *Staphylococcus aureus* (possibly cloxacillin-resistant if previously hospitalised, e.g. premature), β-haemolytic *Streptococcus*, and in septicaemic patients may be Gram negative.
- Infants and older children: *Staphylococcus aureus*, most cloxacillin-sensitive, penicillin-resistant.

Septic arthritis

- < 2 years: 50% no growth, *Staphylococcus aureus*, *H. influenzae* (rare since vaccination introduced), *Streptococcus* spp, *Pneumococcus* spp.
- > 2 years: 50% no growth, 40% *Staphylococcus aureus*, *Streptococcus* spp, *Pneumococcus* spp.

Clinical features

- ↑ temperature, ill, may be septicaemic
- 75% of neonates not ill, feeding well
- Neonate and infant: pseudoparalysis and swelling
- Older child: refusal to weight bear, metaphyseal tenderness
- Joint effusion palpable in peripheral joints, not hip

- ↓ range of all movements, but may be normal in infant and septicaemic/confused patient.

Special investigations
- FBC and differential: ↑ WCC (75%); ↑ ESR (100%), CRP ↑, blood culture positive (acute haematogenous osteomyelitis = 80%; septic arthritis = 30%)
- Radiographs:
  - Older child: normal, excludes other pathology
  - Neonatal hip: metaphyseal rarefaction and/or subluxation always present.
- Isotope bone scan: helpful in localizing sites around hip, pelvis and spine.

Treatment
Acute haematogenous osteomyelitis: cloxacillin 200 mg/kg/day IV for at least 48 hours, then oral flucloxacillin 100 mg/kg/day for 6 weeks if temperature settled. Add fusidic acid 50 mg/kg/day for possible resistant staphylococcus in a previously hospitalized neonate

Septic arthritis: cloxacillin as for AHO. If < 2 years add ampicillin 150 mg/kg/day IV followed by amoxycillin 75 mg/kg/day orally for 3 weeks if *H. influenzae* is cultured. If streptococcus or pneumococcus: amoxil after 48 hours intravenous therapy *if sensitive*.

Open surgical drainage is imperative in all cases of septic arthritis and neonatal osteitis that present with pus in the joint.

In AHO extra-osseous pus (present in 80% of patients) should be drained. Early cases that respond to antibiotics do not require surgery.

Transient synovitis of the hip

Definition
Acute onset of 'irritable hip' with gradual, complete resolution.

Clinical features
- Mean age 6 years. Do not diagnose < 1 yr
- 70% previous URTI, 30% trauma
- Acute onset of hip pain with limp
- Main problem is differentiating from septic arthritis:
  - Not systemically ill, temperature < 38.5 °C
  - WCC < 12 000, ESR < 40
  - Hip movements less restricted, mainly ↓ abduction and internal rotation.

Treatment

Resolution on bedrest and traction clinches the diagnosis.

Skeletal tuberculosis

Incidence

- Rare in comparison to pulmonary tuberculosis: 1:400
- Mainly spine, then hip, knee, foot and ankle, elbow.

Spinal tuberculosis

Clinical features

- Angular kyphus with or without paralysis
- Differential diagnosis:
  i congenital deformity due to hemivertebra or 'unsegmented bar',
  ii neurofibromatosis.

Special investigations

- X-ray: disc space loss with destruction of contiguous vertebrae,
  - Differential: pyogenic spondylitis: disc space loss, but contiguous vertebrae maintain architecture (not destroyed).
- ↑ ESR and positive Mantoux > 90%
- Chest X-ray positive for active or old tuberculosis in 50%.

Treatment

- Antituberculous treatment: rifampicin, isoniazid and pyrazinamide for 9 months (ambulant chemotherapy), add ethionomide/ethambutol if resistance suspected
- Surgery (anterior decompression and strut graft) required for paralysis and if 2 or more vertebrae show total body destruction, for cosmesis and to prevent late onset paraplegia.

Tuberculous arthritis

Clinical features

- Knee, ankle/foot, elbow: monarthritis (effusion + synovitis) ↓ ROM.
- Hip: Trendelenburg, painful limp, ↓ ROM.

Special investigations

- X-ray: features of chronic inflammation: osteopaenia, erosions, joint space narrowing (late)

- Differential: JIA, haemophilia
- ESR, Mantoux and CXR: as for spinal tuberculosis
- Synovial biopsy: histology (85% +e), culture (75% +e).

Treatment

Antituberculous treatment as for spinal tuberculosis. Surgery (biopsy) for diagnosis always; aspiration has a very low yield.

Congenital deformities

Club foot

Definition

Fixed hindfoot equinus and varus, forefoot adduction and cavus.

Aetiology

- 95% idiopathic. Rest: myelomeningocele, arthrogryposis, constriction band.

Treatment

- Serial weekly plaster manipulation: supination and abduction
- At 2 to 3 months carry out residual equinus corrected surgery
- With this technique of manipulation (Ponseti), the more extensive posteromedial release is now seldom performed.

Developmental dysplasia of the hip (DDH)

Spectrum

- Dislocation at birth (Ortolani positive)
- Dysplasia: late dislocation (> 4 months), painful limp in adolescence.

Clinical features

- Neonatal screening: early diagnosis offers easy treatment, and a good prognosis:
  - Ortolani test: a dislocated hip that relocates with a clunk on abduction of the leg
  - Ultrasound at 6 weeks: if there is a family history and in firstborn breech
  - X-ray: only accurate at > 6 weeks.
- Older child:

- ↓ abduction
- Short leg, Trendelenburg limp
- X-ray diagnostic.

Treatment

- < 6/12 Pavlik harness for 3 months
  Treat: Ortolani positive hips
  Ultrasound at 6 weeks showing dysplasia: α-angle < 50°
- 6–18 months: Closed or open reduction
- > 18 months: Open reduction plus pelvic osteotomy (Salter).

Rotational variations in children: intoeing and outtoeing

Rotational variations in children are extremes of normal development. They almost always resolve spontaneously and very seldom require treatment. However, if present after 7 years they will persist into adulthood. Surgery will not have any functional benefit or prevent arthritis.

Assessment

- Gait: foot progression angle (FPA)/angle of gait   N = 10° > 4 yrs
- Thigh foot angle (TFA) assesses tibial torsion   N = 10° > 4 yrs
- Internal rotation of hip (IR)   N = 45° > 7 yrs
- External rotation of hip (ER)   N = 45° > 7 yrs

Normal development (extremes present with intoeing or outtoeing)

- Infant: ↑ ER hip, metatarsal adductus: resolves > 1 yr
- Toddler: intoeing due to tibial torsion (↓ TFA): resolves > 4 yrs
- > 4 yrs: intoeing due to femoral neck anteversion: resolves > 7yrs
- Outtoeing due to femoral neck retroversion: resolves by 7 yrs.

Genu varum and genu valgum

Bow legs and knock knees are normal physiological developmental variations, but pathology, mainly rickets, dysplasia and Blount's disease, should be excluded.

Assessment

- Mechanical axis: centre hip, centre patella, centre ankle: N = 0°
- Anatomical axis: shaft femur, shaft tibia: N = 5° valgus

Normal development

- 0–2 yrs   genu varum (monitor with intercondylar distance)
- 2½ yrs   straight
- 3–7 yrs   genu valgum (monitor with intermalleolar distance)
- ≥ 8 yrs   'straight by 8'.

Investigations

X-ray indicated if:
- Severe or unilateral deformity
- Genu varum persists > 2 yrs to rule out Blount's
- Suspecting rickets
- Syndromic/dysplasia.

Treatment

Genu varum:
    Osteotomy:
        – Persistent physiological varus > 4 yrs
        – Underlying pathology.

Genu valgum:
    Stapling distal medial femoral physis:
        – Persistent physiological genu valgum > 10 yrs.

Perthes' disease

Definition

Avascular necrosis of the femoral head, which heals spontaneously (unlike avascular necrosis due to steroids, post-sepsis or trauma which does not heal).

Pathology

Table 17.8 The classification of Perthes' disease

Stage	X-ray appearance of femoral head
(i) Avascular necrosis	Sclerosis
(ii) Revascularization	Fragmentation
(iii) Healing	Re-ossification

Clinical features

- Mean age 7 years (4–9 yrs)
- Boys:girls 4:1

- Small for age, delayed bone age
- ADHD in 30% of patients
- Painful, Trendelenburg limp, ↓ abduction and internal rotation.

Special investigations

X-ray: AP pelvis and frog lateral hips shows:
- Stage of disease
- Amount of head involved.

Treatment

- Containment: conservative (broomstick plasters) or surgical (femoral or pelvic osteotomy)
- Prognosis is worse if patient presents > 8 yrs and with more than 50% of head involved.

Slipped upper femoral epiphysis (SUFE)

Definition

Posterior slip of femoral head on femur neck during adolescence (9–16 years).

Aetiology

- Unknown
- Definite aetiology very rare, present < 9 years or > 16 years: renal rickets, primary hypothyroidism, pituitary tumour.

Clinical features

- Adolescent, 50% overweight
- Hip pain, often referred to anterior thigh and knee
- Painful, Trendelenburg limp
- On flexion hip goes into external rotation
- Duration of slip: acute < 3 weeks; chronic > 3 weeks
- 50% of acute slips are unstable, i.e. cannot walk even with crutches
- 25% bilateral (50% simultaneously, 50% within 18 months).

Special investigations

X-ray: A–P pelvis and frog lateral hips. Note: lateral shows early, mild slip best.

Treatment

This is with a cannulated screw.

Complications
- Avascular necrosis: occurs in unstable, severe slips
- Chondrolysis: occurs in females with chronic, severe slips.

Flexible or postural flat foot

This is a normal variant in most young children. The condition implies that, during standing, the child has no longitudinal arch due to laxity of the ligaments that stabilize the foot in stance. On tiptoe, a good arch develops as the muscles come into play. The condition usually resolves > 8 years.

Differential diagnosis
- Paralytic flat foot: cerebral palsy and myelomeningocele
- Rigid flat foot: congenital vertical talus and peroneal spastic flat foot of adolescence
- Flexible: benign hypermobility or syndromes with ligament laxity, (eg Marfan's syndrome).

Treatment
- This does not change the natural history.
- If there is medial shoe wear in the child > 8 years: longitudinal arch support.
- Rigid flat feet always require surgical treatment and severe paralytic flat feet benefit from surgery.

Recommended reading
1. Cassidy, JT and Petty, RE. *Textbook of Pediatric Rheumatology* 5th ed. Elsevier. Saunders.
2. Web links:
   http://printo.it
   http://nice.org.uk/Guidance/TA35
   http://www.arthritis.org.za

18 Eyes and vision

R. Grotte

This chapter deals with common eye problems that might present to a paediatric medical officer, with an emphasis on differentiating between those problems that can be resolved with simple treatment and those that require referral to a specialist unit.

Visual assessment

A basic age-appropriate visual assessment should be part of any medical examination and requires only basic tools. An experienced mother will recognize visual problems early, but delayed presentation is often a problem with a first child.

Visual milestones

At birth	Baby blinks at bright light. Will turn away from bright light but towards soft suffused light.
6 weeks	Makes and keeps eye contact. Smiles responsively at parent
3 months	Visually very alert. Particularly preoccupied by nearby human face. Follows toy at 15–25 cm from face
4 months	Visually directed reaching
6 months	Visually insatiable. Reaches out with both hands to grasp interesting objects
12 months	Points with index finger at wanted objects. Picks up small objects, e.g. sweets, crumbs
> 2½ years	The child who speaks can be tested with culturally appropriate picture charts. Older and more sophisticated children can match single letters charts using the letters HOTV. Preschoolers can often read number charts.

Fix-and-follow test

Remember to use an appropriate target. A torchlight does not have good edge contours and is not visually interesting to a baby. A coloured toy is more appropriate, but the best target is the human face. A baby should fix his mother's face when feeding. Fixation should be steady and pursuit movements should be smooth. Assess both eyes initially.

Perform a fix and follow test with each eye covered in turn. Objection to occlusion of 1 eye suggests that vision in the other is defective. If, when the cover is removed from an eye, that eye moves to take up fixation on the target, then a squint is present.

Signs suggesting poor vision

- Lack of response to mother's face
- Wandering eye movements
- Staring at bright lights
- Eye poking.

Probable causes of poor visual responses

- Corneal opacities/scarring
- Cataracts
- Congenital retinal disease
- Brain damage, e.g. perinatal hypoxia, near drowning.

Additionally, children who are very sick or post ictal are likely to show visual inattention, which usually recovers.

> *Practice point:*
>
> Always check the red reflex with an ophthalmoscope. Cataracts or other media opacities will obscure the red reflex.

Amblyopia (lazy eye)

Amblyopia is central suppression of vision. This is a problem unique to young children who are visually immature (< 8 years old) but it has lifelong consequences. Anything interfering with a clear image on the retina, e.g. a cataract, refractive error or ptosis will cause the affected eye to become amblyopic. A squint produces double vision, which is quickly suppressed by the immature brain, damaging binocular vision. Fixation preference for 1 eye implies suppression of the image from the other, causing amblyopia.

> *Practice point:*
>
> Without treatment, vision is permanently impaired. The younger the child the more dense the amblyopia. Prompt treatment (usually by occluding the sound eye) will restore vision.

Strabismus (squint)

A squint exists when the eyes are out of alignment. Normally the corneal light reflection from a hand-held pen torch should be centred equally in the pupils. Squinting eyes are either convergent (esotropia – where light reflex falls temporally) or divergent (exotropia – where light reflex falls nasally). Vertical misalignment is less common. If squint is suspected, cover the fixing eye and watch the other one. If the uncovered eye is squinting it will move to take up fixation. The other eye will now squint under the cover and will also move to take up fixation when the cover is reversed.

Congenital deviations

The eyes of a very young baby may slip out of alignment intermittently. After the age of 6 weeks the eyes should be aligned most of the time. A constant squint or one that persists beyond 12 weeks needs investigation. It is highly unlikely to resolve spontaneously and highly likely to produce dense amblyopia if unilateral.

Acquired deviations

Older children will complain of diplopia.

Differentiate between a paralytic squint (a third, fourth or sixth cranial nerve palsy) and a non-paralytic (concomitant) squint. In paralytic squint the deviation varies with the direction of gaze, being greatest when looking in the direction of action of the paralysed muscle. In non-paralytic (concomitant squint,) the common squint of childhood, the deviation is the same size regardless of position of gaze.

All acquired squints need assessment. An *acquired* cranial nerve palsy needs neurological investigation. An *acquired* concomitant squint needs prompt ophthalmological assessment.

Timeous treatment of the underlying cause (e.g. refractive error) will preserve binocularity.

Occasionally an acquired esotropia is the first sign of a retinoblastoma.

External abnormalities

Congenital abnormalities of the eye and eyelids are often associated with other congenital problems.

Defective eyelids

Eyelids that do not cover and protect the cornea will rapidly lead to blindness from corneal desiccation and ulceration. Corneal protection and lubrication is urgent.

Ptosis (blepharoptosis, drooping eyelid)
- Congenital: due to dystrophy of the levator palebrae superioris
- Neurological: third cranial nerve palsy or sympathetic lesion (Horner's syndrome)
- Mechanical: due to a lid mass, e.g. haemangioma
- In young children this will cause amblyopia if the visual axis is obscured.

Lid lumps
- Inflammation of a meibomian gland in the tarsal plate due to a blocked meibomian duct and retained sebaceous material causes a chalazion or meibomian cyst. Often sterile initially, it may become secondarily infected. If acutely inflamed it will often respond to topical antibiotic ointment and warm compresses. If it does not, it will require incision and curettage from the inside of the eyelid. A small proportion go on to chronic granulomatous inflammation, which produces a painless pea-like swelling in the eyelid and also requires incision and curettage.
- A hordeolum (stye) is a lash follicle infection. Remove the eyelash and treat with antibiotic ointment, e.g. chloramphenicol.
- Haemangiomas of the eyelid are rare, usually present with rapid growth in the first year of life and may occlude the visual axis, causing amblyopia or producing astigmatism. They should be referred for treatment by excision, local steroid or bleomycin injection, or treatment with systemic propranolol, which requires paediatric supervision

Big (enlarging) eye
Congenital glaucoma due to an abnormality of the aqueous drainage channel makes the immature eyeball stretch. Corneal oedema makes the cornea hazy with photophobia and watering. Uncontrolled intraocular pressure destroys the optic nerve. This usually presents around the age of three months or more. It can be unilateral or bilateral and more difficult to spot when bilateral. Referral for surgery is urgent.

Watering eyes (epiphora = tearing)
This is an extremely common complaint in the first months of life due to delayed canalization of the nasolacrimal duct and causes a watery eye without a runny nose. It usually resolves spontaneously. Stagnant tears in the lacrimal sac are prone to infection and the mother should be instructed to express the contents of the sac at least twice a day. A short course of topical antibiotics may be required to clear infection.

A lacrimal abscess requires drainage. Persistent tearing over the age of 12 months is usually cured by probing of the nasolacrimal duct, which requires a general anaesthetic.

> ***Practice point:***
> Watering and photophobia (due to corneal oedema) together with an enlarging eyeball are signs of congenital glaucoma, which requires urgent specialist treatment.

Other causes include corneal or subtarsal foreign bodies and ingrowing eyelashes. All the above cause a watery eye with a runny nose.

Red eyes with purulent discharge

Purulent conjunctivitis
- The cornea should be clear and the iris clearly visible.
- This is usually due to haemophilus, streptococci, pneumococci or staphylococci.
- Treat with broad spectrum antibiotic ointment, e.g. chloramphenicol initially 2 hourly and expect prompt resolution.
- Any grey or yellowish spot on the cornea implies corneal ulceration (which will lead to scarring). A cloudy anterior chamber implies intraocular inflammation. Both require specialist referral.

An especially risky situation exists in hospitals where an unconscious child's eyes are not closed and develop an epithelial defect due to exposure. Secondary infection, particularly if caused by *Pseudomonas*, will rapidly destroy the cornea leading to loss of the eye, unless suspected and treated immediately.

Ophthalmia neonatorum
This is a purulent conjunctivitis in the neonatal period, usually caused by organisms from the mother's birth canal.

Gonococcal infection
- Presents around day 2
- Intensely red eye and copious purulent discharge
- Untreated, progresses to corneal ulceration with severe scarring
- Gram stain of the pus reveals gram negative intracellular diplococci
- Sight-threatening emergency requiring admission.

Treatment

- Irrigate eyes with normal saline every 5 minutes to remove the pus.
- Give a single intramuscular dose of ceftriaxone 50 mg/kg. ☆☆☆☆☆
- Corneal involvement requires 3 day antibiotic cover and urgent ophthalmic referral.

Chlamydial infection

- Commonest cause of opthalmia neonatorum
- Presents around week 2 with sticky eyes and swollen eyelids
- Saline eyewashes and oral erythromycin 10 mg/kg/dose qid for 2 weeks eradicates the organism and prevents chlamydial pneumonitis later. ☆☆☆☆☆

The baby presenting with gonococcal infection should probably be treated for both conditions.

Red eyes with watery discharge

Viral conjunctivitis (epidemic pink eye)

This is most commonly due to an adenovirus. Severity varies from minimal redness with a follicular conjunctival reaction, to a severe pyrexial illness with exudative conjunctival pseudomembranes, usually in very young children. Treatment is supportive. A combined vasoconstrictor and antihistamine eyedrop 6 hourly can be very soothing. Avoid topical steroid eyedrops. ☆☆☆☆☆ The condition is highly contagious.

Herpes simplex (see below) can also produce a follicular conjunctivitis, which is usually unilateral unlike other types of infective conjunctivitis.

Red itchy eyes

Suspect allergic eye disease. Acute rhinoconjunctivitis is the commonest form of allergy and presents with intermittent attacks of redness, watering and itching with lid oedema, conjunctival oedema and follicles, due to an IgE mediated reaction.

Intermittent (seasonal) allergic conjunctivitis (hay fever) is due to pollens and occurs in spring.

Persistent (perennial) allergic conjunctivitis is milder and usually due to house dust mite, animal dander or moulds and spores.

Treat with antihistamine eye drops 6 hourly or if available, 12 hourly olopatidine or ketotifen eye drops, which have additional mast cell stabilizing action.

Severe cases might require topical steroid eye drops, but there is always the danger of unsuspected herpetic infection in which they are strictly contraindicated. Specialist advice is needed.

Vernal conjunctivitis

This type involves a cell mediated response, has a much longer summer season and causes chronically red itchy eyes with white stringy discharge. Pigmented patients develop gray limbal infiltrates and discoloured sclerae. Non-pigmented patients get tarsal cobblestone infiltrates. All require mast cell stabilizing eye drops, e.g. cromoglycate or ketotifen long-term and usually topical steroid eye drops to control inflammation. Specialist supervision is required.

The unilateral red eye

Herpes

Herpes simplex is a virus, which usually causes a unilateral follicular conjunctivitis sometimes with herpetic eyelid vesicles. Corneal involvement starts with an epithelial branching (dendritic) ulcer demonstrated by staining with fluorescein. Patients with corneal involvement should be referred for specialist assessment. Treatment is with acyclovir eye ointment 5 times a day. Topical steroid eye drops are absolutely contraindicated and will exacerbate the ulcer, leading to extensive corneal ulceration and scarring. ☆☆☆☆☞

Phlyctenular conjunctivitis

This presents as a red eye with a watery discharge and an infiltrate that looks like a white or yellowish spot with intense local hyperaemia, commonly at the limbus. It represents a sensitivitiy (Mantoux) reaction to bacteria, usually the tubercle bacillus but occasionally staphylococci. The usual cause is droplet infection of the conjunctival sac by someone with open TB. The phlycten settles well with topical combination steroid and antibiotic eye ointment. Investigate for the source.

The white pupil (leucocoria)

Cataracts (opacities of the lens)

These are the commonest cause of a grey or white opacity seen in the pupil. This is associated with painless, progressive loss of vision and loss of the red reflex. Cataracts may be congenital or acquired, unilateral or bilateral. All require referral for specialist treatment. The younger the child the greater is the urgency. Test for galactosaemia and congenital rubella in babies. Bilateral cataracts are often familial; unilateral ones traumatic.

An acquired leucocoria that is not due to a cataract, particularly one presenting in the second year of life, is very suspicious of a retinoblastoma (a malignant retinal neoplasm that can spread to the brain) and should be examined by a specialist urgently. Retinoblastoma carries an excellent prognosis in industrialised countries, but the prognosis is poor in sub-Saharan Africa, due mainly to late presentation. Increased awareness among primary health workers and clinicians to assess red reflex, is crucial.

The injured eye

Lid lacerations require repair with careful apposition of the lid margins to prevent notching and are usually best treated by an ophthalmologist or plastic surgeon. Involvement of the lacrimal canaliculi requires a stented repair.

Conjunctival lacerations need not be sutured if small, but bear in mind the possibility of associated penetrating globe injuries.

Corneal foreign bodies can be removed with a sterile cotton bud and local anaesthetic if the child is cooperative. A deeply embedded foreign body or a very frightened child will require a general anaesthetic for removal.

Corneal lacerations and other penetrating injuries must be referred urgently for microsurgical repair. Apply a clean eyepad and shield and transfer the patient starved, in preparation for a general anaesthetic.

Bleeding into the anterior chamber (hyphaema) usually results from blunt injury. The eye is usually red and painful, and a blood level may be seen in the anterior chamber. This is best managed in a specialist centre. There may be loss of vision if it is severe. There is a risk of a bigger secondary haemorrhage 4 or 5 days later producing secondary glaucoma. To prevent this:
- Admit child for bedrest until the haemorrhage is resorbed.
- Sedate if necessary.
- Treat with G. atropine 1% bd and G. dexamethasone 1% qid ☆☆☆☆☉
- Tranexamic acid 25 mg/kg orally every 8 hours for 5 days.

Vitreous haemorrhage may be associated with a hyphaema and takes much longer to clear. The fundus cannot be seen clearly and damage to the posterior segment, e.g. retinal detachment must be excluded.

Specialist investigation, e.g. with ultrasound, is indicated. A young child with a vitreous haemorrhage that fails to clear quickly will become amblyopic and start to squint. (Always consider the possibility of shaken baby syndrome or physical abuse in the presence of vitreous and/or retinal haemorrhage.)

The orbit

An orbital haematoma will resolve, but any restricted eye movement or diplopia arouses suspicion of an orbital floor fracture with entrapment of inferior rectus muscle and/or soft tissue. This requires urgent specialist assessment and treatment.

Chemical burns

- Immediate and copious washing with water (wash basin, hose pipe, shower or IV giving set)
- Remove particulate matter from under the lids
- Urgent referral to specialised unit
- Treatment will be aimed at preventing scarring and adhesions.

Recommended reading

1. Baterbury, M, Bowling, B, Murphy, C. *Opthalmology: An illustrated colour text.* 3rd Ed. Churchill Livingston. 2009.
2. Kanski, JJ. *Clinical Opthalmology: A systematic approach.* 6th Ed. Butterworth-Heinemann. 2007.
3. Kaiser, P, Friedman, N, Pineda, R. *The Massachussets Eye and Ear Infirmary Illustrated Manual of Opthalmology* 3rd Ed. Saunders. 2009.

19 Ear, nose and throat problems

G. Copley

The examination of the ENT system in children can be difficult and needs time, reassurance, and careful explanation.

The ear

Impacted wax

> **Practice point:**
>
> Ear wax dissolves best in warm water.

This is common and usually presents as a blocked ear with mild hearing loss. Ear wax can become very hard and dissolves best in warm water.

- Syringe the ear with warm soapy water, which should be exactly at body temperature. If the wax is very dry and hard, then recommend wax softening drops with water or an aqueous-based product ☆☆◊. Olive oil is traditional but does not have any additional beneficial effect ☆☆☺. Use at night for a week and then bring back for repeat syringing.
- Tell the mother NOT to use cotton buds (ear buds), as these usually push the wax further down the canal.

Foreign bodies in the ear canal

Children do not tolerate having the ear probed with hooks or forceps, without anaesthesia.

- Most foreign bodies can be syringed out.
- Drown live insects in vegetable or olive oil prior to syringing. Be careful of impacted organic matter (a peanut or seed), which can swell after failed syringing, further impacting it. If this happens, refer to an ENT specialist for removal with instruments.

Otitis externa (diffuse or 'swimmer's ear')
This is a bacterial, fungal or mixed infection of the skin of the external ear canal.

Clinical features
- Itching, pain, discharge and swelling of the ear canal leading to hearing loss
- The ear is frequently tender when the pinna is manipulated to visualize the canal or ear drum; prescribe analgesia.

Treatment
- Syringe and dry mop as much debris/discharge as possible.
- In mild infections consider an antiseptic eardrop (such as dilute acetic acid). For more severe infections consider an antibiotic/steroid eardrop (or an antifungal when fungal infection is suspected) instilled 3 times daily for a week.
- Oral flucloxacillin 25 mg/kg/dose 4 times a day for 5 days if there is gross inflammation of the ear canal skin.

Otitis externa (furunculosis)
- An infection (a folliculitis or abscess) in the hair-bearing area of the lateral canal skin, frequently caused by *Staphylococcus* spp.
- Gently pack cotton wool that has been soaked in glycerine ichthammol (G&I) solution around the furuncle. Add fresh drops of G&I twice a day until the infection has resolved, then remove the cotton wool.
- Give an antibiotic, e.g. oral flucloxacillin 25 mg/kg/dose 4 times a day for 5 days.

Acute otitis media
This is most frequently associated with an acute viral upper respiratory infection.
- Acute otitis media usually resolves spontaneously with simple analgesia and antipyretics (paracetamol and ibuprofen).
- Commonly the middle ear becomes secondarily infected, usually with either *Streptococcus pneumoniae* or *Haemophilus influenzae* and may require antibiotic therapy, especially when access to health care is difficult or follow up cannot be assured.
- For further information see http://www.sign.ac.uk/pdf/qrg66.pdf.

Clinical features

- Babies and infants are irritable and usually have signs and symptoms of an upper respiratory tract infection (URTI). Ear pulling is common. Older children complain of ear pain.
- The ear drum is usually intact but inflamed and may bulge.
- If the ear drum perforates, a mucopurulent (sometimes blood-stained) discharge may be seen.

Treatment

- Children diagnosed with acute otitis media should NOT routinely be prescribed antibiotics as the initial treatment. ☆☆☆☆☺ In general practice delayed antibiotic treatment is appropriate. The child can be prescribed amoxicillin 80 mg/kg/day 8 hourly for 5 days, which may be collected at parents' discretion after 72 hours, if the symptoms have not improved. ☆☆☆👍
- Prescription of decongestants or antihistamines has no added benefit. ☆☆☆☺

ENT referral is recommended if:
- There is persistent high fever, with signs and symptoms of acute otitis media, despite antibiotic therapy. The child may benefit from a myringotomy and a middle ear aspirate can be submitted for microbial culture and sensitivity.
- If there are signs of mastoiditis.
- If there is a facial nerve paresis.
- If there are intracranial complications.

Active chronic otitis media

If an acute otitis media does not resolve following perforation of the ear drum, the middle ear cleft may become colonized with mixed organisms, usually low pathogenic, saprophytic, coliform type organisms (*Pseudomonas* species and other Gram negative bacilli) and *Staphylococcus* species.

Clinical features

- A painless chronic mucopurulent discharge from the affected ear
- A persistent perforation of the ear drum
- There may be associated hearing loss.

Treatment

- Prevention: avoid getting water in the ear and avoid upper respiratory tract infections.
- First line therapy entails cleaning the ear using dry mopping with a cotton swab on a wooden applicator (NOT commercial cotton buds), followed by instillation of an antiseptic eardrop.
- If there no response after 2 weeks with simple topical therapy this usually means that the topical agent is not getting into the infected middle ear. In longstanding cases this may be due to excessive inflammation with profuse discharge.
- In these cases consider changing to a steroid/antibiotic topical ear drop (quinolone antibiotic with steroid being the least ototoxic). Emphasize frequent aural toilet before each application of topical antibiotics.
- If there is still little improvement consider adding oral antibiotics. It is best if the choice is guided by microbiological culture and antibiotic sensitivity. A swab from as deep down the ear canal as safely possible would be adequate (there are specific thin wire microbiological swabs available for this). Quinolones are the most effective empiric therapy (ciprofloxacin 10 mg/kg/dose 12 hourly for 5 days); however trimethoprim/sulfamethoxazole or amoxicillin/clavulanate is also frequently used. During systemic therapy, topical treatment and ear toilet should be continued.

ENT referral is recommended if:

- The discharge continues despite a repeat course of steroid/antibiotic ear drops and antibiotics.
- There is a lot of granulation tissue in the depths of the ear canal and the ear bleeds when dry mopped (may benefit from cautery).
- The infection is subsequently controlled but the perforation persists because of its 'sealed' margins. The resulting dry perforation is classified as inactive chronic otitis media. Reinfection is common, either during an upper respiratory tract infection or when water gets in the ear. Advise water precautions.
- Once the ear is dry, refer for hearing assessment and possible corrective surgery.

Cholesteatoma

This is a rare condition in which the tympanic membrane epidermis becomes invaginated and entrapped in the middle ear cleft. This may become secondarily infected and can damage the ear drum and the ossicles and erodes bone over the facial nerve and the inner ear. Another serious potential complication is acute-on-chronic mastoiditis with intracranial sepsis.

This is potentially the most dangerous of the middle ear disorders. Because this condition is difficult to diagnose and needs specialist management all suspected cases should be referred.

Clinical features

- A chronically discharging ear that does not dry up with topical eardrops and antibiotics. The discharge is often foul smelling
- Marked hearing loss
- Ear pain.

Otitis media with effusion (glue ear)

An effusion of mucus may persist in the middle ear after resolution of an acute or subacute infection behind an intact tympanic membrane. There is Eustachian tube dysfunction with inadequate aeration of the middle ear (adenoidal hypertrophy can contribute to this problem). The effusion causes a mild conductive hearing loss.

Clinical features

- Hearing loss and delayed speech development.
- The dull immobile eardrum may or may not be retracted medially.
- Tympanometry (if available) will produce a 'flat' curve.

Treatment

- Antibiotics are not recommended for an uninfected middle ear. ☆☆☆☆☹
- If the history is suggestive of recent onset then, after diagnosis, observe for 6 weeks before referral. If the history is suggestive of long-standing effusion (i.e. speech is affected) then refer earlier.
- Refer for specialist examination and assessment of hearing. Suspected recent onset effusions will undergo a period of active observation before insertion of ventilation tubes if audiometry confirms a significant hearing loss. ☆☆☆👍

Mastoiditis

This is a rare complication of otitis media. Infection trapped in the mastoid air cells may result in osteitis in the surrounding mastoid bone, which frequently spreads to form a subperiosteal abscess. Mastoiditis has the potential for serious intracranial complications.

Complications of acute mastoiditis
- Intracranial sepsis (meningitis, subdural empyema, brain abscess)
- Internal jugular vein thrombophlebitis.

Clinical features
- In the early stages there is pain and tenderness in the post auricular region or mastoid tip.
- The child is unwell, feverish and irritable.
- Signs of middle ear infection differentiate mastoiditis from a post-auricular node lymphadenitis.

Treatment
- Refer *urgently* to an ENT specialist.
- If referral will be delayed commence intravenous ampicillin and cloxacillin.
- If there are symptoms and signs of intracranial sepsis add ceftriaxone.
- Analgesia (paracetamol and ibuprofen).

Hearing loss in children

Hearing loss is the most common congenital abnormality with a general incidence of 1:1 000 births, but with higher incidence in some countries, e.g. significant bilateral hearing loss occurs in up to 6:1 000 births in South Africa. If hearing loss is detected late this affects communication and language and has severe consequences for the cognitive and socio-emotional development of the child. Any suspicion of hearing loss in children should be treated seriously and all children should be investigated by an audiologist as soon as possible for early diagnosis. If hearing loss is confirmed, intensive rehabilitation including hearing aids, speech therapy and special schooling improves outcomes.

Risk factors
- An illness or condition requiring admission of 48 hours or more to a neonatal ICU.
- Stigmata or other findings associated with a syndrome known to include a sensorineural and or conductive hearing loss.
- Family history of permanent childhood sensorineural hearing loss.
- Craniofacial anomalies, including those with morphological abnormalities of the pinna and ear canal.
- *In utero* infection such as cytomegalovirus, herpes, toxoplasmosis, rubella, HIV, or malaria.

Clinical features
- A parent/caregiver suspects that the child cannot hear properly.
- A poor response or no response to sound.
- Delayed or poor speech development.

Investigation
- It is safe, cheap, quick and simple to test the hearing of all children from birth using otoacoustic emission testing ☆☆◐. Ideally all neonates should have a hearing screen.
- From 4 years of age pure-tone audiometry can be used.
- Specific investigations for genetic and intrauterine causes may include chromosomal analysis, TORCH group serology or viral culture for CMV and rubella, as well as X-rays of the skull or long bones.
- Urine may also be tested for blood and protein (Alport's syndrome) or mucopolysaccharides.
- Ophthalmic assessment may reveal cataracts and retinopathy in congenital rubella or heterochromic irises in Waardenburg's syndrome.

The nose

Nasal obstruction in the neonate

Neonates are obligate nasal breathers. If nasal obstruction is present at birth (from choanal atresia), strenuous and unsuccessful respiratory efforts will be present with marked chest recession. The infant may become cyanosed. These signs will be relieved with crying or with insertion of an oral airway.

Facial moulding during birth may cause the nasal septum to buckle and result in swelling of the septal and turbinate mucosa. If significant obstruction develops, use a combination of decongestant nasal drops and a topical steroid (can use steroid eye drops).

Choanal atresia

Bilateral choanal atresia is a rare congenital cause of complete nasal obstruction in the neonate.
- Attempts to pass a feeding or suction tube through the nasal cavities into the nasopharynx will be met with obstruction.
- Use a small oral airway to support breathing.
- Feed via an orogastric tube.
- Refer for urgent ENT opinion.

Acute rhinosinusitis

This is usually preceded by a viral upper respiratory tract infection.

Clinical features
- Facial pain, headache, fever and malaise.
- Purulent nasal and postnasal discharge, nasal obstruction with loss of vocal resonance.

Cellulitis of the soft tissues of the cheeks usually results from dental infection rather than sinus problems.

Treatment
- The majority are viral in aetiology and respond to symptomatic treatment.
- Topical nasal decongestants such as oxymetazoline drops for 5 days, analgesics, antipyretics, and steam inhalations will provide relief.
- If symptoms persist beyond 5 days then consider oral amoxicillin for 5 days. If there is still no resolution, extend antibiotic therapy for an additional 5 days, preferably based on culture of a deep nasal swab.

Complications
- Orbital sepsis is a rare complication, occurring when infection spreads from the ethmoid sinus. The vision is at risk. Refer urgently to ENT or ophthalmology. If there is any delay, start IV ampicillin, cloxacillin and metronidazole.
- If there are symptoms and signs of intracranial sepsis ceftriaxone and vancomycin provide adequate intracranial penetration, making them a good first-line choice.

Chronic rhinosinusitis

This is a constellation of symptoms arising from a spectrum of aetiologies that, by definition, should have been present for more than 3 months. A careful history and examination of the ears, nose and throat help in making the diagnosis.

Clinical features
- Persistent bilateral purulent nasal discharge
- Nasal obstruction and snoring
- Loss of sense of smell
- Look for signs and symptoms of reactive airways (allergic rhinitis, asthma)
- Adenotonsillar hypertrophy.

Treatment

- No one treatment regimen exists for chronic rhinosinusitis.
- Look for and treat the underlying cause as well as treating symptoms.
- If an allergy is suspected attempt to identify the cause and advocate avoidance and consider antihistamine therapy.
- Treat any associated asthma.
- If a purulent nasal discharge is present then consider oral co-amoxiclav for 5 days, if still no resolution extend antibiotic therapy for an additional 5 days.
- Use a topical nasal decongestant (oxymetazoline < 6 years 0.025%, > 6 years 0.05% solution each nostril 2 to 3 drops twice daily) for 5 days.
- Use a topical steroid nasal spray (beclomethasone) in each nostril twice a day for a month.
- If the discharge and/or obstruction persists despite treatment refer the child for an ENT assessment.

> ***Practice point:***
>
> A child with unilateral smelly nasal discharge probably has a foreign body in that cavity.

Nose bleeds (epistaxis)

In children, bleeding usually occurs at the front of the septum (the partition between the nasal cavities). Precipitating factors include inflammation of mucosa (e.g. a viral upper respiratory tract infection, allergy, or vestibular infection) or minor trauma (e.g. digital trauma or sporting activities).

Treatment

- Reassure the patient; bed rest with head up 45 degrees.
- Compress the nose for 5 to 10 minutes.
- If the bleeding cannot be controlled by compression then gently slide a nasal tampon into the problematic cavity and refer.
- If bleeding is controlled prescribe a topical nasal decongestant (oxymetazoline < 6 years 0.025%, > 6 years 0.05% solution each nostril 2 to 3 drops twice daily) for 5 days.
- Attend to the underlying problem, e.g. treat infection and discourage the habit of picking.

Enlarged adenoids

Adenoids are present at birth and then begin to enlarge. They, along with the tonsils, continue to grow until individuals are aged 5-7 years. They play an important role in the development of the immune system. Enlarged adenoids may become symptomatic, with snoring, nasal airway obstruction, and obstructed breathing during sleep, when children are aged approximately 18-24 months. By the time children reach school age, the adenoids normally begin to shrink, and, by the time children reach the preteen or teenage years, the adenoids are usually quite small. It is common for children to develop snoring, with or without upper airways obstruction, usually associated with rhinosinusitis, but this can progress to an obstructive sleep syndrome. Adenoidal hypertrophy can also be a predisposing cause of middle ear effusions and infections with subsequent hearing loss.

Clinical features
- Persistently blocked nose
- Mouth breathing and snoring
- Sometimes associated with enuresis
- Restlessness and sleep deprivation can result in behavioural problems.

Treatment
- Look for and treat any other cause for chronic nasal obstruction, e.g. allergic rhinitis, chronic rhinosinusitis or foreign body.
- No good evidence supports any curative medical therapy for chronic infection of the adenoids.
- Some studies indicate benefit from using topical nasal steroids in children with adenoid hypertrophy. ☆☆◐
- In a child with nasal obstructive symptoms, with or without presumed allergic rhinitis, a trial of topical nasal steroid spray and saline spray may be considered.

Indications for adenoidectomy
- A lateral X-ray of the nasopharynx can be useful to confirm the presence of adenoid hypertrophy but is unreliable for assessing the degree of obstruction. The severity of symptoms determines the need for adenoidectomy.
- Chronic upper airway obstruction, especially obstructive sleep apnoea, and/or chronic mouth breathing with palatal and dental deformity.
- Recurrent or persistent middle ear problems.

The throat

Tonsillitis

Do not rely on clinical examination to differentiate between viral and bacterial sore throat. There is no evidence that bacterial sore throats are more severe than viral ones or that the duration of the illness is significantly different in either case. The precise diagnosis may be of academic interest, or possibly clinically relevant in more severe cases. The most common single organism identified is group A ß-haemolytic *Streptococcus*, which has the potential to cause immunological complications, e.g. rheumatic fever, glomerulonephritis. It may be necessary to prescribe antibiotics in these cases to prevent complications.

Clinical features
- Fever, sore throat and difficulty in swallowing.
- The tonsils are swollen and inflamed.
- The tonsilar crypts may contain debris and pus.
- Cervical adenopathy is frequently present.

Treatment
- When a sore throat is mild, or associated with a viral upper respiratory tract infection (cough and nasal discharge) only supportive treatment and analgesia are necessary. ☆☆☆☊
- If you suspect a bacterial pharyngitis/tonsillitis consider oral penicillin for 5 days.
- For frequent episodes under 3 years of age: consider pneumococcal vaccine (if unvaccinated) or try a long-term course of low dose antibiotics.

Indications for tonsillectomy
- Significant recurrent tonsillitis, i.e. 5 or more episodes of definite tonsillitis per year for the preceding 2 years
- Significant upper airway obstruction with or without obstructive sleep apnoea (in combination with adenoidectomy).
- A unilaterally enlarged tonsil (think of lymphomas), or persistent throat infection with cervical lymphadenitis (think of TB). Send tonsils for histology.
- One or more episodes of peritonsillar abscess (quinsy).

> **Practice point:**
>
> Acute pseudomembranous tonsillitis/pharyngitis is uncommon and the differential diagnosis should include diphtheria, leukaemia, and glandular fever.

Laryngeal stridor

The presence of stridor in a child is indicative of pathology causing airway obstruction. Urgent diagnosis is essential.

Acute stridor

- If the child has been well and the onset of stridor is sudden then always consider the possibility of foreign body inhalation.
- For the child who is unwell, usually with an upper respiratory tract infection, then laryngotracheobronchiolitis is the most common cause.
- Consider a possible retropharyngeal abscess; a lateral neck X-ray can be helpful.
- Refer urgently to a hospital paediatric service for definitive diagnosis and management.
- If the airway obstruction is life threatening support the airway with an endotracheal tube.

> **Practice point:**
>
> The quickest and safest way to secure a compromised airway is by an experienced anaethetist placing an endotracheal tube in theatre.

Chronic stridor

- Laryngomalacia is the most common cause of stridor in infants. Its inspiratory component varies in rhythm and in intensity, with alterations in the depth of respiration, or when changing position, or when the infant becomes excited.
- Rarer causes include recurrent laryngeal nerve palsies, congenital laryngeal cysts, haemangiomas, congenital laryngeal stenosis, tracheal stenosis, and vascular rings.
- Recurrent respiratory papillomatosis is usually associated with hoarseness.

- Refer all infants/children with chronic stridor to a hospital respiratory or ENT service.
- A definitive diagnosis requires laryngoscopy.
- Lateral and AP neck X-rays, chest X-rays, airway studies and a barium swallow (vascular ring) are ancillary investigations.

Drooling

- Children who drool usually have a neuromuscular disorder that impairs the control of mouth closure and of swallowing.
- Speech therapy and the removal of tonsils and adenoids may benefit mouth closure.
- Drooling tends to diminish with age.
- If it persists in a child of school-going age, relocation of the salivary gland ducts from the front to the back of the mouth will usually resolve the problem.
- Refer children with significant drooling to an ENT specialist for assessment.

Recommended reading

1. Middle ear infections http://emedicine.medscape.com/article/860227-overview
2. Otitis media with effusion http://www.nice.org.uk/guidance/CG60/nice guidance/pdf/english
3. Rhinosinusitis http://emedicine.medscape.com/article/ 861646-treatment
4. Adenoid hypertrophy http://emedicine.medscape.com/article/872216-treatment
5. Tonsillitis http://www.sign.ac.uk/pdf/sign34.pdf
6. Stridor http://emedicine.medscape.com/article/995267-overview
7. Obstructive sleep apnoea http://emedicine.medscape. com/article/1002803-overview

20 Fluids, electrolytes and acid-base

H. Buys, R. Diedericks

A basic approach to fluid requirements is important because the body is made up of about 60% water, and death and serious morbidity may ensue if the balance between input and output is disturbed. The special fluid needs of complex conditions such as total parenteral nutrition, diabetic ketoacidosis, complex cardiac and renal failure and neonatal needs are not considered here.

Maintenance fluids

Total body water is distributed between 2 main fluid compartments that interact dynamically via semi-permeable membranes. Abnormal fluid shifts between the compartments occur in ill patients.

Figure 20.1 Body water compartments and composition

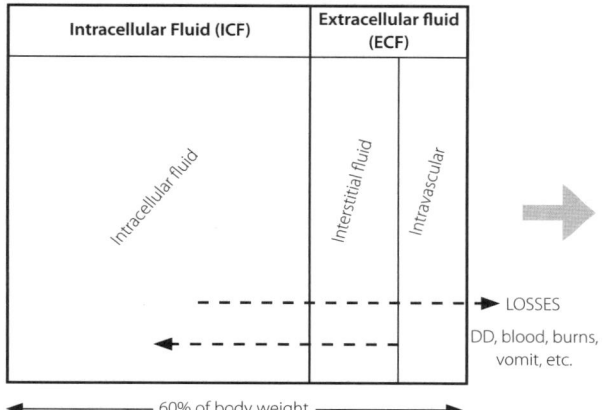

> **Practice point:**
>
> Losses from the intravascular space may occur rapidly leading to death from intravascular collapse (e.g. gastroenteritis, septic shock, bleeding and burns in young infants and children) in the absence of clinical dehydration. These conditions are potentially lethal, but eminently treatable, causes of hypovolaemia without dehydration.

- Maintenance fluids should be given enterally wherever possible. Intravenous fluids are only indicated in a minority of patients where the *nil per os* order is absolute.
- A useful guide to maintenance fluid requirements is derived from the Holliday-Segar calculator that works on the premise that the metabolic rate of a well child requires 1 ml of water for each kcal (multiply by 4.185 to convert to kJ) used (Table 20.1).
- Replacement fluids should be added where there are abnormal losses.
- Fluid restriction to approximately 50–60% of maintenance should be adhered to where there is a risk of inadequate excretion, e.g. with inappropriate ADH secretion leading to hyponatraemia (e.g. pneumonia, meningoencephalitis, post surgery) or renal failure. In these situations measurement of serum and urinary sodium concentrations would be useful to help guide fluid therapy.

> **Practice points:**
>
> - Children who are unwell require less fluid and should have their fluid requirements carefully worked out to avoid iatrogenic hyponatraemia.
> - Whatever the clinical situation, repeated review of the patient's clinical progress should dictate fluid calculations to minimize errors.

Table 20.1 Normal maintenance fluid requirements

Body weight	Energy needs/ metabolic rate kcal/kg	Maintenance fluids in ml/*day*	Maintenance fluids/ *hour* in ml/kg ('4,2,1' rule)
First 10 kg	100	100 ml/kg	**4**
11–20 kg	50	1 000 ml + 50 ml/kg for each kg > 10 and < 20 kg	40 ml PLUS **2** ml/kg for each kg >10kg
> 20 kg	20	1 500 ml + 20 ml/kg for each kg > 20 kg	60 ml PLUS **1** ml/kg for each kg > 20 kg

Note:
- *For infants under the age of 3 months: 150 ml/kg/day*
-              *over   the age of 3 months: 120 ml/kg/day*
- *Obese infants and children should have their needs calculated according to their ideal weights on the 50th percentile on weight-for-age charts. Fat does not store water!*

Replacement fluids

Resuscitation fluids

Hypovolaemic shock compromises cerebral and other organ perfusion and intravascular perfusion must be urgently restored.

Suitable resuscitation fluids: 0.9% saline, modified Ringer's lactate (Plasmalyte L®) and Ringer's lactate are appropriate to replenish the intravascular space (sodium content 154, 131, 131 mmol/l respectively).

Dose: 20 ml/kg by rapid infusion with a syringe via the intravenous or intraosseous route as a starting dose. More should be given in 5 ml/kg aliquots until tissue perfusion has been restored. (Figure 20.2 on next page.)

> ***Practice points:***
>
> - The main aim of the sequence is to restore perfusion and normal blood pressure rapidly, since this greatly enhances the chances of survival.
> - Delays in effective management increase mortality.
> - Low blood pressure is a late sign of shock.
> - It is imperative to urgently restore intravascular volume. An enlarging liver and basal crackles suggest that inotropic support may be required to improve perfusion – refer patient after initial stabilization.
> - Colloids are expensive and offer no advantage. ☆☆☆☺

Figure 20.2 The management of hypovolaemic shock

HYPOVOLAEMIC SHOCK IS A LIFE-THREATENING EMERGENCY	
STEP 1	Recognize poor perfusion and other signs of shock • depressed LOC • mottled cool/cold peripheries • poor/weak peripheral pulses • decreased capillary refill time (> 3 s) • reduced urine output
STEP 2	**A**irway • check airway patency, suction any vomitus/secretions **B**reathing • give high concentration O_2 via face mask
STEP 3	**C**irculation • establish vascular access or intraosseous access if no venous access after 2 good attempts • give 20 ml/kg Ringer's lactate or 0.9% saline by rapid infusion using a syringe and a 3-way tap • ensure no gallop, hepatomegaly, basal creps (i.e. no cardiac failure) • repeat Ringer's 20 ml/kg if still shocked (or 5 ml/kg aliquots x 4 is safer – reassess and give more if still shocked)
STEP 4	**D-E-F-G**: **D**on't **E**ver **F**orget **G**lucose Check Visidex and correct hypoglycaemia (glucose < 3 mmol/l)
STEP 5	Reassess ABC and response so far
STEP 6	If still shocked • give more Ringer's 20 ml/kg (by now 60 ml/kg given) • give first dose of ceftriaxone 80 mg/kg stat to cover for sepsis (by now 15–20 minutes have passed)

Within 15 minutes

• Call your Level 2 Unit to discuss further
• Contact Flying Squad to effect transfer
• Start IV fluid infusion ½ DD at 20 ml/kg/hour

At Level 3 Unit
• Start inotropes: dopamine at 10 mcg/kg/min (3 mg/kg in 50 ml 5% dextrose water at 10 ml/hour (=10 mcg/kg/minute))
• Admit to ICU

—APLS; Han et al, *Pediatrics*

The management of hypovolaemic shock in severely malnourished children

Extreme caution should be exercised in any severely malnourished child requiring IV fluids because of the risk of fluid overload, congestive cardiac failure and death. Hypovolaemic shock is one situation where IV fluids cannot be avoided and where inadequate fluid resuscitation will increase mortality in any patient. The initial approach is the same as in normally nourished children but the bolus aliquots and rate of infusion should be modified in the following manner:

Table 20.2 An A, B, C approach is essential

1st bolus:	15 ml/kg 0.9% saline or Ringer's lactate over 30 minutes. Reassess carefully, if still shocked.
2nd bolus:	15 ml/kg 0.9% saline or Ringer's lactate over 30 minutes. Reassess carefully, if still shocked.
3rd bolus:	15 ml/kg 0.9% saline or Ringer's lactate over 30 minutes.

> ***Practice points:***
>
> - Signs of intravascular overload during resuscitation include an increased heart and respiratory rate, puffiness of the eyelids and an enlarging liver. If these develop the bolus should be aborted and the child should be reassessed and further management urgently discussed with a senior colleague.
> - The signs of deteriorating shock and impending congestive cardiac failure may be difficult to distinguish by the inexperienced observer – ask for help!
> - Once perfusion has been restored, the enteral route should be used to rehydrate the dehydrated child over 24 hours.
> - Hypoglycaemia should be excluded and managed in the usual way if present.
> - Antibiotic cover should not be forgotten (see WHO Ten Steps in Chapter 5, Growth and nutrition, page 157).

Rehydration fluids

Fluid boluses with plasma expanders restore the intravascular space. Rehydration fluids are needed to restore the interstitial compartment. It is important to use solutions with sufficient sodium concentration to prevent hyponatraemia.

- In acute *gastroenteritis*, half Darrows dextrose is appropriate (½ DD has 60 mmol/l [Na$^+$]) if the intravenous route is used, or oral rehydration solution ([Na$^+$] ~ 60 mmol/l) for enteral replacement.

- Home-based sugar salt solution is suitable for oral replacement ($[Na^+]$ ~ 60 mmol/l).

> NB: Recipe for home-based sugar salt solution (SSS)
> 8 level teaspoons sugar + ½ level teaspoon salt + 1 litre cooled boiled water

- Where *vomiting* is the main source of fluid loss, rehydration fluid (0.45% NaCl and 5% dextrose) with added potassium is appropriate. Half DD is *not* suitable.
- Rehydration fluids should be given via the enteral route wherever possible.
- Rapid rehydration over 4 hours is effective in most dehydrated patients but should not be employed in situations of severe malnutrition, cardiac failure, severe pneumonia, encephalopathy, hypernatraemic dehydration and infants less than 3 months of age. In these patients, slower rehydration over 24 hours or even 48 hours should be used.

Dose of ½ DD IV or ORS via NG infusion for *rapid rehydration* over 4 hours:

IMCI 'Some' dehydration (5% dry)   12.5 ml/kg/hour
(50 ml/kg over 4 hours)

IMCI 'Severe' dehydration (10% or more dry)   25 ml/kg/hour
(100 ml/kg over 4 hours)

Table 20.3 Signs of dehydration

Signs	Some (5%)	Severe (10%)	Shock (danger signs)
Consciousness	Normal	Lethargic	Unresponsive
Pulse rate	Normal	Rapid	Rapid/bradycardia
Pulse volume	Normal	Weak	Feeble, impalpable
Skin turgor	Skin pinch slow	Skin pinch very slow	Mottled, cold
Eyes	Sunken	Very sunken	Dull
Anterior fontanelle	Sunken	Very sunken	–
Respiration	Deep	Rapid and deep	Laboured, irregular
Mucous membranes	Dry	Parched	Variable
Thirst	Present	Intense	Drinks poorly, uninterested
Weight Loss	< 5%	5–10%	Variable

> **Practice points:**
>
> - Neonates, malnourished infants and fat infants, as well as those with hypernatraemia, are often mis-assessed and require astute vigilance. Dehydration is often over-estimated in wasted infants and under-estimated where infants are obese, oedematous or hypernatraemic.
> - Shock may occur in the absence of dehydration or weight loss.

Ongoing losses

- Losses need to be replaced by equal volumes of fluid of similar composition. Stool losses vary from normal losses of <10 ml/kg to over 200 ml/kg/day in severe diarrhoea. For moderate losses add 30 ml/kg/day to maintenance requirements, but more should be given if needed. For those taking by mouth IMCI recommends 50–100 ml ORS after each loose stool for those under 2 years, and 100–200 ml after each loose stool for those over 2 years.
- Home-based sugar salt solution is suitable for oral replacement ($[Na^+] \sim 60$ mmol/l).
- Small frequent volumes of home based sugar salt solution – as little as a teaspoon (5 ml) a minute – can be effective in preventing dehydration even in vomiting infants.
- Administer ½ DD intravenously if oral replacement not possible.
- Rehydration fluid (0.45% saline and 5% dextrose) with added potassium (20 mmol/l) is used to replace gastric losses associated with vomiting. Start at 5 ml/kg per vomit replacement. This solution may also be used for children *without* diarrhoea who are unable to take fluids enterally.

> **Practice points:**
>
> Breast feeding should never be stopped and oral feeding should be encouraged for other infants and children once perfusion is restored. This can result in improved weight gain and earlier discharge from hospital.
>
> - Children should be weighed 6 hourly to improve accuracy in estimating the degree of dehydration and severity of losses, as weight is the only objective measure of gains or losses in overall fluid.

Acid-base disturbances

Disturbances in fluid balance are often accompanied by disturbances in acid-base and electrolyte balance, which can only be fully appreciated in conjunction with full laboratory data interpretation. Plasma pH is accepted as normal if its measured laboratory value falls within the range of 7.35 – 7.45. Hence in blood gas analysis:

- pH < 7.35 = acidaemia
- pH > 7.45 = alkalaemia
- Base excess (BE) and HCO_3^- reflect the metabolic component
- pCO_2 reflects the respiratory component

This approach reflects the bicarbonate/carbon dioxide system. The pH in bodily fluids is controlled by buffer systems involving the lungs, kidneys and cellular mechanisms; primary disturbances in each of these 3 systems trigger compensatory responses in the other 2:

Table 20.4 Interpretation of blood gas parameters

	pH	Primary problem	Compensation
Metabolic acidosis	pH < 7.35	HCO_3^- < 18 mmol/l (BE negative)	+/– ↓pCO_2
Respiratory acidosis	pH < 7.35	pCO_2 > 45 mm Hg (6 kPa)	+/– ↑HCO_3^-
Metabolic alkalosis	pH > 7.45	HCO_3^- > 25 mmol/l (BE positive)	+/– ↑pCO_2
Respiratory alkalosis	pH > 7.45	pCO_2 < 32 mm Hg (4.3 kPa)	+/– ↓HCO_3^-

During acute compensation, the direction of change of the pCO_2 and HCO_3^- is typically the same; however where mixed respiratory and metabolic abnormalities occur, the pCO_2 and HCO_3^- change in opposite directions. (Figure 20.3)

> ***Practice points:***
> - Overcorrection of the pH does not occur in physiological compensation.
> - One of the most common causes of acidosis in a sick infant or child is hypovolaemic shock, and regardless of the cause, tissue perfusion should be urgently restored.
> - Other causes of acidosis should also be considered and dealt with – fluid boluses may not be appropriate, e.g. cardiogenic shock in myocarditis.

- There is another approach to understanding acid-base disorders – the strong ion approach (Stewart's Strong Ion Theory) – whereby the effects of strong ions also powerfully influence pH. The degree to which electrolytes dissociate in solution determines whether they are called 'strong ions' like Na^+, Cl^- in the intravascular compartment and K^+ and Mg^{2+} intracellularly, or 'weak ions' like HCO_3^-, PO_4^{3-} and protein. Electrical neutrality is the rule, and thus changes in relative concentrations of the serum strong ions like chloride and sodium may have a big effect on acid-base. These relationships are of practical significance when giving large volume resuscitation fluids, e.g. 0.9% sodium chloride solution. Refer to recent texts on physiology for more detail.

Figure 20.3 Acid-base disturbance

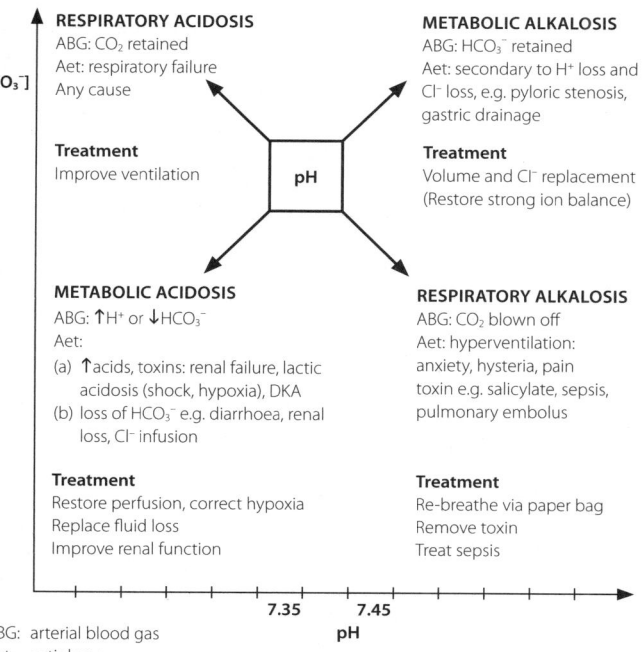

[HCO_3^-]

RESPIRATORY ACIDOSIS
ABG: CO_2 retained
Aet: respiratory failure
Any cause

Treatment
Improve ventilation

METABOLIC ALKALOSIS
ABG: HCO_3^- retained
Aet: secondary to H^+ loss and Cl^- loss, e.g. pyloric stenosis, gastric drainage

Treatment
Volume and Cl^- replacement
(Restore strong ion balance)

METABOLIC ACIDOSIS
ABG: ↑H^+ or ↓HCO_3^-
Aet:
(a) ↑acids, toxins: renal failure, lactic acidosis (shock, hypoxia), DKA
(b) loss of HCO_3^- e.g. diarrhoea, renal loss, Cl^- infusion

Treatment
Restore perfusion, correct hypoxia
Replace fluid loss
Improve renal function

RESPIRATORY ALKALOSIS
ABG: CO_2 blown off
Aet: hyperventilation: anxiety, hysteria, pain toxin e.g. salicylate, sepsis, pulmonary embolus

Treatment
Re-breathe via paper bag
Remove toxin
Treat sepsis

7.35   7.45
pH

ABG: arterial blood gas
Aet: aetiology

Diagram adapted from Siggaard-Andersen 1971 and Brenner and Rector 2004

Common acid-base disturbances

Metabolic acidosis

Metabolic acidosis is the most commonly encountered acid-base disturbance in clinical practice and indicates a serious disruption of normal homeostasis by an underlying disease process. The most consistent findings include:

$$pH < 7.35 \text{ (acidaemia)} \quad \text{Base deficit} \quad \downarrow HCO_3^-$$

Electrochemical neutrality is the rule in normal health where the sum of the serum cations (Na^+, K^+, Mg^{++}, Ca^{++}) and the sum of the anions (HCO_3^-, Cl^-, PO_4^{3-}, albumin, organic acids) should equate. The serum anion gap is a calculated measure that is employed to define the disease process in a metabolic acidosis; it is determined by the following calculation:

$$Serum\ anion\ gap = Na^+ - (HCO_3^- + Cl^-)$$

There is a normal anion gap of 3–11 mEq/l as a result of the negative charge carried by albumin. Any value > 16 mEq/l indicates a seriously ill infant or child with a severe metabolic acidosis who has an abnormal accumulation of acids or toxin. A lower level may be abnormal in a child with low albumin.

Metabolic acidosis can be divided into *high anion gap* and *normal anion gap* acidosis. There is either a *gain of strong acids (usually organic)* or a *loss of HCO_3^-* through the gut or kidneys. During shock and tissue anoxia, metabolism is incomplete (anaerobic) and leads to the generation of ketoacids and lactic acid via the partial oxidation of carbohydrates and fat.

Table 20.5 Metabolic acidosis

High anion gap (> 16 mEq/l) (normochloraemic)	Normal anion gap (3–11 mEq/l) (hyperchloraemic)
Added *endogenous* acids: • Lactic acid (shock, seizures) • Local tissue hypoxia, mitochondrial toxicity) • Ketone bodies (DKA) • Inborn errors of metabolism	Loss of HCO_3^-: • Diarrhoea • Renal tubular acidosis (RTA)
Added *exogenous* acids: • Ethanol poisoning • Aspirin ingestion • Carbon monoxide poisoning • Iron poisoning	Failure to excrete H^+: • Renal failure • Saline infusion (added Cl^-)

Special investigations to consider are:
- Blood tests:
  — Serum electrolytes – Na^+, K^+, HCO_3^-, Cl^-, albumin, (calculate the anion gap)
  — Urea and creatinine (assess renal function)
  — Arterial blood gas – in practice a venous blood gas is acceptable if oxygenation is not the prime concern (to assess pH, HCO_3^-, BE and pCO_2)
  — Blood glucose ± ketones in diabetic ketoacidosis (DKA)
  — Full blood count, blood culture, C-reactive protein (septicaemia)
  — Lactate measurement (elevated in hypoxia, poor perfusion, septic shock – type A lactic acidosis, and in type B lactic acidosis – associated with toxins, inherited metabolic disorders and systemic disease processes)
  — Toxicology as indicated.
- Urine tests:
  — Urine dipstick for glycosuria, ketonuria (DKA), protein and pH (in acidaemia urinary pH should be < 5 ; if > 5 then consider renal tubular acidosis (RTA) or salicylate ingestion).

Management

A metabolic acidosis is reversed by managing the underlying condition, urgently restoring intravascular volume, improving tissue perfusion, and correcting hypoxia and electrolyte imbalances.

> ### *Practice points:*
>
> - Saline-induced hyperchloraemic acidosis may be problematic following the use of large volumes of 0.9% saline during fluid resuscitation and may be less severe if Ringer's lactate is used as the volume expander. A fluid cocktail with additional sodium bicarbonate but devoid of chloride may be considered if a severe metabolic acidosis persists *after* intravascular perfusion has been restored.
> - In the case of DKA, fluid resuscitation, insulin and potassium replacement are needed; insulin is essential to allow utilization of glucose, and stop the acidosis and production of alternate fuels in the form of ketone bodies. See Chapter 14, Endocrinology.

Metabolic alkalosis

Characterized by: pH > 7.45 (alkalaemia)   Base excess   ↑HCO_3^-
Common causes include: persistent vomiting (e.g. pyloric stenosis)
prolonged nasogastric drainage
cystic fibrosis
potassium depletion
furosemide use
Management: rehydration with either 0.9% saline + K^+ (up to 40 mmol/l) + 5% glucose
OR 0.45% saline and 5% dextrose (rehydration fluid) + K^+
AND replace losses ml for ml.

> *Practice point*
>
> In the case of persistent vomiting and a metabolic alkalosis, lactate or bicarbonate-containing fluids are not suitable replacement fluids, as the restoration of strong ion balance cannot be achieved.

Respiratory acidosis

- Characterised by: pH < 7.35 (acidaemia)   ↑pCO_2
- Causes include:
  - inadequate ventilation (pneumonia, airway obstruction, restricted chest)
  - central hypoventilation.

  Symptoms relate to CO_2 retention:
  - bounding pulses, depressed level of consciousness,
  - papilloedema, increased respiratory effort.
- Management involves improving ventilation and treating the underlying condition.

Respiratory alkalosis

- Characterized by: pH > 7.45 (alkalaemia)   ↓pCO_2
- Causes include: hyperventilation due to anxiety, cardiac failure, pulmonary emboli, fever
- Symptoms relate to decreased ionised calcium: tetany, spasms, paraesthesia, depressed level of consciousness and light-headedness.

Hypoglycaemia

Correcting hypoglycaemia in sick children in the emergency room is imperative at all primary, secondary or tertiary units. (see also Hypoglycaemia p. 369, Chapter 14, Endocrinology). Because the brain is only able to utilize glucose as an energy source, hypoglycaemia is a potent cause of brain damage, seizures, confusion, apnoea (in young infants) and death at any age. The sooner it is detected and managed the better the neurological outcome.

1. *For practical purposes assume hypoglycaemia if the Visidex® is < 3 mmol/l.*
2. *Give a bolus of either:*
   a) *5 ml/kg 10% dextrose if available OR*
   b) *1 ml/kg 50% dextrose water DILUTED 1:4 with sterile water for injection. i.e. add 4 'volumes' of water to 1 'volume' of 50% dextrose – this creates a 10% dextrose solution OR*
   c) *5 ml/kg 10% dextrose (remove 20 ml from a 200 ml bag of 5% dextrose and add 20 ml 50% dextrose to the remaining 180 ml)*
3. *The dextrose bolus should be followed by at least a 5% dextrose-containing maintenance infusion (e.g. paediatric maintenance solution, ½ DD, or 0.45% saline and 5% dextrose solution).*
4. *A higher dextrose concentration is occasionally needed. A 10% dextrose-containing infusion can readily be made by removing 20 ml from a 200 ml bag of either paediatric maintenance solution, or ½DD or 0.45% saline and 5% dextrose solution and replacing this with 20 ml of 50% dextrose water.*
5. *Check the Visidex® every 15 minutes initially until stable.*

Practice points:

- It is also important to establish why hypoglycaemia has occurred; if it occurs in the face of a low intake then one must increase glucose provision (or it will simply recur).
- Hypoglycaemia may be a sign of an underlying endocrine abnormality. If it occurs when the patient is receiving a normal or high intake, further tests may be indicated at the time of presentation – discuss with senior doctor. (See Hypoglycaemia p. 369, Chapter 14, Endocrinology.)
- 50% dextrose should *never* be given undiluted.
- Persistent hyperglycaemia should also be avoided.

Electrolyte abnormalities

Daily electrolyte requirement

Sodium 3 mmol/kg   Potassium 2 mmol/kg   Chloride 2 mmol/kg

Glucose is also needed to provide about 20% of caloric requirement to prevent catabolism.

Deliberate supplementation of electrolytes is only usually necessary if feeds are withheld; hence the importance of maintaining enteral nutrition in sick infants and children regardless of aetiology. Supplementation in sick children is usually guided by interpretation of laboratory parameters in the context of the child's clinical condition and maintenance requirements.

Hypernatraemia

Normal serum sodium is 135–145 mmol/l. Hypernatraemia is defined as a serum sodium > 150 mmol/l. Sodium is the predominant cation responsible for the tonicity of plasma. Serum osmolality is calculated as follows:

$$\text{Serum osmolality} = [2 \times Na^+] + \text{glucose} + \text{urea}$$

Using normal values:

$$[2 \times 135] + 4 + 4 = 278\ mOsm/kg \quad \text{(range: 280–295)}$$

Hence if there is hypernatraemia, there will be hyperosmolarity leading to intense cellular dehydration, which in the case of the brain leads to shrinkage and shearing of blood vessels with resultant haemorrhagic encephalopathy and cerebral venous thrombosis.

Figure 20.4 Management of hypernatraemia (see next page)

> ***Practice points:***
> - Rapid correction leads to rapid fluid shifts and cerebral oedema (the signs of which include lethargy, headache, confusion, vomiting, seizures, and coma).
> - Rapid correction can only be done under exceptional circumstances and with specialist input.
> - Pure water deficit occurs with diabetes insipidus; use water via NG infusion and consult with paediatric endocrinologist.

Chapter 20: Fluids, electrolytes and acid-base 475

Figure 20.4 Management of hypernatraemia

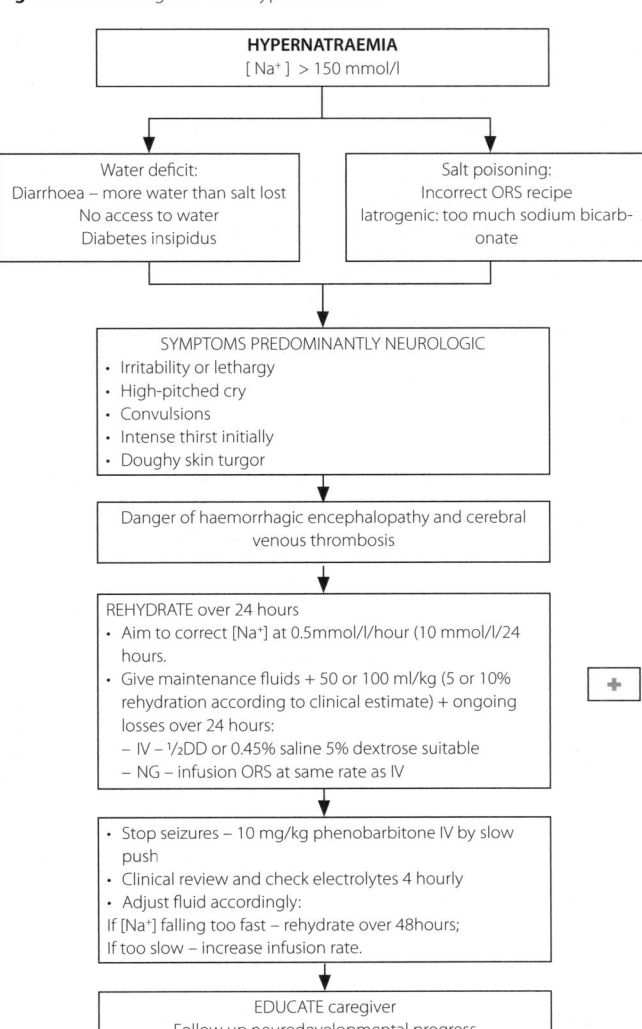

Hyponatraemia

Hyponatraemia is defined as serum sodium < 135 mmol/l and may be asymptomatic or mildly or severely symptomatic. Severe acute hyponatraemia can precipitate abnormal fluid shifts leading to cerebral oedema – the main causes are considered in Figure 20.5. One of the most common causes of hyponatraemia is the iatrogenic administration of hypotonic fluids at normal maintenance rates that are not adjusted and reduced for the abnormal fluid handling and requirements of the sick child. Great care should be taken when prescribing these fluids; paediatric maintenance solution (a hypotonic solution) is no longer recommended for routine use because of these associated dangers.

Figure 20.5 Management of hyponatraemia (see p. 478)

> *Practice points:*
>
> - Emergency treatment of hyponatraemia is only used when there is acute symptomatic hyponatraemia, i.e. signs of cerebral oedema. After the emergency dose of hypertonic saline has been given, the rate of sodium correction should not exceed 10 mmol/l/24 hours.
> - Chronic hyponatraemia should never be corrected rapidly.
> - Rapid correction of chronic hyponatraemia is associated with the risk of central pontine myelinolysis and subsequent permanent brain damage and quadriplegia.
> - Generally one should aim to correct serum sodium concentrations at 0.5 mmol/l/hour, raising the sodium by no more than 10–12 mmol/l/24 hours.
> - Slow correction should be done over 48–72 hours using the following formula:
>
> > Using 3% or 5% hypertonic saline:
> >
> > $$\text{Infusion rate in ml/hour} = \frac{2 \times \text{weight (kg)}}{\% \text{ saline infused}}$$
> >
> > Number of hours of infusion $= 2 \times (140 - \text{serum sodium})$
> >
> > Adjustment of rate should be done if the serum sodium is increasing too rapidly.
>
> - 0.9% saline has 0.15 mmol/ml Na$^+$
> - 3% saline has 0.5 mmol/ml Na$^+$
> - 5 % saline has 0.9 mmol/ml Na$^+$

Hyperkalaemia and hypokalaemia

The normal serum potassium level is 3.5 – 4.5 mmol/l.
The commonest clinical scenario associated with hyperkalaemia is acute hypovolaemic pre-renal impairment. Diarrhoeal disease is the commonest cause of hypokalaemia. (Figures 20.6 and 20.7).

Figure 20.6 Management of hypokalaemia (see p. 480)

> *Practice points:*
>
> - The maximum safe concentration of potassium for any intravenous fluid cocktail is 40 mmol/l.
> - *NEVER EVER* give KCl by intravenous bolus – this causes cardiac arrest!

Figure 20.7 The management of hyperkalaemia ☺☆ (see p. 481)

> *Practice points:*
>
> - Since Kexelate® may be difficult to retain rectally in a child with diarrhoea, the oral route may be used.
> - Mix the solution with 1 ml/kg sorbitol; exclude intestinal obstruction before oral administration.
> - Insulin should be used with caution as children are exquisitely sensitive to insulin; the risk of hypoglycaemia is high and should be anticipated and managed aggressively.
> - The duration of action of even the shortest acting insulin is 2–3 hours, and a satisfactory rate of glucose administration must be maintained over this period to avoid hypoglycaemia. (See above.)

Disorders of calcium, phosphate and magnesium homeostasis

Disturbances of calcium, magnesium and phosphate are often considered together and can be associated with life threatening events.

Calcium

(normal: 2.25 – 2.27 mmol/l)
Serum calcium levels are maintained within narrow limits under the regulatory influences of PTH, calcitonin and vitamin D acting on bone,

(continued on page 486)

Figure 20.5 Management of hyponatraemia

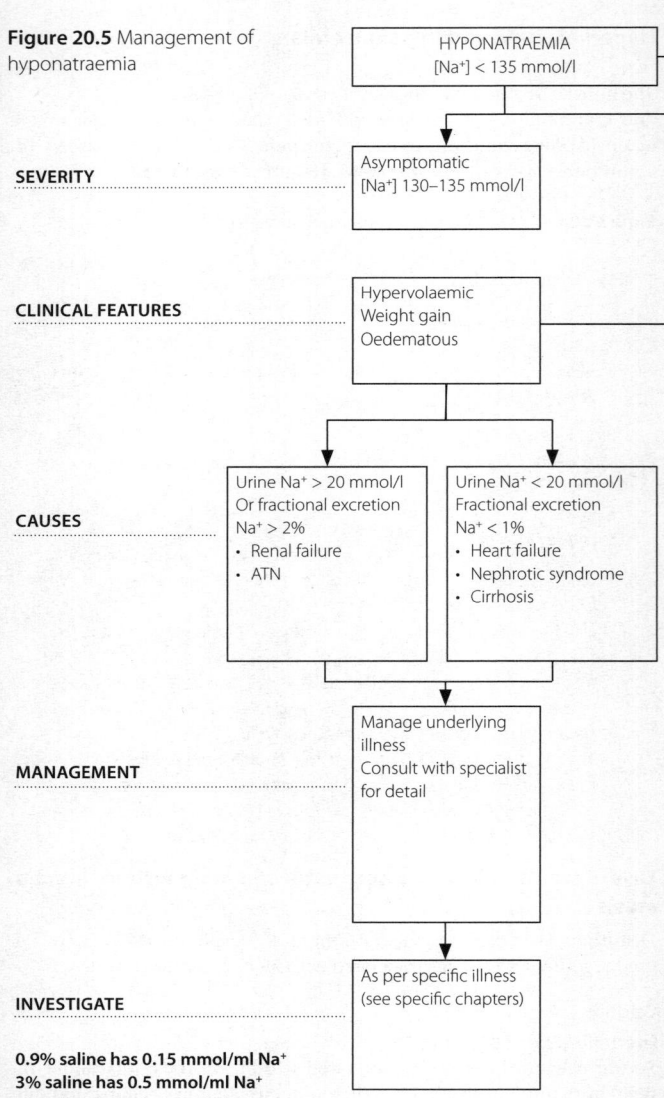

0.9% saline has 0.15 mmol/ml Na⁺
3% saline has 0.5 mmol/ml Na⁺
5% saline has 0.9 mmol/ml Na⁺

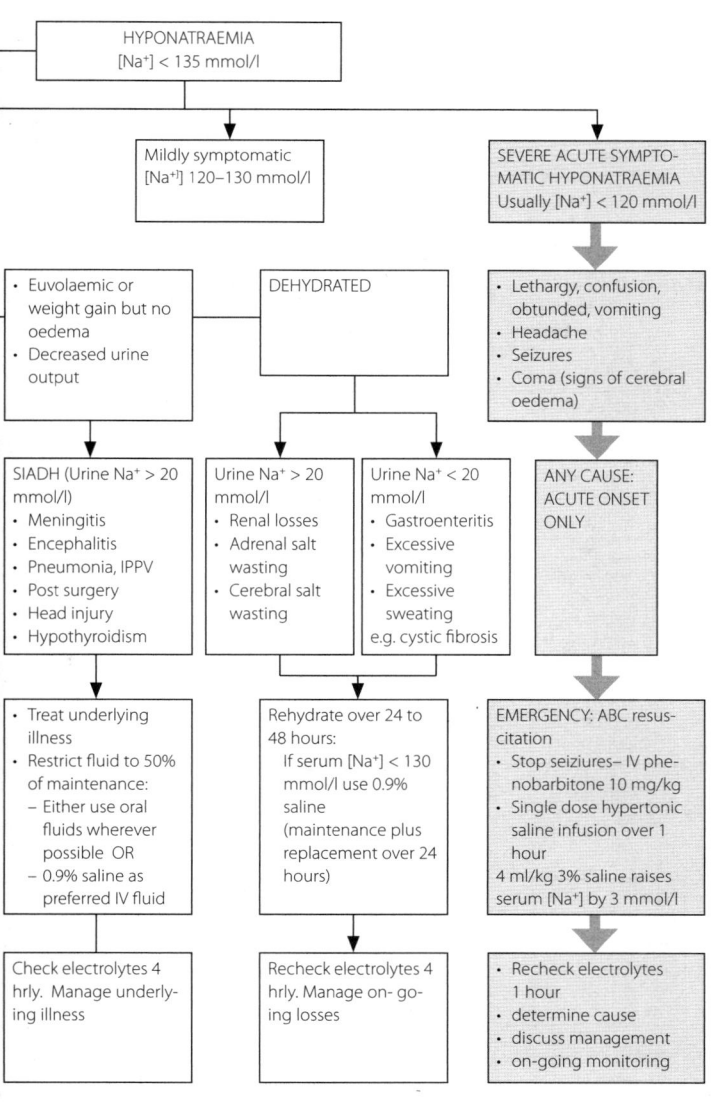

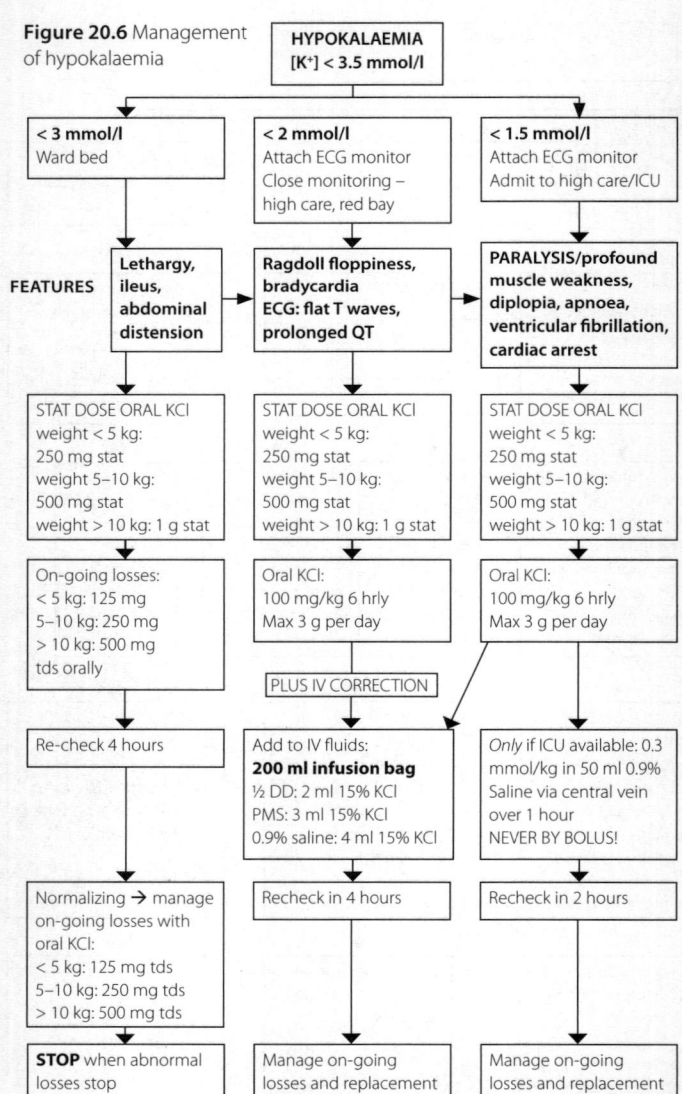

Figure 20.6 Management of hypokalaemia

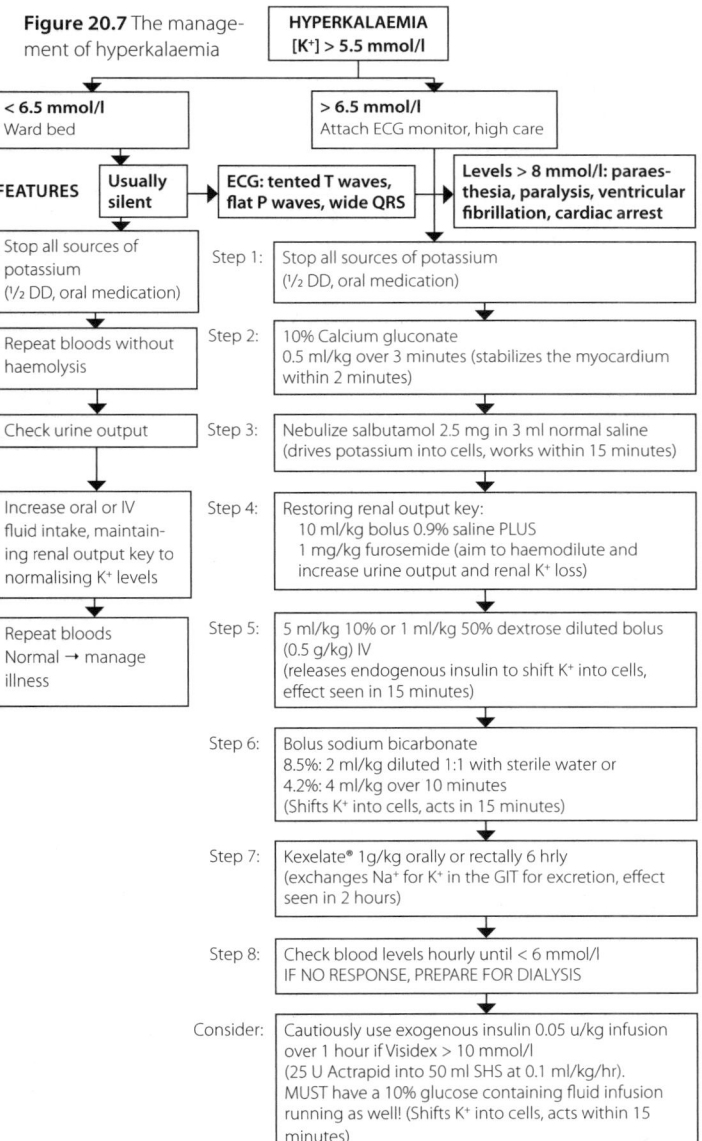

Figure 20.7 The management of hyperkalaemia

Figure 20.8 Summary of calcium, phosphate and magnesium disorders

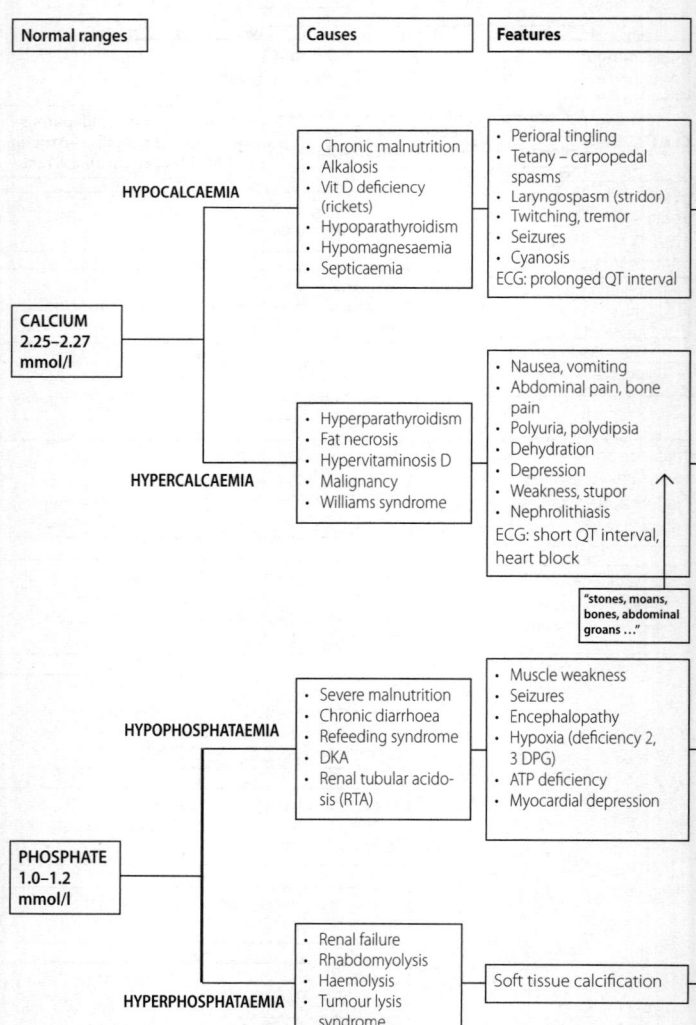

Normal ranges		Causes	Features
CALCIUM 2.25–2.27 mmol/l	HYPOCALCAEMIA	• Chronic malnutrition • Alkalosis • Vit D deficiency (rickets) • Hypoparathyroidism • Hypomagnesaemia • Septicaemia	• Perioral tingling • Tetany – carpopedal spasms • Laryngospasm (stridor) • Twitching, tremor • Seizures • Cyanosis ECG: prolonged QT interval
	HYPERCALCAEMIA	• Hyperparathyroidism • Fat necrosis • Hypervitaminosis D • Malignancy • Williams syndrome	• Nausea, vomiting • Abdominal pain, bone pain • Polyuria, polydipsia • Dehydration • Depression • Weakness, stupor • Nephrolithiasis ECG: short QT interval, heart block "stones, moans, bones, abdominal groans …"
PHOSPHATE 1.0–1.2 mmol/l	HYPOPHOSPHATAEMIA	• Severe malnutrition • Chronic diarrhoea • Refeeding syndrome • DKA • Renal tubular acidosis (RTA)	• Muscle weakness • Seizures • Encephalopathy • Hypoxia (deficiency 2, 3 DPG) • ATP deficiency • Myocardial depression
	HYPERPHOSPHATAEMIA	• Renal failure • Rhabdomyolysis • Haemolysis • Tumour lysis syndrome	Soft tissue calcification

| **Emergency management** | **Notes** |

Levels < 1.9 mmol/l corrected

- For acute symptomatic hypocalcaemia
  Under ECG control:
  10% calcium gluconate 1–2 ml/kg over 10 minutes (max 20 ml)
- Chronic hypocalcaemia: Refer Growth and nutrition and Endocrinology chapters

Risk of bradycardia if bolus too rapid.
Calcium salts cause severe tissue necrosis in the event of extravasation. Replace magnesium first if also low.

Levels > 2.9 mmol/l

Promote hydration and renal excretion:
1. 0.9% saline infusion at 1½ maintenance fluid requirement.
2. Furosemide 1mg/kg 6 hrly once hydrated.
DISCUSS URGENTLY with paediatric endocrinologist

Refer early/seek expert advice!
Need to investigate cause promptly,
Refer Endocrinology chapter

Levels < 0.8 mmol/l

- IV Infusion:
  Add to IV fluids, not to exceed 40 mmol/l [K$^+$]
  Potassium hydrogen phosphate contains:
  2 mmol/ml potassium and
  1 mmol/ml phosphate OR
- Oral replacement dose:
  1 mmol phosphate/kg/day in 3 doses
  Joules solution 1 mmol/ml or
  Phosphate Sandoz effervescent tablet 16 mmol/tablet

Oral phosphates can lead to diarrhoea

Levels > 2.5 mmol/l

- Volume expansion to increase renal excretion
- Dialysis
- Reduce dietary sources
- Calcium carbonate binding with meals
  30 mg/kg/day tds with meals
  (1 tablet = 168 mg elemental calcium)

Calcium carbonate does not bind if not given with meals

(Continued on next page)

| Normal ranges | Causes | Features |

MAGNESIUM 0,7–1.0 mmol/l

HYPOMAGNESAEMIA
- Chronic diarrhoea
- Malabsorption
- Severe malnutrition
- Short bowel syndrome
- DKA, renal tubular acidosis, drugs
- Toxins, e.g. fluoride

- Same as hypocalcaemia
- Neuromuscular irritability
- Cardiac arrhythmias, e.g. Torsade de pointes

HYPERMAGNESAEMIA
- Renal failure
- Iatrogenic

- Hypotension
- Weakness
- Paralysis
- Loss of deep tendon reflexes
- Bradycardia

ECG: prolonged QT, heart block

Emergency management

Levels < 0.5 mmol/l

- IV Magnesium sulphate 50% solution
  0.1– 0.2 ml/kg diluted in 20 ml normal saline, infuse over 20 minutes
  can repeat 6 hrly but first check levels and deep tendon reflexes OR
- IMI stat dose 0.2 ml/kg into anterolateral thigh muscle if no IV access OR
- Oral if asymptomatic:
  magnesium chloride 10% solution
  25-50 mg/kg 6 hrly (440 mg/5 ml syrup)

Notes: Avoid excessive doses. Check deep tendon reflexes first.
Children with Torsade de pointes often also have associated hypokalaemia – replace potassium as well

Levels > 2 mmol/l

- Stop oral magnesium intake
- Calcium gluconate 10% solution: 0,5 ml/kg IV over 10 minutes– risk of bradycardia if too fast
- Dialysis if all else fails

Uncommon condition

intestine and kidneys. Levels fluctuate with serum pH and albumin levels; half of the calcium is bound by albumin, the other half is ionised and active. Calcium disturbances and management are summarised in the flowchart (Figure 20.8).

Phosphate

(normal: 1 – 1.2 mmol/l)
Phosphate is a major intracellular anion essential for the structure and optimal functioning of important enzymes such as ATP and 2, 3, DPG. Hence disturbances can have profound effects on cellular metabolism (Figure 20.8).

Magnesium

(normal: 0.7–1.0 mmol/l)
Magnesium is another major intracellular metalloenzyme. Serum levels can fall dramatically with chronic renal tubular disorders and persistent diarrhoeal stool losses. Hypomagnesaemia is also often associated with hypocalcaemia and hypokalaemia. Conversely, hypermagnesaemia is uncommon and occasionally seen as an iatrogenic complication (Figure 20.8).

21 Surgical problems

A. Millar

Problems of the newborn

Surgery is indicated for the following congenital abnormalities:
- Diaphragmatic hernia if lung hypoplasia is compatible with life
- Omphalocele and gastroschisis
- Oesophageal atresia and tracheo-oesophageal fistula
- Intestinal obstruction (atresia, stenosis, aganglionosis, meconium ileus)
- Ano-rectal malformations.

Surgery is contraindicated for:
- Congenital anomalies that cannot be corrected or that are incompatible with life.

Clinical presentation

- Most conditions present with respiratory distress, intestinal obstruction or obvious surface defects.
- If one anomaly is obvious, always look for others (e.g. VATER association: **v**ertebral, **a**no-rectal, **t**racheo-o**e**sophageal defects, **r**adial aplasia, renal and heart defects).

Factors that influence survival

Uncontrollable:
- Degree of prematurity
- Significance of multiple abnormalities.

Controllable: the chance of success is increased by:
- Early diagnosis, especially *in utero*.
- Prompt specialist referral
- Care prior to and in transit
- Meticulous perioperative care
- Correct timing of appropriate surgery.

Diaphragmatic hernia (congenital)

Abdominal contents may enter the thorax through a postero-lateral defect in the diaphragm. This is frequently on the left side (85%).

Clinical presentation
- Respiratory distress is common. There is apparent dextrocardia with heart sounds more prominent on the right.
- Bowel sounds may be audible in the chest.
- The abdomen is small and scaphoid.

Diagnosis
- Antenatal ultrasound may detect the lesion *in utero*.
- Chest X-ray shows the deviated mediastinum and air-filled bowel in the hemithorax.
- Differential diagnosis includes a large pnuemothorax, cystic adenomatoid malformation, eventration of the diaphragm and an air-filled duplication cyst.

Management
Survival depends on the degree of lung hypoplasia, and a 'trial of life' is attempted before surgery is contemplated. This includes:
- Gastric decompression
- Respiratory support (low pressure oscillation, permissive hypercarbia if ventilation needed)
- Constant observation for a pneumothorax.

Surgery is delayed until the infant is ready to be weaned off the ventilator. The phase of pre-operative stabilization may take days.
- Surgery involves reduction of the abdominal contents from the chest and repair of the defect, which requires a patch if large.
- Prognosis depends on the degree of lung hypoplasia and associated cardiac and genetic anomalies.

Exomphalos (unruptured)

Clinical presentation
- *Minor*: abdominal wall defect (less than 4 cm) with bowel contained within a sac of peritoneum and amnion.
- *Major*: abdominal wall defect (more than 4 cm) with bowel and liver contained within the sac.

Management

- Decompress the stomach with a nasogastric tube. Enclose the trunk, legs and exomphalos with plastic bag or film to prevent heat and fluid loss and transport the infant to a surgical unit.
- Most cases require a primary repair.
- Where there is a large defect in a small or unfit baby, non-operative treatment using antiseptic ointments on the sac is indicated. Delay repair for months if necessary.

> ***Warnings:***
>
> Exclude hypoglycaemia, which may last for several weeks in an infant with the Beckwith-Wiedemann syndrome (macroglossia, gigantism and exomphalos).

Gastroschisis and ruptured exomphalos

Clinical presentation

- *Gastroschisis*: an evisceration of bowel through a small defect to the right of the umbilicus. The bowel is thickened and oedematous and no membranes are present.
- *Ruptured exomphalos*: a large central defect in the abdominal wall with evidence of membrane rupture at delivery. The liver may lie outside the abdominal cavity.

Management

- Cover the defect with plastic film or place the baby from the nipples down in a plastic bag. Control heat and fluid loss, particularly during transport.
- Primary closure is usually attempted. However, as prelimary treatment, a preformed silo can be placed in the nursery. Beware of impairment of respiration and venous return (abdominal compartment syndrome). Failure of primary closure requires the placement of a silo (Silastic or PVC IV-fluid bag cut to size), The bowel should be progressively reduced and the abdominal wall defect repaired within five to seven days to avoid local sepsis. The mean time to full enteral tolerance is ~30 days.

Intestinal obstruction

Common causes are listed in Table 21.1.

Table 21.1 Causes of neonatal intestinal obstruction

High	Low
Oesophageal atresia	Distal small bowel or colonic atresia/stenosis
Hypertrophic pyloric stenosis	Meconium ileus (fibrocystic disease)
Duodenal atresia or stenosis	Hirschsprung's disease
Malrotation with volvulus	Meconium plug syndrome
Proximal small bowel atresia/stenosis	Ano-rectal malformation
	Complicated inguinal hernia

Clinical presentation

- Bile-stained or persistent non-bile-stained vomiting implies intestinal obstruction until disproved.

High obstruction:
- *Before birth*: history of polyhydramnios
- *At birth*: gastric contents exceed 20 ml
- *After birth*: vomiting is prominent.

Low obstruction:
- Abdominal distension is prominent.
- The passage of meconium is delayed.
- The term baby normally passes a large meconium stool within 24 hours of birth.

Investigations

- *Antenatal ultrasound*: for polyhydramnios, oligohydramnios, growth retardation, or a previous history of an abnormality.
- *X-ray of abdomen*: essential for all suspected cases of obstruction.
- *Barium meal*: needed for bilious vomiting and for incomplete proximal obstruction.
- *Barium enema*: may be required for distal obstruction.

Management

- Resuscitate and rehydrate if necessary.
- Insert a nasogastric tube and apply suction.
- Transfer to a surgical unit.
- Define the type and level.
- Surgical correction of the obstruction.

Oesophageal atresia

- Polyhydramnios antenatally; persistent drooling after birth

- A chest X-ray shows the nasogastric tube coiled up in the oesophageal pouch
- If a feed is inadvertently given, it is regurgitated immediately
- A nasogastric feeding tube (12 French gauge) cannot be passed into the stomach.

Management
- Insert a Replogle tube in the upper oesophagus. Constantly aspirate it to maintain an empty pouch.
- Place the infant in a 15° head-up position to prevent reflux through a tracheo-oesophageal fistula (present in > 90%).
- Assess and if necessary manage other congenital abnormalities.
- Treat pneumonia if present.

Surgery
- Extrapleural thoractomy (thoracoscopic repair an alternative)
- Closure of tracheo-oesophageal fistula
- Repair of oesophagus: this is done in stages if the gap is too wide. The infant is fed via a gastrostomy until oesophageal continuity has been restored.

Duodenal atresia
- Vomiting soon after birth; stomach aspirate exceeds 20 ml
- Antenatal ultrasound and abdominal X-ray show fluid levels in the stomach and duodenum ('double bubble'). No distal gas is seen unless there is a fenestrated membrane or stenosis.

Malrotation
- The posterior fixation of the mid-gut mesentery is narrow, predisposing the bowel to undergo volvulus.
- Initially feeding may be normal, followed by bile-stained vomiting, or the infant may present with intermittent bile-stained vomiting.
- Abdominal X-ray shows a high obstruction of the small bowel in 80% of cases. It may be normal in 20%. Barium meal shows malrotation and obstruction in the distal duodenum.

Proximal small-bowel obstruction
- Polyhydramnios and vomiting are characteristic clinical features.
- Abdominal X-ray shows fluid levels in loops of distended small bowel.

Distal small-bowel obstruction

- Abdominal distension and an abnormal stooling pattern
- Many fluid levels on abdominal X-ray. No gas in the distal bowel (prone view). A barium enema confirms the level of obstruction if proximal to the caecum and the patency of the colon (colon atresia is present in < 5% of small-bowel atresias).

Meconium ileus

- There may be a family history of cystic fibrosis.
- The abdomen is distended from birth with palpable loops of bowel.
- Vomiting is not a significant early feature.
- Abdominal X-ray shows a 'ground-glass' abdomen with dilated loops of bowel. A few fluid levels may be seen. A barium enema may show a microcolon.
- Obstruction is due to multiple inspissated mucous pellets in the distal ileum and usually a large loop of dilated bowel filled with tenacious tar-like meconium. This loop may undergo volvulus and perforation.

Management

- Half-strength gastrografin enemas if there is no peritonitis or volvulus
- *Surgery*: if enemas are unsuccessful, a laparotomy is done.

Hirschsprung's disease

Presentation

- Neonatal intestinal obstruction
- Bowel dysfunction is common, e.g. intermittent constipation with feed refusal and vomiting
- Abdominal distension
- Explosive decompression may occur on rectal examination.

Diagnosis

- *Barium enema*: a transition zone is seen between the innervated and dilated proximal bowel and the narrow aganglionic distal bowel.
- *Suction biopsy of the rectum*: histology shows absent ganglia and increased parasympathetic nerve fibres in the muscularis mucosa.

Management

- Decompress the bowel with rectal wash-outs.
- *Surgery*: a colostomy is done proximal to the aganglionic bowel confirmed by frozen section histopathology

- Six to 9 months later a definitive 'pull-through' procedure is done.
- If the presentation is early, an 'endo-anal pull-through' may be done in the neonatal period without prior colostomy. Laparoscopic assistance may be needed.

Meconium plug syndrome

- Characteristic features are abdominal distension and a delay in stooling.
- Contributing factors include prematurity, sepsis, infant of diabetic mother, maternal sedation or antihypertensive therapy before birth, hypothyroidism and cystic fibrosis.
- Hirschsprung's disease *must be excluded* ultimately by biopsy.

Management

- A barium enema identifies the plug.
- The plug can often be dislodged with a half-strength gastrografin enema. If this fails, a laparotomy is done to form a stoma. At the same time the distal bowel is biopsied to exclude Hirschsprung's disease.

Ano-rectal malformations/imperforate anus

Careful examination of the ano-rectal area is necessary in all newborns to exclude malformations. Meconium on the napkin does not exclude an ano-rectal anomaly.

High lesions are associated with rectourethral fistulae in males (meconium in urine) and rectovaginal fistulae in females. Low lesions may have fistulae to the perineum and anal pits.

Diagnosis

Abdominal X-ray (lateral invertogram or prone lateral):
- *Low lesion*: the gas shadow in the rectum is below the inferior tip of the ischium.
- *High/intermediate lesion*: the gas is above this level or there is gas in the bladder. The X-ray may have to be delayed for 24 hours to obtain a satisfactory image.
- Ultrasound examination and a micturating cysto-urethrogram may be needed to exclude other abnormalities, particularly urinary tract defects and tethering of the spinal cord (MRI preferred).

Treatment

- Anal stenosis may be treated with simple dilatation. Other lesions require surgery.

Cleft lip and palate

This is a common congenital anomaly in which the lip and/or the palate is cleft along the lines of embryological fusion. There is a family history in 20% of cases. Cleft lip and cleft lip and palate are genetically distinct from the isolated cleft palate.

Approximately 5% of patients present with a cleft lip and palate, 25% with an isolated cleft lip and 25% with an isolated cleft palate. Associated anomalies are found in 20%. The remaining uvula can be grooved (submucous cleft palate) and may be associated with early otitis media.

Management
- *Cleft lip*: encourage breastfeeding; if not possible, use expressed breast milk. Refer to a plastic surgeon; surgery between 3 and 6 months. In a few cases surgery can be done a few days after birth.
- *Cleft palate*: encourage breastfeeding and avoid nasogastric feeding unless the infant is too weak to feed normally. An adapted teat may be required for a wide cleft or Pierre Robin syndrome (micrognathia, small tongue, cleft palate).
- *Cleft lip and palate*: feed the baby with expressed breast milk via a nasogastric tube. Refer to orthodontist for special feeding plate and to a plastic surgeon; surgery at 3 to 6 months.
- Early surgery minimizes the risk of middle-ear infection. In bilateral clefts or very wide clefts of the palate, the repair may have to be accomplished in stages and may be delayed until sufficient tissue has developed.

Post-operative management
- Inpatient for 3 days and is fed with a teaspoon for about 10 days. During that time the infant's arms must be restrained to prevent a finger being pushed through the repaired tissues.
- Revision surgery may be needed for the lip and nose before school and secondary surgery may be necessary at 9 to 11 years for a palatal fistula, nasal speech or bone graft of the alveolus. Cosmetic correction of the nose is done at about 16 years.

Abscess

Pus under pressure results in pain, swelling and loss of function. All soft tissue and lymph node drainage areas are affected.

Neonatal breast

- Do not manipulate or massage normally enlarged breasts. This may result in infection and abscess formation.

Treatment

- Peripheral dependent incision and drainage. Prescribe a broad-spectrum antibiotic, e.g. amoxycillin/clavulanic acid to prevent necrotizing fasciitis and breast bud damage.

Abdominal wall

- A deep intramuscular abscess can mimic intra-abdominal pathology. Incise and drain.

Psoas muscle

- Common in boys and presents with pain, fever, a limp and fixed flexion of the hip without gastrointestinal symptoms. A mass may be palpable in the iliac fossa. Confirm the diagnosis with ultrasound.

Treatment

- At surgery, locate by aspirating pus with a needle and syringe after an extraperitoneal exposure of the muscle. Incise and drain. The abscess is situated in pale oedematous muscle.

Deep external iliac nodes

- Suppurative adenitis presents in a similar way to psoas abscess. Healing septic lesions may be seen on the skin of the leg, perineum, or abdomen on the affected side.
- The treatment is similar to that for a psoas abscess.

Liver

- A pyogenic abscess is 5 times more common than an amoebic one. Presents with fever, pain in the right upper quadrant and tender hepatomegaly. Confirm the diagnosis with ultrasound and with the complement-fixation or monoclonal antibody tests for amoebiasis.

Treatment

- Give antibiotics, e.g. cloxacillin, aminoglycoside and metronidazole. If signs and symptoms worsen or persist despite 2 days of therapy, percutaneous, laparoscopic or surgical drainage is necessary. This is needed in 60–70% of cases overall and for most left lobe abscesses.

Peri-anal abscess

Seen in the first year of life, mainly in males. Usually a fistula develops from the level of the anal columns to the site of the peri-anal abscess after incision and drainage.

Anal fissure

(See constipation, p. 147.)

This is the most common cause of fresh, painful bleeding from the rectum in infants. Identify the fissure by inspection. A rectal examination, anal stretch and removal of the faecaloma may have to be done under general anaesthesia. Prescribe a stool softener such as lactulose. Nitric oxide paste may be a useful supplementary treatment.

Appendicitis

Presentation

- Anorexia, nausea, vomiting, abdominal pain and disturbance of stooling pattern. Localized signs of inflammation in the right iliac fossa, right flank, or pelvis. Evidence of a systemic response with pyrexia, tachycardia, and raised white blood cell count
- X-ray abdomen: Localized ileus, faecolith, scoliosis concave to right and blurring of soft tissue definition.
- Ultrasound scan may show localized, inflammatory oedema and fluid.
- Exclude urinary tract infection and renal colic. In girls with high fever and a vaginal discharge, exclude a primary peritonitis by blood culture and gram stain of the discharge (usually *Pneumococcus*).

Management

Full resuscitation is essential before appendectomy. Prophylactic antibiotics, e.g. metronidazole plus gentamicin plus penicillin are recommended to prevent wound infection and to control spread of abdominal sepsis.

Ascariasis

Presentation

- *Age four to ten years*: heavy infestation can cause bolus obstruction with colic, vomiting, and palpable masses.

- *Abdominal X-ray and ultrasound scan*: whorls of worms and partial bowel obstruction.

Management
- Bed-rest, intravenous fluids, nasogastric tube, analgesia, antispasmodics, e.g. hyoscine butylbromide.
- 95% of cases resolve within 24 hours.
- A vermifuge, e.g. albendazole or piperizine is administered only when asymptomatic.
- Beware of complications: impaction necrosis producing a tender mass; or volvulus – a tender mass with shock. Urgent laparotomy is needed in these cases.

Complications
- *Biliary ascariasis*: this presents with biliary colic. With heavy intestinal infestation worms may enter the liver. The majority (95%) resolve on conservative treatment. Monitor with ultrasound. Cholangitis, liver abscess, biliary strictures can occur.
- The worms can be identified with endoscopic retrograde cholangio-pancreatography (ERCP) or magnetic resonance cholangio-pancreatography (MRCP) and extracted endoscopically if symptoms fail to resolve or if the worms are still present after four weeks. Conduct surgical exploration if ERCP fails or is unavailable.
- *Pancreatitis*: generalized pain with raised serum amylase. Treatment: resuscitation and supportive therapy.
- *Intussusception*: see p. 502.
- *Appendicitis*: see previous page.

Biliary atresia

Clinical presentation
- Pale stools, dark urine and jaundice in neonates indicate obstructive hyperbilirubinaemia of which biliary atresia is an important and potentially correctable cause.
- Differentiate from other causes of conjugated hyperbilirubinemia, particularly the neonatal hepatitis syndrome:
  - Typical findings: acholic stools indicate obstruction. Haematology and liver-function tests demonstrate cholestatic jaundice.
  - Ultrasound and radioisotope imaging indicate liver and biliary structure and function, but may be falsely negative.
  - Definitive diagnosis is by open-liver biopsy and cholangiography.

Treatment

- A porto-enterostomy (Kasai procedure) enables bile to flow into the gut in > 50% of cases if operated on before 10 weeks.

> **Warning:**
>
> A delay in the diagnosis of biliary atresia can result in progressive biliary cirrhosis. It also diminishes the efficacy of the Kasai operation. Up to 80% of all cases become candidates for liver transplantation.

Branchial arch and cleft remnants

These include cysts that may become infected, fistulae or sinuses and cartilaginous skin tags. The commonest, pre-auricular skin tags require cosmetic excision only. Fistulae and sinuses will require careful excision and should be referred. If infected, treat with an antibiotic (e.g. amoxycillin/clavulanic acid, cephalosporin).

Cervical lymphadenopathy

- Causes of cervical nodes include viral infection, bacterial lymphadenitis and tuberculosis. Rarer causes include neoplasia (usually lymphoma) and mycobacterium-avium-intracellulare-scrofulaceum complex (MAIS). This is unilateral, has a subacute course and a negative Mantoux. It does not respond to anti-TB therapy and requires excision for a cure.

Management

- Exclude systemic, regional and local disease.
- Treat acute infections with antibiotics empirically if no local cause is identified.
- If the size does not decrease within 2 weeks, investigate with full blood count, erythrocyte sedimentation rate, chest X-ray and Mantoux.
- *Indications for excision biopsy*: long history, more than 2.5 cm diameter, firm/hard, matted or failure to respond to antibiotics within 2 weeks.

Circumcision

In the newborn the foreskin adheres to the penis and cannot be retracted fully. This is not an indication for circumcision. Do not retract the fore-

skin forcibly. By 5 years there is still a 15–20% chance of adherence and by 12 years only a 1% chance.
- The only medical indication for circumcision is phimosis caused by recurrent balanoposthitis.
- Mild phimosis responds to topical hydrocortisone cream 1% for 10 days.
- If circumcision is contemplated, it is best delayed until the infant is out of napkins.
- Absolute contraindications: hypospadias, napkin eczema.

Complications are more likely to occur with Plastibell® circumcisions done as an outpatient procedure. They include bleeding, infection, coronal fistula, removal of excess skin, meatal ulceration, and stenosis.

Cystic hygroma

This consists of multiple fluid-filled endothelial-lined cysts. Usually evident from birth in the cervico-facial region. The cysts often surround vital structures in the neck. Refer early as spontaneous resolution is unlikely. Complications such as infection and tissue oedema causing obstructed airways may be lethal.

Management
- Do not aspirate.
- Careful surgical excision may be done in stages.
- Sclerosant injections are effective in selected cases.

Ectopia vesicae (bladder exstrophy)

The anterior abdominal wall below the umbilicus is deficient and the bladder lies open and exposed. The anus is placed anteriorly. There is an epispadias or a bifid clitoris and wide separation of the symphysis pubis. Exomphalos is common. Early closure is necessary, so refer immediately.

Fused labia

This results from a delicate incomplete fusion of the labia minora in the midline, due to a low level of oestrogen or to infection. Wetting problems or 'absent vagina' are frequent reasons for referral.

Management
- Apply an oestrogen cream locally. If this fails, the labia should be separated under sedation or general anaesthesia. Re-apply the cream to prevent a recurrence.

Cutaneous vascular lesions

These are very common (1 in 3 children) and few require a medical opinion. The natural history, prognosis and treatment depend on the type of lesion, but because of overlap, classification may be difficult. Several weeks may elapse before the allocation to a particular group can be confirmed. When proliferating lesions are near a vital organ, they may impair its function (e.g. airway, eyesight). Other problems include haemorrhage, ulceration, infection, recurrent trauma and increased regional growth. Very large lesions may cause systemic complications such as consumptive coagulopathy, thrombocytopenia and congestive heart failure.

Clinical presentation
- *Macular stain*: 'stork bite', 'salmon patch', 'naevus flammeus'. These flat pink blemishes are present at birth and account for 30–40% of the total. They are seen on the upper eyelids, forehead, chin or scalp. They blanch on pressure and become suffused during crying. They fade and disappear within a year.
- *Haemangioma*: 'strawberry naevus'. Commonest rapidly growing tumour of infancy. A bright red nodule appears within weeks of birth and enlarges rapidly because of endothelial proliferation. Multiple lesions may be present anywhere on the body. By 5 years 50% have resolved, and at 7 years 90%. Only complicated lesions need treatment (see below).
- *Vascular malformation*: this structural abnormality of low-flow capillary or venous tissue may have an arterial component to cause an arteriovenous malformation, e.g. 'port-wine stain'. Present from birth as a flat, dark red stain and does not proliferate or involute. Its growth parallels that of the child. Laser treatment is effective (see below).
- *Vascular lesion with mesodermal elements*: includes haemangiomatous and vascular malformations with or without a lymphatic component. It can be cystic or cavernous to cause a large puffy swelling in the deep soft tissues or muscles. The haemangiomatous element may proliferate and then involute.

Treatment

- Most vascular lesions do not require treatment. Many disappear and the natural history must be explained to the parents, who need this reassurance.
- If amenable to surgery, the lesion may be excised; alternatively intralesional steroid injection (e.g. triamcinolone) may be used.
- Port-wine stains and ulcerated capillary haemangiomata have been treated successfully with pulsed-dye laser therapy. The former respond best in the first year of life.
- Steroids are recommended for large lesions that are technically impracticable to excise. Give prednisolone 4 to 6 mg/kg/day for 3 weeks. If the lesion regresses, continue treatment for 3 months and then tail off the dosage over 4 to 6 weeks. Approximately 50% fail to respond to steroid treatment. Interferon, propranolol and vincristine has been used with success in some cases.
- Other methods of treatment include ligation of a feeding vessel, e.g. hepatic artery for liver haemangioma, and embolization of a feeding vessel with radiological guidance.

Hernia

Hydrocoele

- Present at birth and may be unilateral or bilateral. Fluid enters a narrowly patent processus vaginalis and is trapped within the tunica vaginalis testis.
- The fingers are able to 'get above' this palpable scrotal swelling. The scrotum transilluminates brightly with cold light.

Indications for herniotomy

Perform a herniotomy when the hydrocoele:
- Is huge and tense
- Persists beyond 12 months of age
- Develops later in childhood or is associated with an abnormal testis.

Fluid hernia

- This implies a widely patent fluid-filled processus vaginalis with fluctuations in the size of the scrotum. Elective herniotomy is indicated, as it is unlikely to resolve spontaneously and a bowel-containing hernia may develop.

Inguinal hernia

At any age requires surgical treatment without delay.
- The younger the patient, the greater the incidence of complications.
- An irreducible hernia with evidence of strangulation (local oedema being the first sign) requires immediate surgery.
- For an irreducible hernia without strangulation, a single attempt may be made under sedation to reduce it manually. If successful, a repair is done after 24–48 hours. If unsuccessful, operate immediately.

> ***Practice point – warning:***
>
> In females a gonad is commonly found in the hernial sac. If a Fallopian tube is not observed, the gonad should be examined and biopsied at surgery to exclude androgen insensitivity (testicular feminizing syndrome). Do chromosomal sexing prior to surgery if the hernias are bilateral and contain a gonad. The passage of a thin probe into the vagina confirms its presence and a length of more than 3 cm signifies female sex.

Para-umbilical and supra-umbilical hernias

- These do not regress, frequently strangulate, and should be repaired.

Umbilical hernia

- This usually regresses spontaneously and rarely strangulates. Repair at 5 years of age if there are no signs of closure.
- Complications may occur if the hernia is associated with pica (sand-eating) as putty-like intestinal contents become entrapped in the hernia. The hernia usually reduces on bed rest and sedation. Treat iron deficiency and repair electively.

Hypospadias and chordee

Meatal obstruction does not occur and circumcision is contraindicated. May be corrected surgically from the age of 1 year and should be completed before school-going age.

Intussusception

- This occurs mostly in the ileocaecal region as a result of lymphoid hyperplasia. In children over 2 years old consider lead-point pathology as a cause, e.g. Meckel's diverticulum, hamartoma, duplication cyst or lymphoma.

Clinical presentation
- Sudden onset of colic and vomiting in a previously healthy infant less than 2 years old.
- An abdominal mass – may also be palpable on rectal examination.
- Bloody mucoid stools and intestinal obstruction occur later.

Investigation
- An ultrasound scan shows the intussusception as a 'target' on transverse scan and a 'Swiss roll' on longitudinal scan. Contrast enema will confirm or exclude the diagnosis.

Management
- *Early uncomplicated case*: pneumatic reduction. Precede by resuscitation if necessary, and by sedation (e.g. pethidine 1 mg/kg IM).
- Contraindications to attempted reduction include a tender mass, peritonitis, poor general condition, symptoms for more than 36 hours, marked small-bowel obstruction (distension: abdominal X-ray shows multiple fluid levels).
- Resuscitation and laparotomy if pneumatic reduction fails or is contraindicated.
- A manual reduction may still be successful; if not, a bowel resection is necessary.

Macroglossia (enlarged tongue)

This may be encountered with Beckwith-Wiedemann syndrome, Down's syndrome and hypothyroidism or infiltrated with lymphangiomatous, haemangiomatous or neurofibromatous involvement.

Management
- Partial glossectomy if the tongue cannot be accommodated comfortably in the mouth. Beware of severe post-operative oedema and airway obstruction.

Meatal stenosis

A pinhole meatus with a thin stream on micturition. This usually results from an inappropriately timed circumcision or from a healed meatal ulcer.

Management
- Generous meatotomy.

Parotid enlargement

Inflammatory causes
- Parotitis
- Viral, e.g. mumps
- Acute suppurative: often associated with trauma to the meatus of the parotid duct during teething or sucking. Commonly seen in AIDS.
- *Treatment*: a broad-spectrum antibiotic, e.g. amoxycillin/clavulanic acid
- Recurrent parotitis: unilateral mild symptoms, 4–10 years of age. Due to rupture of acini and chemical inflammation (sialectasis). Spontaneous resolution at puberty.

Other causes
- Lymph-node enlargement within the gland capsule, e.g. pyogenic (common in AIDS), TB, lymphoma. Also autoimmune disease, starvation, mesodermal malformation, haemangioma, first branchial arch cyst, and tumour.

Management
- Identify the cause by biopsy if necessary. Hamartoma or haemangioma requires a conservative approach because of the danger of facial nerve damage. Refer tumours to a specialist centre.

Pyloric stenosis
- The incidence in the first 6 weeks of life is 1 in 500 infants. Male to female ratio is 4:1.

Clinical presentation
- Persistent non-bile-stained forceful vomiting develops after some weeks of normal feeding. Constipation or green mucoid 'hunger' stools may be present.

Complications
- *Metabolic*: dehydration, hyponatraemia, hypochloraemia, hypokalaemia, metabolic alkalosis, jaundice.

- *Haematemesis*: due to gastritis, Mallory-Weiss tear, or oesophagitis.
- *Infections*: chest and urinary tract.

Diagnosis
- *Clinical*: empty the stomach with a nasogastric tube. Test feed. Look for epigastric peristalsis and feel for the 'olive' tumour with the left hand. It is typically firm, and intermittently palpable to the right of rectus sheath below the liver. Ultrasound and barium meal are used if the diagnosis is doubtful.

Management
- Rehydrate and correct metabolic and electrolyte abnormalities. (See Chapter 20, Fluids, electrolytes and acid-base).
- Treat infection.
- Give Vitamin K 1 mg IM.
- Pyloromyotomy.

Sublingual cysts

All cysts in the floor of the mouth need referral for surgical treatment, either deroofing and marsupialization or complete excision.

Rectal prolapse

Partial-thickness prolapse is commonly due to faulty bowel habits. Attend to constipation (p. 147). Full-thickness prolapse should be differentiated from a prolapsed intussusception (which is sausage-shaped, severely congested, and has a sulcus between the anal canal and the intussusception) and prolapse of a rectal polyp.
- Identify a possible underlying cause such as cystic fibrosis, whooping cough, proctocolitis, *Trichuris* infestation, neurologic causes (e.g. spina bifida), and anatomic causes (e.g. exstrophy of the bladder).

Management
- *Emergency management*: reduce the prolapse under sedation and strap the buttocks for 48 hours. Definitive treatment is needed if there is a relapse after strapping.
- *Sclerosant*: submucous injection of 5% phenol in almond oil.
- Thiersch circum-anal suture using No. 1 gauge absorbable suture. This may be complicated by pain and sepsis.
- Formal reconstruction or amputation is rarely required.

Acute scrotum

Aetiology
- Torsion of the testis is the most common cause at all ages.
- Other causes in order of frequency are:
  - Epididymo-orchitis
  - Torsion of a testicular appendage
  - Idiopathic scrotal oedema
  - Funiculitis (infected material may descend into the scrotum via a patent processus vaginalis)
  - Scrotal cellulitis.

Always exclude a strangulated inguinal hernia by confirming that the swelling is scrotal rather than inguino-scrotal.

Management
- A confident clinical diagnosis is difficult. Urgent surgical exploration is advocated.
- After correction of a torsion and fixation of the testis, the opposite side must be explored and fixed.

Sternomastoid tumour

Torticollis from *in utero* positional moulding corrects itself in the first few months of life. In infants a firm mass is noted in the sternomastoid muscle. The head is turned away from, but tilted towards, the affected side. In older children facial hemi-hypoplasia and plagiocephaly may result from fibrosis and shortening of the muscle.

Management
- Diligent passive stretching is successful in nearly all cases.
- In older children exclude a squint or a cervical spine deformity.
- If passive stretching fails, division of the sternomastoid muscle and deep fascia of the neck may be required. Post-operative physiotherapy is essential.

Tongue tie

This does not interfere with feeding or speech and seldom requires surgical correction.

Management

- If at 2 years the child is unable to protrude the tongue beyond the incisors and the tongue is indented in midline by frenulum tethering, perform a release under general anaesthesia.

Undescended testis

This is a testis that has never been in the scrotum, nor can it be manipulated to the bottom of the sac. This differentiates a true undescended testis from a retractile one.

Management

- No place for hormone therapy.
- Surgery is indicated to improve fertility, to prevent complications such as hernia and torsion, to monitor for later malignant change (30–50 times greater incidence in intra-abdominal testis; 10 times greater incidence in palpable testes), and for psychological reasons.
- Orchidopexy during the second year of life. Long-term follow-up.

Umbilicus

- *Omphalitis*: see p. 67.
- *Granuloma*: pale pink swelling in the umbilical stump due to incomplete healing following separation of the cord. Treat with local excision or cauterization with silver nitrate
- *Polyp 'cherry tumour'*: vitelline mucosal remnant
- *Patent vitello-intestinal duct*: faeculent discharge
- *Patent urachus*: watery discharge.

Management

A sinogram will identify any deeper fistulous connection. Most require umbilical exploration to exclude an attached Meckel band.

Recommended reading

1. Beasley, SW, Hutson, JM, Auldist, A. *Essential Paediatric Surgery*. Hodder Arnold. 1996
2. *Newborn Surgery*. 2nd Ed. Puri, P (Ed) Hodder Arnold. 2003.
3. *Ashcraft's Pediatric Surgery* 5th Ed. Holcomb III, GW, Murphy, JP. Saunders (Eds). Elsevier. 2010.

22 Palliative care and pain management

L.G. Reynolds, J. Thomas

Palliative care

Child health practitioners must always act in the best interests of the child. When it is not possible or appropriate to save the child's life or restore optimal health, the central purpose of care shifts from curative to palliative care. While this may (or may not) imply withholding or stopping curative care, palliative care is not limited to end of life care. Nor is it 'passive' care: pursue the goals of palliative care as actively as you do the goals of curative care.

Figure 22.1 A model of modern integrated palliative care services

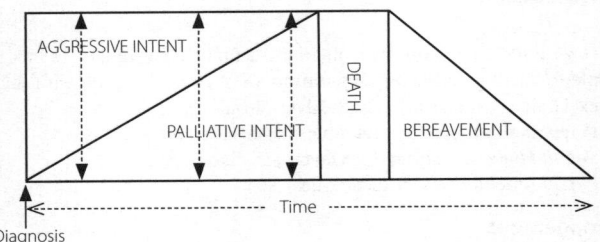

Definition

According to the World Health Organization (WHO) palliative care:
- Incorporates the active total care of the child's body, mind and spirit and support for the family
- Begins when illness is diagnosed
- Alleviates a child's physical, psychological, and social distress
- Requires a broad multidisciplinary approach (includes family and community resources)
- Can be provided anywhere.

Good decisions about palliative care

Basic requirements for good decisions about palliative care involve:
- Good up-to-date information, clearly recorded in the patient's notes:
  - Clinical information to minimize uncertainty about the diagnosis and prognosis
  - Information about the patient's family and their social, cultural and religious networks.
- Good, open communication:
  - Between colleagues, within the team, with the child and family.
- Continuity of care. Keep membership of the team constant.

Palliative care as the main goal

It is sometimes difficult to know whether it is appropriate to withhold or withdraw life saving care. In other words, to recognize when the main goal shifts to palliative care. The difficulty is compounded when the following are present:
- Clinical uncertainty about the diagnosis and prognosis
- Different views within the team about which options are in the child's best interests
- Disagreement with the parents (or among family).

When may life-saving care reasonably be withheld or withdrawn?

The Royal College of Paediatrics and Child Health (United Kingdom) established 5 situations in which it may be acceptable to withdraw or withhold life-saving care.

1. The brain dead child. Brain death must be diagnosed by 2 experienced doctors according to accepted criteria. A child who is brain dead is clinically dead.
2. The permanent vegetative state. Following a severe insult to the brain the child is permanently incapable of any meaningful relations with the outside world. A permanent vegetative state exists when the patient has been in a persistent vegetative state for longer than 1 year. Exclude a 'locked-in' state or severe paralytic disease.
3. The 'no chance' situation. The child is severely ill and not responding to optimal therapy. Continuing treatment is futile; it prolongs suffering.
4. The 'no purpose' situation. The child may survive with appropriate treatment, but will be left with severe physical or mental impairment and an unbearable quality of life.
5. The 'unbearable' situation. The child and family feel that in the face

of progressive and irreversible illness further treatment would be unbearable. They want a particular treatment withdrawn or refuse further treatment irrespective of the medical opinion.

> ***Practice point:***
>
> Dealing with uncertainty
>
> Uncertainty about the prognosis is often present and legitimate. It is then necessary to continue life saving care together with palliative care. The patient's response to treatment will bring more clarity. Always involve trusted and experienced professional colleagues in clinical assessments about prognosis and therapeutic options. Hospital ethics teams, if available, can be useful. The following is a useful 'ethics' check:
>
> A decision is morally acceptable if it complies with 5 characteristics (ideal observer theory):
> - Omniscience: the decision has included all the readily available and relevant facts
> - Omnipercipience: the decision has empathetically taken into account the feelings of all of those involved
> - Disinterest: the decision is not based on vested interests
> - Dispassion: the decision is not made under conditions in which emotions obscure critical thinking
> - Consistency: similar cases are decided similarly.

Good practice in making palliative care plans

A good palliative care plan meets the specific and detailed needs of an individual patient.

Pay careful attention to detail. Use all available knowledge of the patient to anticipate problems and questions that may arise. Formulate an active plan for each.

Essential issues to consider for active management:
- Cardio-pulmonary resuscitation (CPR). Would it serve the child's best interests? Where CPR is not appropriate, clear instructions such as 'do not give CPR' and 'do not intubate' are better than simple 'do not resuscitate' orders. An 'allow natural death' order (the abbreviation 'AND' may be more suitable on the ward notes) may be useful.
- Control of pain and discomfort (especially dyspnoea: a horrible, undertreated symptom)

- Psychosocial needs. Include the family and community resources and networks available to the child and family.
- Nutrition. What are the nutritional needs of the child and what level of intervention (or inaction) is needed or justified? Dying children are generally overfed and over-dripped at the end of life because doctors feel supplying these are essential and nurses struggle not to feed 3 hourly. In the face of gastroparesis, which occurs at the end of life, continued regular feeds can cause gastric distension and abdominal discomfort. The advantages of decreasing and eventually stopping feeds are less gastric discomfort, fewer secretions and induction of ketosis, which has analgesic properties in itself and leads to the release of endorphins.
- Hydration. Is he or she at risk of dehydration and what intervention is needed/justified? Over-hydration at the end of life can increase respiratory secretions and cause cerebral oedema, which aggravates pain and dyspnoea.
- Oxygen. Is there risk of hypoxia and is monitoring required/justified? Supplemental oxygen has been shown not always to be of benefit at the end of life even with hypoxia. Treat the patient not the sats machine. Treat dyspnoea with low dose morphine (one-third to one-half of the pain dose).
- Blood tests. Will these affect management?
- Blood products. Will a transfusion benefit the child in this situation? Treat the patient not the Hb and the platelet count (or the gallop!).
- Antimicrobials. When to give? What are the implications? Will giving them simply defer the same decision to withhold later?
- Appropriate airway management. Should the child be referred for intensive care (if available)? Even in children who would not be considered good ICU candidates sometimes where acute reversible airway obstruction is causing considerable distress and anxiety that cannot be quickly relieved by symptom control drugs (morphine or benzodiazepines), short term intubation (maybe to buy time for steroids to work for example) may be indicated.

Most of these questions apply to all patients, but extraordinary measures are needed in palliative care. Consider each issue in turn as a team. Encourage everyone to state their views and take them seriously. Aim for consensus. Weigh benefits against burdens *and* the dictum that 'good palliative care neither hastens nor postpones death'.

Communicating decisions

Inadequate communication destroys good palliative care. A multidisciplinary 'round table' discussion may help the team gain deeper insight into the patient's situation.

Record the discussion and who was present. Write notes and orders clearly in the appropriate place, sign them legibly, and date them. Meet again to review. Palliative care plans may be changed.

Talking with the family

Parents should always participate in the care and decision-making. They need the best available information to understand the child's condition, the prognosis, and the available therapeutic options. Avoid jargon. Communicate simply and in mother tongue. They need sufficient time on their own to discuss the issues to their satisfaction. Be available to help. They also need to ask questions and voice problems.

A senior doctor, with a senior member of the nursing team and the social worker, should meet the parents as often as necessary. Speak frankly, openly and honestly. Be sensitive to verbal and non-verbal clues to distressing thoughts or feelings. Check what they already know and how much more they would like to know. Give a 'warning' before you break bad news. Don't be scared of silences, lulls in conversation or emotional outbursts. Families may need these to assimilate what they have been told. Involve extended family and friends.

Talking with the child

As small children grow older they steadily develop the capacity to understand, express themselves and decide on their care. Such children are said to be *competent*.
- Inform and educate children about their condition but let them guide you in how much they want to know and what concerns them.
- Communicate appropriately for their age.
- Listen carefully to their views and opinions.
- Answer questions gently, frankly and honestly.
- Allow them the capacity to make their own decisions.

Practical management of pain in children

Historically, pain in children has been poorly managed. Neonates, infants, and children feel and remember pain, and suffer because of this. The neuro-hormonal effects of pain can be attenuated or ablated by timely and adequate treatment, which will improve surgical outcome and reduce hospital stay. Repeated procedures produce local hyperalgesia, and long-term alterations in behavioural responses to pain have been reported in ex-neonatal ICU infants. The ability to feel pain is a protective mechanism to avoid injury, but pathological pain requires treatment. Anxiety in children significantly aggravates pain, and this is of particular relevance when performing procedures.

Assessment and measurement of pain

Especially in the pre- or non-verbal child, recognizing and assessing pain in children is notoriously difficult. It is important to be aware of the normal behaviour and physiological parameters for various age groups.

Physiological parameters are the most frequently used for non-verbal children, those on ventilators, and those who are mentally challenged. Increases in heart rate, blood pressure, and sweating will reflect painful sensations. Adaptation in chronic pain however may mask physiological manifestations.

Behavioural features may include grimacing, crying, screaming, and physical withdrawal, but other indicators may be anorexia, sleep disturbances, retrogressive behaviour, inattention, and a reluctance to play. The FLACC scale, which uses a combination of behavioural responses, is a useful tool in the non-verbal child.

Visual analogue scales are commonly used as pain rating scales in the older age groups but are not successful in younger children, those with minimal education, and those with a different interpretation of the conventional understanding of the scale. Caution should be used when using the Wong Baker Faces Scale, as the pain face may be interpreted as a sad face. The Revised Faces Scale may be better.

Parental interviews are vital in assessing a child's pain, as their knowledge of their child's pain responses will complement the treatment plan.

A tactile and visual scale is an important recognition that watching and touching the child (the body language) will give the health professional a very good indication of pain and discomfort being experienced.

> ***Practice points:***
>
> - Clinical examination and simple measures (hugs, comfort, dummies, food) will differentiate pain from separational anxiety, sleep deprivation, hunger, or hypoglycaemia.
> - It may take as little as the documentation of 'Is the child in pain – yes or no' to draw attention to the problem and improve quality of care. The presence or absence of pain should be regarded as the fifth vital sign in observations of children.

Principles of treatment

- Communicate with the child and his/her parents. Discuss the planned procedure and clarify the roles of the patient and parents.
- Provide a safe environment for the sedated child, both before and after the procedure. Prevent pain when it is predictable (pre-emptive analgesia), and allay anxiety.
- Dose of analgesic should be calculated per kilogram of body weight.
- Postoperative pain, in general, is treated better than pain during procedures for medical interventions.
- Children who have needle or mask phobias may benefit from psychotherapy and by learning coping skills.
- Neonates, both premature and full term, feel and appreciate painful stimuli, and should be treated accordingly. Management of procedural pain in neonatal ICUs worldwide is still problematic, although postoperative pain control in this group is improving.
- Local anaesthetics should be used whenever possible.

Procedural pain

- Procedures may vary from simple application of dressings to insertion of intercostal drains. There are also those procedures that require a quiet still child, where there is minimal pain, compared with those where there is considerable discomfort. Regardless of what is to be done, the same principles should apply.
- Aim for a child free of pain and discomfort, not anxious, and in a safe environment.
- The progression from mild sedation or analgesia to general anaesthesia is not easily divisible into discrete stages, and practitioners who use drugs with respiratory and haemodynamic consequences must be able to rescue their patient from these events.
- Drugs preferred for procedures are short-acting, with rapid onset and off-set.
- However, most of these agents are more potent than the longer-acting drugs commonly available in South Africa at present and practitioners using them must be experienced in resuscitation and airway management. A state of 'conscious sedation' is virtually impossible to achieve in younger children, and even if achieved, may be disorientating and frightening.
- Vascular access is not mandatory when oral, nasal, rectal or intramuscular drugs are administered. However, when repeated administration is necessary or intravenous drugs are used, intravenous access is preferred. If intravenous access is not achieved, an

experienced person, and all the necessary equipment should be immediately at hand.

Pain management of the ill child

The ill child with pyrexia, a headache, otitis media, tonsillitis and pharyngitis, stomach cramps with vomiting and diarrhoea, may all benefit from some form of analgesia and/or antispasmodic. When children present for their immunizations, pre-emptive paracetamol and topical Emla® 1 hour before the procedure may be very beneficial. When children undergo lumbar puncture, an anti-inflammatory, with paracetamol, and local anaesthetic prior to the event is very successful. Non-steroidal anti-inflammatories (NSAIDs) should be used with caution in the dehydrated, hypovolaemic child who is not passing urine, as renal damage may occur.

Management of the trauma/postoperative child

- Pre-emptive, balanced analgesia is optimal. In the trauma child, prior to doing a procedure, an anxiolytic with the analgesia and sedation may be advantageous. Topical agents in the form of Emla®, lignocaine + adrenaline + cocaine (LAC), tetracaine + adrenaline + cocaine (TAC), ice (beware of hypothermia), and melaleuca hydrogel (Burnshield®) may be used, as well as providing oral or intravenous supplementary medication.
- Nerve and regional blocks for acute injury and postoperative management are very effective and are becoming increasingly popular, but do require special expertise.
- Commonly used opioids include tilidine HCl (Valoron®), morphine, tramadol and codeine (only oral use in South Africa). Codeine is becoming increasingly unpopular as it has a very wide bio-availability and up to 30% of people in some studies may not have the necessary enzyme to metabolize it to morphine, which is its active metabolite. Some experts are suggesting we use low dose morphine instead of codeine for this reason. Co-administration of paracetamol may facilitate a reduced dose of opioid. Pethidine should not be used as regular medication for longer than 24 hours because of the accumulation of metabolic products (nor-meperidine) which causes convulsions.
- Avoid IMI injections where possible in children.

Drug therapies

- Decide what is required for the child: analgesia, sedation, anxiolysis and/or amnesia. The choice of agents will depend on what is being done, by whom, when and where.

- The choice of drug should be the right drug, at the right time, with the right dose, for the right reasons, and via the right route for the right patient.
- Start with simple analgesics, and work up toward multimodal balanced analgesia. The WHO Step Ladder approach is useful, with the additional option of an anxiolytic when it is necessary.
- Local anaesthesia should be used whenever possible.
- Mild pain: paracetamol, NSAIDs
- Moderate pain: paracetamol, NSAIDs, codeine
- Severe and postoperative pain: strong opioids, e.g. morphine, plus paracetamol and/or NSAIDs, especially in protracted pain or neuropathic pain, adjuncts (α_2-agonists, e.g. clonidine, antidepressants, anticonvulsants, anxiolytics) are often very useful.

What to look for in preparations

- Ease of dosage: mg/ml/dose
- Formulation: syrup, suspension or suppository versus tablet or capsule
- Registration of the drug in South Africa, for age limits and indications
- Taste: compliance, method of administration
- Alcohol and sugar content
- Preservative and colorants: some drugs, e.g. Vallergan Forte®, still contain tartrazine.
- Safety: caps, toxicity.

Treatment modalities

Pharmacological

Opioids have been used for paediatric pain for many years, and their side effects, especially respiratory depression, have made clinicians cautious about using any of them for pain in children. However, much research has been published, clarifying the preferred drugs and their dosage regimes necessary in infants and children.

Drugs commonly used in South African children today include the following:
- Opioids:
  - Morphine
  - Tilidine HCl
  - Codeine
  - Fentanyl
- Non-opioid analgesics:
  - Paracetamol is a good analgesic and antipyretic but has poor

anti-inflammatory activity. Intravenous paracetamol, Perfalgan®, is available for those children in whom the oral or rectal route cannot/should not be used.
— NSAIDs: diclofenac, ibuprofen, mefanamic acid. Although this group of drugs is not recommended for children under 1 year, or < 10 kg, it has been used successfully and safely in this group. Avoid in asthmatics, those with a bleeding disorder, gastric irritation, and (actual or anticipated) poor renal function.
- Clonidine has the advantage of moderate sedation, anxiolysis, and analgesia.
- Anxiolytics:
  — Benzodiazepines: midazolam, lorazepam, diazepam.
  — Clonidine
  — Hydroxyzine.
- Anaesthetic agents:
  — Ketamine has a dose-dependent effect ranging from mild analgesia at low dose to general anaesthesia at high doses. The effects also depend on the route of administration: immediate effect with intravenous and slower onset with oral or rectal.
- Sedatives with no analgesic effects:
  — Trimeprazine (Vallergan®) in some preparations has tartrazine, so do not administer in tartrazine-sensitive children.
  — Promethazine (Phenergan®) has good antihistamine effects. It is not recommended for use in children under 2 years of age.

Non-pharmacological

- Complementary modalities such as reflexology, aromatherapy, and massage have been proven to have significant benefits in ill children. Caution should be shown with the use of herbal preparations, as many of these agents taken via the enteral route have anti-platelet activity.
- The use of oral sucrose, preferably with a dummy, in young infants provides good analgesia for simple procedures. Breastfeeding provides the same advantages during venesection and drip insertion.
- Virtual reality has shown increasing popularity in providing distraction for change of dressing procedures in burned children.
- Transcutaneous electrical nerve stimulation, acupuncture and hypnosis have a limited use in younger children.

Weaning from opioids and benzodiazepines

When children have been on opioids and benzodiazepines for longer than 1 week, a planned wean from these drugs is essential to avoid the possibility of withdrawal symptoms. The period for weaning is directly proportional to the length of time of drug administration. A quick wean involves reducing the daily dose by 30% per day (i.e a 3-day wean). When the exposure has been for a long period (e.g. 1 month), weaning should be 7–10% reduction of the daily dose per day. Alternatively, the drug may be changed to a longer-acting one (e.g. methadone instead of morphine), and then the weaning process continued.

Conclusion

'Pain is soul-destroying. No patient should have to endure intense pain unnecessarily. The quality of mercy is essential to the practice of medicine. Here of all places it should not be strained.' These words encompass our collective responsibility as medical practitioners in treating our children with responsibility, care, and compassion.

List of drugs

Clonidine	1–6 mcg/kg/dose PO 8–12-hourly 3–5 mcg/kg/dose 2.5 mcg/kg/dose for premed single dose
Diclofenac	1 mg/kg/dose 8–12-hourly PO, PR. 1–3 mg/kg/day
Fentanyl	1–3 mcg/kg/dose IVI stat Infusion: 1–5 mcg/kg/hr in theatre or ICU
Flumazenil (Anexate®)	5 mcg kg IVI every 60 secs to maximum total 40 mcg/kg (max 2 mg) Infusion: 2–10 mcg/kg/hr
Indomethacin	0.5–1 mg/kg/dose 8-hourly po, pr
Ketamine	IVI: sedation+analgesia: 0.25–0.5 mg/kg/dose 　　　anaesthesia: bolus: 1–2 mg/kg/dose 　　　Infusion: 10–20 mcg/kg/min 　　　　　　　　1–4 mg/kg/hour IMI: sedation+analgesia: 2–4 mg/kg/dose 　　　anaesthesia: 7–10 mg/kg/dose PO: sedation+analgesia: 2–6 mg/kg/dose 　　　anaesthesia: 10 mg/kg/dose
Ketoprofen	1–2 mg/kg dose 6–12-hourly PO, IVI, IMI, PR
Ketorolac	Oral: 0.2 mg/kg/dose (max 10 mg) (max 0.8 mg/kg/day)
Lorazepam	0.02–0.06 mg/kg/dose 8–24-hourly PO　　0.05–0.2 mg/kg/dose slow IVI Infusion: 0.01–0.1 mg/kg/hour

Mefanamic acid	10 mg/kg/dose PO 8-hourly		
Methadone	0.1–0.2 mg/kg/dose 6–12-hourly PO, SC, IMI		
Midazolam	Sedation:	PO:	0.25–0.5 mg/kg/dose
		IVI:	0.1 mg/kg/dose
		IMI:	0.1 mg/kg/dose
		intranasal:	0.2 mg/kg/dose
	infusion:	0.1–0.2 mg/kg/hr	
	Anticonvulsant: 0.2 mg/kg/dose IVI		
Morphine	IVI:	0.1 mg/kg/dose 4–6 hourly	
	IMI:	0.2 mg/kg/dose 4–6 hourly	
	PO:	0.3–0.4 mg/kg/dose 4–6 hourly	
	Infusion:	5–40 mcg/kg/hour. Draw up 0.5 mg/kg of morphine sulphate in 50 ml normal saline. Run and 0.5–4 ml/hour, which will deliver 5–40 mcg/kg/hour. (1 ml = 10 mcg/kg morphine)	
	PCA:	20 mcg/kg bolus with 5 minute lock-out time. If a background infusion is used, the dose for this is 5 mcg/kg/hour.	
	Slow-release morphine: 0.6 mg/kg/dose 12-hourly, increasing every 48 hrs if required.		
Naloxone	For opioid overdose: 0.1 mg/kg/dose (max 2mg) IVI, IMI, SC, intratracheal.		
	Infusion: 0.01 mg/kg/hour		
Pethidine	IVI: 0.5–1 mg/kg/dose		
	IMI: 0.5–2 mg/kg dose		
Tilidine HCl (Valoron® drops)	1 mg/kg/dose 6 hourly. For the dose in drops, take the child's body weight in kg and divide by 2.5. (Each drop contains 2.5 mg of Valoron®)		

Recommended reading

1. Amery, J. *Children's Palliative Care in Africa*. 1st edition. Oxford University Press. 2009.
2. Anand KJS, Johnston CC, Oberlander TF, Taddio A, Lehr VT, Walco GA. Analgesia and Local Anaesthesia during Invasive Procedures in the Neonate. *Clin Ther*. 2005; 27.
3. Cooper P. *Ethical issues in child health*. In: *Child Health for All*. 4th edition, pp 490–495. Oxford University Press. South Africa. 2007.
4. Ducharme C, Carnevale FA, Clermont M-S, Shea S. A prospective study of adverse reactions to the weaning of opioids and benzodiazepines among critically ill children. *Intensive Crit Care Nurs*. 2005. 21:179–186.
5. Finley GA. Pharmacological Management of Procedure Pain. Chapter 4. *Acute and Procedure Pain in Infants and Children*. Finley and McGrath. 2001.
6. Goldman A, Hain R, Liben S. *Oxford Textbook of Palliative Care for Children*. 1st edition, Oxford University Press. 2006.

7 Jassal et al. *Basic symptom control in paediatric palliative care*. The Rainbow Children's Hospice Guidelines. 7th edition 2008. Available www.rainbows.co.uk
8 Krauss B, Green SM. Sedation and Analgesia for Procedures in Children. *New Eng J. Med.* 342: 938–945. March 2000.
9 Reynolds L. *Consent and competence in paediatrics*. Ibid. pp. 503–507.
10 Roux P. *Death, dying and palliative care*. Ibid. pp 496–502.
11 Thomas J, Rode H. *Practical Management of Paediatric Burns*. SAMA Health and Medical Publishing Group. Cape Town, South Africa. 2006.
12 Thomas J. Pain Management. *Handbook of Paediatrics for Developing Countries*. 6th edition. Oxford (Southern Africa). Editor Vincent Harrison. 2005.
13 *Withholding or Withdrawing Life Sustaining Treatment in Children: A Framework for Practice*. Second edition. Royal College of Paediatrics and Child Health 2004. Available on-line at: http//www.repch.ac.uk/Publications-list-by-title
14 Wong D. *Pain assessment in children*. Pediatric pain management and Sedation Handbook. Yaster, Crane et al. Moseby. 1997.

23 Procedures

J. Karpelowsky

Successful procedures depend on adequate preparation. Time taken to ensure the appropriate size equipment, adequate securing devices, and staff to aid in restraint of the child where appropriate cannot be over emphasised. This is stressed throughout the chapter, which describes a variety of useful methods. Because analgesia and sedation are critical issues pertinent to most of these procedures please also read Chapter 22, Palliative care and pain management for more information.

General principles
- Use as few procedures as possible to obtain the required information.
- Discuss indications, possible failure and risks with parents and patient.
- Reassure and comfort the child before, during and after the event.
- Use appropriate analgesia and sedation (see Chapter 22, Palliative care and pain management).
- Ensure sterility of the procedure.
- Wear adequate barrier protection and use sharps containers to prevent transmission of communicable diseases

Restraint
Often needed; however, appropriate sedation, analgesia, or anaesthesia may minimize the need for these. Methods depend on the age and cooperation of the child as well as the proposed undertaking. They include:
- Wrapping the body in a sheet
- Holding the child in the optimum position (e.g. by an experienced nurse for lumbar puncture)
- Splinting a limb
- Restraining an arm or leg to the bed with tie-downs.

A successful outcome can be assured only if attention is given to optimum restraint, adequate exposure, good lighting, operator comfort and effective analgesia and sedation.

Abdominal paracentesis (e.g. ascitic tap)

- Ensure the bladder is empty.
- Position the child supine, with the upper body slightly raised and rotated by about 30 degrees to the left or right.
- Puncture sites would be on the dependant side in the lower quadrants approximately one quarter to one third of the way from the anterior superior iliac spine to the umbilicus (Figure 23.1).
- Anaesthetize the skin. Insert an IV cannula into this site and push it into the abdominal cavity by making a 1 cm wide Z-track through the subcutaneous tissue. This minimizes the risk of subsequent leakage.
- Watch for a flash back of fluid and when achieved withdraw the needle into the cannula prior to inserting it further.
- Aspirate the required amount of fluid and withdraw the needle.

Figure 23.1 Sites for abdominal paracentesis

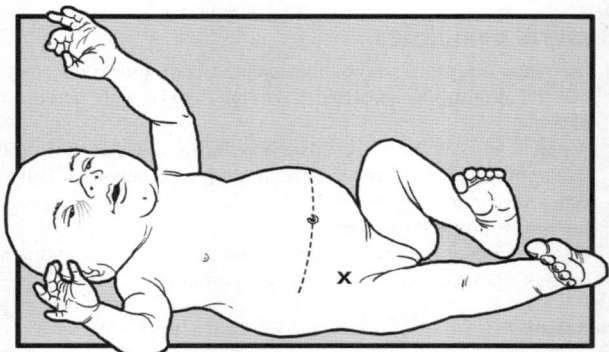

Dangers

- Intestinal perforation
- Bladder perforation
- Shock and syncope if too large a volume (> 1 l) is removed rapidly.
- Infection and peritonitis (ascitic fluid is an ideal culture medium).

Blood collection

Before taking blood ensure that:
- You have decided on the tests to be done.

- The correct tubes are available.
- The amount to be taken is known.
- The laboratory has been consulted about special tests.
- The correctly labelled specimen reaches the laboratory in the required time.

Venipuncture

Common sites: antecubital fossa, external jugular, dorsum of hand or foot and scalp veins.
Less common and more hazardous sites: internal jugular and femoral veins.

External jugular

- The vein lies superficially in the line from the angle of mandible to mid-clavicle (Figure 23.2). Place the restrained infant supine on a table with the head and neck extended, by placing a support under the child's shoulders, and turned 45–60° from the midline to expose the vein. It is easily seen, especially during crying. This site should be avoided in children with a bleeding diasthesis.

Figure 23.2 Vascular anatomy of the neck

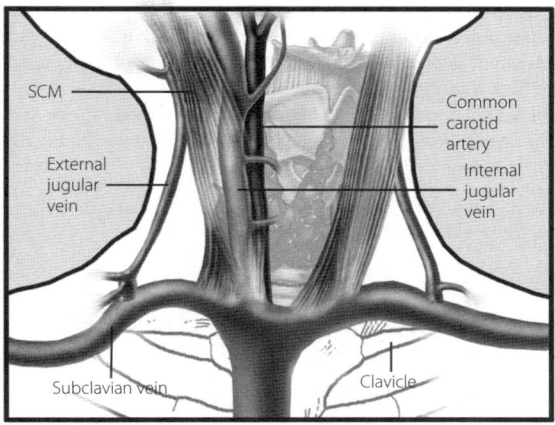

SCM – sternocleidomastoid muscle

> ***Practice point:***
>
> Dangers of using the external jugular:
> - Causes fear and distress-should be used as a last resort
> - Damage to other structures (see 'internal jugular')
> - Impairment of the airway and of respiration
> - Local haematoma (if not compressed after the procedure, especially in a crying child). Do not perform if there is a coagulopathy.

Femoral vein

- Use this only when other sites are inaccessible. The vein is situated below the inguinal ligament and medial to the artery (Figure 23.3). Just below the inguinal ligament, the relationship of structures from medial to lateral is vein, artery, nerve.
- Place the restrained infant on a table. An assistant at the infant's head holds the legs firmly with the knees and hips abducted and externally rotated.
- The femoral artery is palpable just below the inguinal ligament and the vein lies medial to the pulsation. Angle the needle at 30° to the surface, point towards the umbilicus and insert it (with suction applied) through the skin at a point a few millimetres medial to the arterial pulsation and just below the inguinal ligament. Advance it until blood is obtained. Withdraw the needle and apply local pressure for 5 minutes.
- If the artery is inadvertently penetrated, take blood rapidly and withdraw needle. Potential harm has already been done. Apply pressure to the site for at least 5 minutes.

> ***Practice point:***
>
> Danger of using the femoral vein:
> - Local infection, e.g. osteomyelitis of femoral head or septic arthritis
> - Arterial spasm may occasionally lead to gangrene
> - Haematoma: venous or arterial leakage especially in coagulopathic patients
> - Arteriovenous fistulae and femoral nerve damage
> - Pulmonary embolus.

Figure 23.3 Anatomy of the femoral triangle

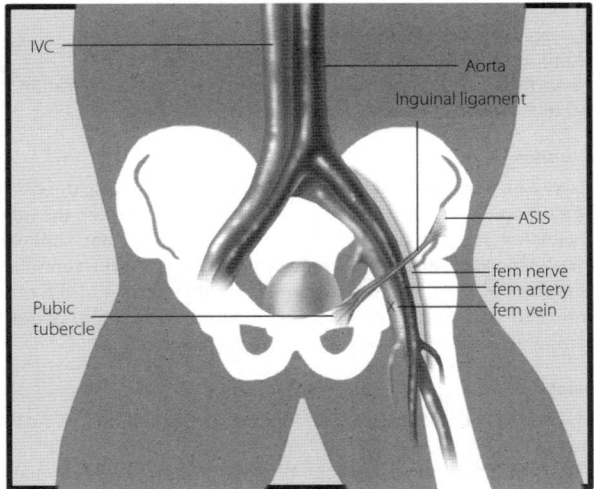

IVC – Inferior vena cava
ASIS – Anterior superior iliac spine
fem – Femoral
X – Marks the spot for puncture

Arterial puncture

- In infants the radial, dorsalis pedis, and posterior tibial arteries may be used. The radial artery is preferred because of the open palmar anastomosis with the ulnar artery so that arterio-spasm after puncture is unlikely to cause distal ischaemia.
- Provide analgesia, clean the area and palpate the artery with the tips of the index and third fingers. Insert a 25 gauge needle into the vessel between the fingertips at an angle of 45° to 60° towards the patient (the needle often penetrates both walls of the vessel).
- Apply suction and withdraw slowly. As the needle re-enters the artery, blood is obtained.
- Withdraw the needle and compress the site for 5 minutes.

Intravenous (IV) line placement

Indications
- Emergency resuscitation and rehydration
- Continuous IV fluids or alimentation solutions
- Intermittent antibiotic therapy or blood product administration
- Administration of other IV pharmaceutical products.

Venous sites
- *Limb veins:* suitable ones are found in the cubital fossa, the dorsum of a foot or hand, the inner forearm or wrist and between the medial malleolus and the anterior tibial tendon (the greater saphenous vein). If possible avoid joints as movement may kink the cannula.
- *Scalp veins:* suitable ones are situated at the hairline of the central forehead and posterior, above or anterior to the ears. Avoid the temporal artery. It can be identified by its pulsations.

Preparation
- Placement requires optimal conditions (p. 521) so do not rush the procedure.
- Ensure that the appropriate administration sets have been connected and filled with the correct IV fluid and appropriate size cannulae are available.
- Strapping must be precut and at hand, and splints or restraining devices must be readily available. Scalp hair may need to be shaved. Remove hair only from the selected site and take care not to nick the skin. Where possible obtain permission from parents beforehand.
- Try to wait until 2 people are available, 1 for restraint, as it is frustrating to achieve venous access and then lose it due to movement of the child.

> ### *Practice point:*
>
> - Promoting venous distension – the basic principle is to obstruct venous flow but not arterial flow:
> - *Scalp veins*: place an elastic band around the head above the eyebrows.
> - *Peripheral veins*: ensure that the limb has been adequately pre-warmed and have an assistant compress the limb lightly above the selected site. One pitfall often seen is too tight a compression around the limb.

Placement of needle or catheter

- Over-the-needle catheters are more suitable. Ideally scalp vein/butterfly needles should not be used. *Sizes*: newborn and infants 24 gauge, others: 22 gauge.
- Clean the site and insert the catheter through the skin directly into the vein. Flow-back of blood can be seen and the distended vein usually collapses. Advance the cannula over the needle into the vein and attach the drip tubing, if good flow occurs, immobilize it with strapping. Set the flow to the selected rate. Further immobilization or splinting may be needed to ensure the drip's survival.

Intraosseous route (under 6 years of age)

- In an emergency, e.g. shock, attempt IV access but only 1–2 attempts; use the intraosseous route early. Do not waste time with several failed attempts in a shocked patient. Early use of an intraosseous line in a shocked patient can be life saving.
- The most suitable site is 1–2 cm below the tibial tuberosity on the medial flat aspect of the tibia (Figure 23.4). Ideally an intraosseous needle should be used. If that is not available then a needle with a stylet such as a lumbar puncture or marrow puncture needle should be used. The wide bore needle (15–18 gauge) is an absolute last resort.
- Hold the needle perpendicular to the skin and advance to the bone, then with a twisting movement push it into the flat part of the tibia until a 'give' is felt; the needle is now in the bone marrow. Do not advance it further.
- Fluid must be introduced under pressure (use a 20 ml syringe attached via a 3-way tap to the IV tubing as a 'push-in' or a sphygmomanometer cuff wrapped around a collapsible IV plastic fluid container). Fluid tends not to run in spontaneously and must be syringed in.
- Observe carefully for extravasation.
- The dosage and volume of drugs and fluid are the same as for direct IV infusion. Any drug or fluid can be given via the intraosseous route.
- Secure the needle so that the site is visible and circumferential dressings are avoided. Useful to add a connector.

Figure 23.4 Site of intraosseous infusion

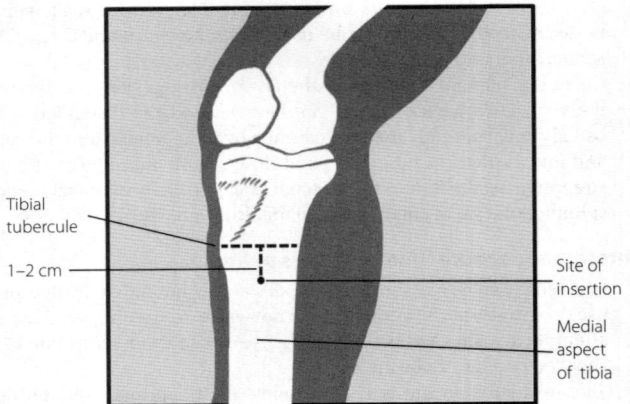

Cut-down technique

- The best site is the great saphenous vein which runs anterior to the medial malleolus and halfway between it and the anterior tibial tendon. Other sites are the basilic vein (ulnar side) or cephalic vein (radial side) in the antecubital fossa.
- Restrain the child and clean, drape and anaesthetize the area.
- Apply a tourniquet tightly enough to occlude venous return below the knee.
- Make a transverse incision (Figure 23.5). Blunt dissect with a curved mosquito haemostat parallel to the vessel towards the tibia.
- Identify the vein and free it with further blunt dissection.
- Place a haemostat beneath the vessel and pull through two 5.0 silk suture stays. Do not tie. The vein is held taut by the distal guide suture.
- A small lateral venotomy or v-shaped incision in the vessel wall should be created. Insert a short bevelled catheter tip of suitable size into the vessel and advance it for 5–8 cm.
- Tie the proximal suture around the vein and catheter. Leave elongated ends for ease of removal later. Remove the tourniquet and the distal guide suture.
- Apply local pressure to stop oozing of blood. Anchor the catheter firmly to the skin and close the incision on each side of the catheter with 5.0 sutures.
- Place folded gauze over the incision and strap it lightly. Use the same technique for the antecubital fossa.

Figure 23.5 Method for great saphenous cut-down

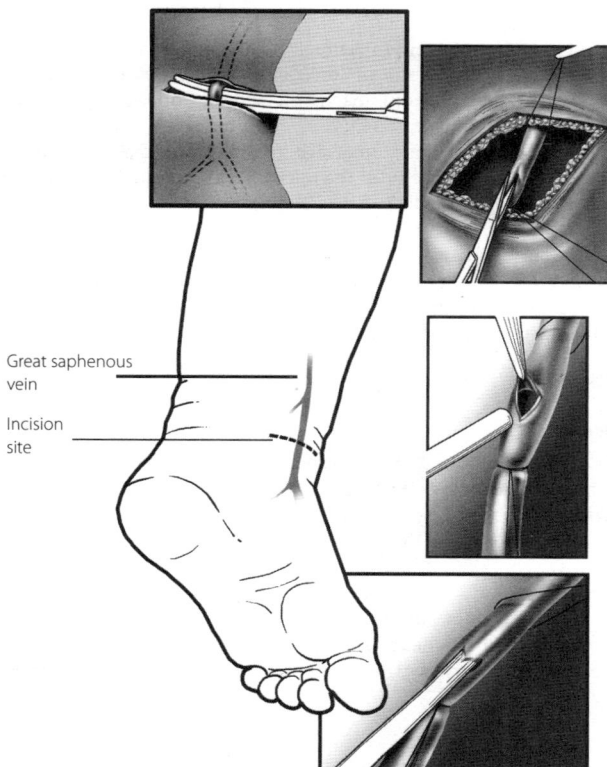

Injections

- Body weight and muscular development rather than age determine the volume to be injected:
  - < 2.5 kg – 5 kg: maximum 0.5 ml/site
  - 5 kg–10 kg: maximum 1.5 ml/site
  - > 10.0 kg: maximum 2.0 ml/site

- Consider the nature of the substance (e.g. iron dextran complex, Imferon®) and do not inject more than 1 ml per site in children under 3 years of age.
- Rotate sites if more than 1 injection is to be given.
- Record the time and site of injection. This applies especially to gentamicin, subcutaneous insulin in diabetes and subcutaneous adrenaline in asthmatic patients.
- Expel air from the syringe out of sight of the child and clean the area with alcohol. Insert needle at the appropriate site, pull back syringe plunger to ensure needle is not in a vessel, and inject smoothly and evenly.
- Give intramuscular injections, e.g. penicillin and Imferon®, deeply into the muscle to prevent abscess formation. To prevent staining of the skin with drugs such as Imferon®, the needle should follow a Z-track through the subcutaneous tissues.

Injection sites

Intradermal
- For example, Mantoux test for tuberculosis. Note angle and placement of the needle. A successful injection must raise a weal in the skin.
- *Site*: ventral surface of the left forearm.

Subcutaneous
- For example insulin, adrenaline. Note angle and placement of needle into the tissue just beneath the skin.
- *Sites*: limbs and trunk where loose tissue space under the skin is obvious.

Intramuscular
Should not be used in coagulopathic patients.

Vastus lateralis:
- This area of the thigh is generally the only permissible site for intramuscular injections in neonates and young infants. The injection should be given at the junction of the upper third and lower two-thirds of the thigh.
- *Never* use the antero-medial area, which contains vital structures such as the femoral vein, artery and nerve.
- Grasp the leg as shown (Figure 23.6) and insert the needle vertically into the compressed muscle of the mid-lateral anterior thigh.

Figure 23.6 Intramuscular injection: vastus lateralis

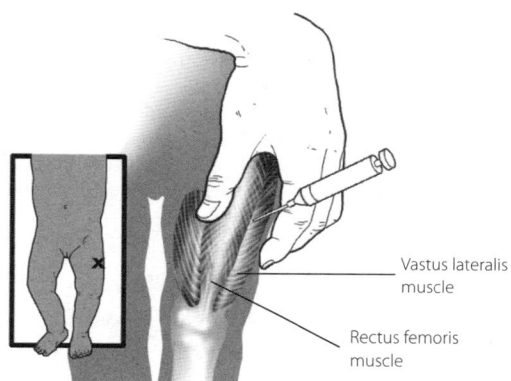

Posterior lateral gluteal:
- This area (upper and outer quadrant) is permissible for intramuscular injection *over* 6 years of age. The site is located by an imaginary line between the posterior superior iliac spine and the head of the greater trochanter (Figure 23.7). Insert the needle lateral to this line to avoid the sciatic nerve or superior gluteal artery and vein.

Figure 23.7 Intramuscular injection: posterolateral aspect of the gluteal area

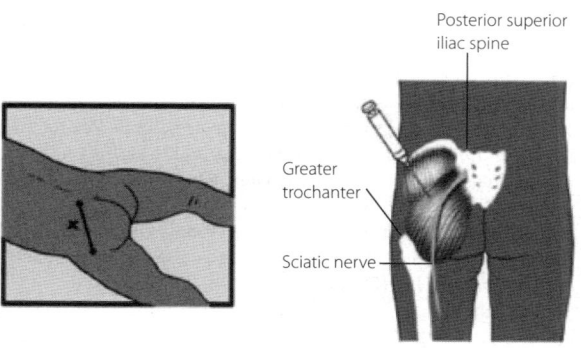

The mid-deltoid:
- This area in the lateral aspect of the upper arm (Figure 23.8) is generally used only for immunizations.
- It may be used in other instances if no other area is available (e.g. in burns).
- The volume should never exceed 1 ml and repeated injections and large quantities of medication are not recommended
- The injection site is identified by the acromion and the axilla as shown. Compress muscle mass prior to inserting needle.

Figure 23.8 Intramuscular injection: mid-deltoid area

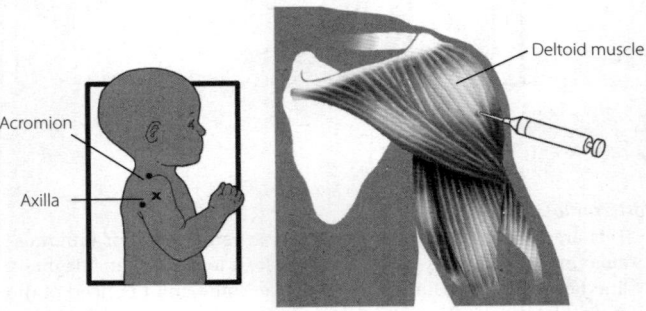

Lumbar puncture

Technique

- Proper positioning and restraint are critical for a successful tap.
- The lateral recumbent position is employed in older infants and children. The operator's line of vision should be on the same horizontal and vertical planes as the puncture site. The lumbar spine must be curved, but avoid pressure flexion of the neck while flexing the back. Hold the shoulders rather than the head and neck.
- Ensure that all items – needles, stylets, manometers, and tubes – are available.
- The site of the puncture is the interspace between L3–4 or L4–5. A line joining the highest points of the two iliac crests passes just above the fourth lumbar spine (Figure 23.9).
- After cleaning and anaesthetizing the skin and tissue down to the laminae, insert a short bevelled needle with stylet in the midline between L3 and L4. Maintain the bevel in the long axis of the dura

to part and not transect the fibres. Loss of resistance is felt as the needle penetrates the ligamentum flavum. The next 'pop' occurs as the needle penetrates the dura. Remove the stylet and if no fluid emerges, turn the needle through 90°. If the 'tap' is dry, replace the stylet and advance the needle a little further. Check again for fluid.

- The distance between the skin and subarachnoid space is 1.5–2.5 cm in infants, 5 cm in 3- to 5-year-olds, and 6–8 cm in adolescents. Measure the cerebrospinal fluid pressure with a manometer if the child is not crying or struggling. The normal pressure is 60–160 mm. If opening pressures are very high, seek neurosurgical advice

> ***Practice point:***
>
> Dangers:
> - Any indication of raised intracranial pressure, especially an *altered level of consciousness* is a *contraindication* to lumbar puncture. Absence of papilloedema is not a reliable sign of raised intracranial pressure.
> - Coning may occur immediately or a few hours later due to persistent leakage of spinal fluid.
> - Caution in the coagulopathic patient
> - Introduction of infection
> - Breakage of needle
> - Introduction of dermis resulting in a dermoid (non-styletted needle)
> - Nerve or cord damage.

Figure 23.9 Recumbent position for lumbar tap

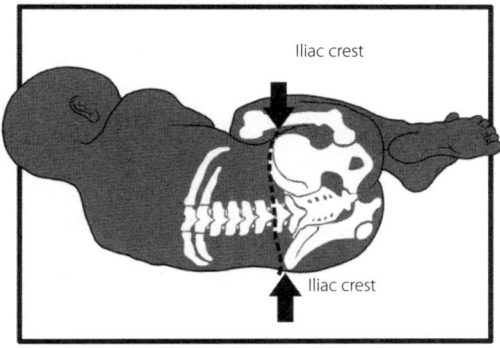

Nasogastric intubation

Indications
- Instil a feed, electrolyte solution or medications.
- Remove gastric contents (toxin/poison).
- Remove amniotic fluid in neonate.
- Remove excessive air, e.g. post-operative decompression.
- Obtain diagnostic material, e.g. to diagnose tuberculosis.

Technique
- Explain the procedure to an older child who should be sitting up. Place a young child or infant supine and have an assistant restrain the patient and flex the head slightly.
- Select the appropriate tube. Determine the length to be passed by measuring the distance from the ear lobe to the mid point between the umbilicus and xyphisternum. Mark the tube at the selected length.
- Lubricate the lower 3–4 cm of the tube with KY jelly or water and pass it through a nostril towards the occiput (not vertex). If resistance is encountered, withdraw the tube and try the other nostril. If still unsuccessful, have the child swallow vigorously (if old enough) and continue even if gagging occurs. Withdraw immediately if there is severe coughing, choking, or cyanosis.
- Introduce the selected length and fix the tube lightly to the cheek. Place the bell of your stethoscope over the umbilicus and inject air (5–10 ml) rapidly into the tube. A gurgling noise indicates that the tip is in the stomach or lower oesophagus. Strap the tube firmly to the upper lip and cheek.
- Alternatively aspirate the tube and test the contents with litmus (blue to pink indicates acid). If no fluid is obtained, advance the tube 3 cm and try again. If still unsuccessful and you are sure that the tube is in the stomach, inject 3 ml 0.9% saline. Withdraw tube if this causes coughing, spluttering or cyanosis.

> ***Practice point:***
>
> Dangers:
> - Vomiting with aspiration during the procedure
> - Ulceration or infection of nasal mucosa or epistaxis
> - Placement of the tube in tracheobronchial tree
> - Otitis media or sinusitis following prolonged use
> - Coiling or knotting of the tube so that it cannot be removed.

Pleural drainage

Emergency drainage
- This is indicated when a tension pneumothorax is suspected on clinical grounds in a hypoxaemic or shocked child.
- Clean the area and introduce a sterile IV cannula (16–20 gauge) perpendicularly into the second intercostal space in the mid clavicular line. A gush of air should be encountered releasing the tension pneumthorax, enabling elective drainage.

Elective drainage
- This is indicated to drain air or liquids from the pleural cavity in children who are not *in extremis*. Sedate and use local anaesthesia to skin and muscle. General anaesthesia may be preferable.
- Do not enter via the pectoral muscles, as bleeding and subsequent ugly scars are common. Make a 0.5–1 cm skin incision over the 4th or 5th intercostal space in the mid-axillary line. Dissect to the parietal pleura with a curved artery forceps over the top of the rib to avoid the neurovascular bundle. Close the forceps and holding it 3– 4 cm from the tip, push it through the pleura. Open the forceps to enlarge the hole and to release air. Insert a tube drain. Close the wound with a suture.
- *Never use a trochar.* Suitable tubes: neonate 10 French gauge (F); infant 10–14 F; child (two to eight years) 14–18 F
- Place 1 or 2 swabs loosely over it and retain them with thin plaster strips. Secure the tube with tape to the abdomen to prevent traction and dislodgement. Use an underwater seal if breathing is spontaneous. The tube should not be more than 1 cm below the water surface.

Fine needle aspiration biopsy

Basic guidelines

(Adapted from FNA Protocol formulated by Prof Colleen Wright, Anatomical Pathology, Stellenbosch University)

Consent

Parental written consent is essential for superficial and deep organ aspirates in paediatric patients.

Anaesthaesia

- No local anaesthetic required
- Sedation in children (oral sedation and paracetamol)
- Topical anaesthetic (Emla® cream) may be used
- Local anaesthetic for deep organ aspirates only (pleura, peritoneum).

Position

- If possible, lie the patient down
- Thyroid – pillow under shoulders to extend neck
- Small supraclavicular nodes – sitting
- If at all possible avoid aspirating from muscle, particularly sternocleidomastoid.

Equipment

(Liaise with your local histopathology laboratory.)

Needle	–	Older children – 23 g (blue)
		Small children, skin nodules – 26 g (brown)
Syringe	–	10 cc
Slides	–	Glass slides with *ground glass* edges: patient details (name, surname and folder number must be written in pencil on the frosted portion of the slides)
Fixative	–	Cytology fixative – *never* hairspray
TB culture medium	–	Bactec® bottles
		MGIT tube

Alcohol swab, small cotton wool ball

Procedure

- Always perform a minimum of 2 needle passes.
- Always use sterile needle and syringe for each pass.
- Each pass yields 2 slides:
  - 1 air dried for Diff Quik® stain (cytoplasmic)
  - 1 spray fixed for Papanicolaou stain (nuclear)
- Average aspirate should always yield 4 slides.
- Stabilize mass with 1 hand and introduce needle.
- Maintain 1–2 cc suction throughout aspirate.
- Aspirate using cutting motion until material appears in HUB of needle.
- Release suction before withdrawing needle.
- Place cotton wool on insertion site and ask assistant to apply pressure.

- Remove needle from syringe, introduce 5–10 cc air into syringe, re-attach needle and, holding needle onto syringe, use air to express material in needle onto glass slide.
- Touch needle tip on glass slide during above, 1 cm from frosted end.
- Place second slide parallel to first, and, maintaining gentle pressure, pull 2 slides apart.
- Spray fix bottom slide with fixative from distance of about 30 cm until wet.
- Repeat above procedure.

TB culture

Rinse needle and syringe in TB culture medium

Cysts

Always empty cyst – send *all* fluid to laboratory.

Bloody aspirates

If blood aspirated, remove needle, apply pressure for 1 minute, repeat aspirate using new needle and syringe. Try smaller needle. If still bloody, try aspirating using no suction at all.

If still bloody, consider vascular lesion, e.g. Kaposi's sarcoma, haemangioma.

Thoracentesis

- Locate the fluid by physical examination, percussion, X-ray or ultrasound where available.
- The site of the puncture is usually in the posterior axillary line at the base of the thorax. With loculated fluid the site of puncture is over the area of maximum dullness but ideally ultrasound location should be used. Clean the area and use a local anaesthetic.
- With the restrained patient in a sitting position, insert a needle into the pleural cavity just over the superior margin of the rib to avoid the intercostal vessels that course below the inferior margin of the rib above.
- Advance the needle while aspirating to confirm when the fluid has been reached. Withdraw the required volume of fluid. Remove the needle and apply a dressing. IV cannulas diminish the risk of lung laceration and may also be used.

> ***Practice point:***
>
> Dangers:
> - Pneumothorax from lung laceration
> - Pulmonary oedema from rapid withdrawal of too large a volume of fluid
> - Damage to the heart, liver, major blood vessels, air embolus
> - Introduction of infection
> - Syncope from the pleuro-pulmonary reflex.

Urine collection

Cleanse external genitalia with soap and water, and then dry with sterile swabs. Apply a disposable sterile plastic bag with a non-irritating adhesive over the penis or onto the perineum. Leave exposed and collect voided urine immediately. Bag samples are often contaminated. Negative cultures exclude a urinary tract infection. This method is widely used for obtaining routine specimens in infancy.

'Clean catch'

- This method can be used in children over 3 years of age. The glans (and foreskin if present) or perineum must be thoroughly cleaned with soap and water and/or dilute antiseptic and dried. A midstream catch is then collected during voiding with the foreskin drawn back or the labia held apart. Running water into the basin or wetting the lower abdomen may stimulate voiding.

Bladder catheterization

- This can introduce infection so the specimen *must* be important enough to warrant the procedure. Catheterization is done under sterile conditions with gloves, careful cleaning (see above). The foreskin should be drawn back. In infants the foreskin should be retracted just enough to enable visualization of the meatus but not fully retracted over the glans. In females the labia should be grasped and drawn towards the operator, exposing the urethra. Pass a lubricated thin catheter or an 8 F feeding tube into the urethral meatus and advance it gently until urine is obtained. Collect this in a sterile tube and withdraw the catheter. An indwelling catheter is hazardous.

Suprapubic aspiration

- This is indicated in a child under 2 years of age if urinalysis is urgent, the perineum is excoriated, or a previous culture was of doubtful significance.

- The full bladder extends into the abdomen and is therefore accessible. Change and feed the infant. After 30 minutes check whether the napkin is dry and the bladder full.
- The infant is laid supine and immobilized in a frog position by an assistant. The lower abdomen is cleaned. The aspiration site is located in the midline 1–2 cm above the symphysis pubis.
- Hold the needle and syringe 10–20° to the skin (pointing towards the pelvis). Insert the needle through the abdominal wall while gently aspirating the syringe. Bladder entry occurs after 1–2.5 cm of advancement.
- If no urine is obtained, repeat with a further 10–15° angulation, aiming into the pelvis. If unsuccessful, cease further attempts. When cleaning the abdomen, be prepared for a midstream 'catch' specimen, as urine is often voided at this stage.

> ***Practice point:***
>
> Dangers:
> - Introduction of infection
> - Local haematoma
> - Bowel perforation and peritonitis.

Endotracheal intubation

Choice of tube

- Apart from the moribund child who does not respond to any stimulus, appropriate anaesthesia should be used when performing endotracheal intubation.
- Always use drugs that you are familiar with.
- A combination of a hypnotic, e.g. ketamine, propofol or etomidate should be used with or without a paralysing agent.
- The lumen of the subglottis is roughly elliptical and is wider in the antero-posterior (AP) diameter. A round tube that fills the AP diameter will damage the mucosa laterally. Post-intubation croup and laryngeal strictures requiring long-term tracheostomy may result.
- Use Table 23.1 as a guide for tube choice. The table indicates the largest tube for initial intubation. In the absence of this table, choose a tube that is slightly smaller than the child's fifth (pinkie) finger. The length for nasal intubation is the length of a curved line from the top of the sternum to the external canthus of the eye and touching the pinna of the ear.

- In younger children an uncuffed tube may be adequate in providing an adequate seal. In children, however, when an uncuffed tube has too big an air leak, rather than using a tube that just fits through the vocal cords to minimise this leak, the use of a cuffed tube with low pressure insufflation would be preferable.

Oral intubation

- This is the preferred method for emergency intubation.
- Cricoid pressure should be applied by gently holding the cricoid cartilage (the cartilage just below the thyroid cartilage or Adam's apple) between thumb and index finger and pushing posteriorly.
- For per oral-laryngeal intubation, one needs to see the vocal cords in order to pass the endotracheal tube (ETT) into the larynx.
- Slightly extend the head. For a good view, use the largest laryngoscope blade that fits comfortably into the mouth (Mackintosh no. 3).
- Put the tip of the blade anterior to the epiglottis. Apply traction along the long axis of the handle to pull the base of the tongue anteriorly and bring the vocal cords into view.
- Common errors: overextension of the head and trying to look for the cords immediately; start by looking for the epiglottis.

Nasal intubation

- Should be used with caution in the coagulopathic patient as it may cause severe nose bleeds
- Is contraindicated in base of skull fractures
- Place the patient's head in the neutral position, facing directly forward
- Pass the ETT through the nose into the back of the throat
- Insert the laryngoscope into the mouth
- Identify the ETT and grasp it about 2 cm from its tip with a McGill forceps
- Pass the tip of the ETT along the posterior surface of the epiglottis into the trachea.

> ***Practice point:***
>
> Useful tip: gently push on the larynx in the following manner: Backwards; Upwards and to the Right; Push (BURP) in order to better visualize the vocal cords.

Precautions

Observe the following in order to avoid ETT-induced injuries:

- Use the smallest tube that suffices for breathing and the removal of secretions.
- Ensure that air leaks past the tube when the airway pressure is about 15 cm water (1.5 kPa). *Always record the tube size and whether or not a leak is present following intubation.* The leak may subsequently become sealed off by oedema or mucus. In this case the ETT need not be changed.
- Replace an occlusive-fitting ETT as soon as possible with a smaller one. Railroad the replacement: pass a long firm plastic introducer down the ETT until it sits within the trachea, then withdraw the tube over the introducer, taking care that the introducer does not pull out of the trachea. Re-intubate the child by passing the smaller ETT over the introducer. Keep the tip of the bevel on the inside of the curve of the introducer (i.e anterior), this ensures that the tip of bevel never projects and thus does not catch in the nose or larynx.
- Avoid tapered ETTs (Cole*, Enderby*) as they can be wedged too tightly in the larynx, particularly during movement under anaesthesia.

Table 23.1 Endotracheal tubes for oral and nasal intubation according to age and weight

(*for older children cuffed endotracheal tubes may be needed)

Largest tube for initial intubation				
Age	Weight (kg)	Diameter (mm)	Length (cm)	
			Oral	Nasal
Preterm	> 2	2.5	8.5	9.5
Term	> 3.5	3.0	9.0	10
6 months	> 6	3.5	10.5	12
1 year	> 8	4.0	12	1.5
2 years	> 10	4.5	13	14
3 years	> 12	4.5	13.5	15.5
4 years	> 14	5.0	14	16
5 years	> 16	5.5	14.5	16.5
6 years	> 17	5.5	15	17
7 years	> 18	6.0	15.5	17.5
8 years	> 20	6.0*	15.5	18
9 years	> 22	6.5*	16	19
10 years	> 24	7.0*	16.5	19.5
11 years	> 26	7.5*	17	20
12 years	> 30	7.5*	18	21

Technique and principles of acute peritoneal dialysis

Peritoneal dialysis (PD) catheter placement

- Acute (p. 236) or chronic renal failure may require dialysis. Transfer the child to a paediatric renal centre if possible. Failing this, request a surgeon to insert a Tenckhoff® catheter. If neither is possible insert a PD catheter.
- Give analgesia/sedation e.g. midazolam/morphine (p. 516).
- Lay the child supine on a flat surface.
- Insert a urinary catheter and empty the bladder.
- Using a strict aseptic technique, clean the abdominal wall from umbilicus to pubis.
- Place the PD catheter on the abdomen in the midline, with its tip just below the symphysis pubis. Mark the upper end on the skin. Aim to insert the catheter just below the umbilicus or halfway between the umbilicus and the anterior superior iliac spine.
- Inject a local anaesthetic into this point below the umbilicus. Ensure that the skin and subcutaneous tissue down to the peritoneum is anaesthetised.
- Insert a Jelco® cannula (usually size 18Fr) into the marked spot in the midline at right angles to the skin. Push it through the subcutaneous tissue and peritoneal membrane. Withdraw the needle into its plastic covering so you do not pierce bowel and advance the cannula into the peritoneal cavity. Now remove the needle and leave the cannula in situ.
- Run in at least 30–50 ml/kg of normal saline or Dialysate® to distend the abdomen. If the fluid doesn't flow easily, withdraw the cannula slightly as it may be abutting on the bowels. If a local bulge appears, the cannula is in the subcutaneous tissues – not the peritoneal cavity. Stop the infusion and resite the cannula.
- Monitor oxygen saturation as respiration can be compromised when the abdomen distends with fluid.
- Insert the guide-wire through the cannula into the abdomen and direct it towards the pelvis. Remove the cannula but leave the wire.
- Enlarge the entry site of the wire with a large bore needle, but ensure that the aperture is not too big, otherwise it will leak.
- Slide the PD catheter (Cohen/Cook®) over the wire. Grip its tip at the skin surface and rotate it through the opening into the abdomen. Push firmly on the catheter and guide it into the pelvis. Now remove the wire. Fluid should drain easily from the catheter. Collect some fluid for microbiological investigations.

- Attach plastic tubing (or transfer set) with a Y connection to the catheter and allow fluid to drain.
- Strap the PD catheter securely to the abdominal wall.
  - Take care not to lose the wire.
  - A stick-type catheter or peel-away Tenckhoff® (or even double lumen central line in desperate situations) may be similarly inserted.
- Replace the PD catheter with a Tenckhoff® after 5 days if dialysis is still required.

Principles of peritoneal dialysis

- Peritoneal dialysis fluid contains electrolytes, an osmotic agent (glucose) and an acid buffer (bicarbonate or lactate).
- Volumes of 20 to 50 mls/kg are used. Use small volumes if there is respiratory compromise.
- The glucose strength of dialyzing fluid ranges from 1.5% through 2.5% to 4.25%. Increase glucose strength by 0.5% for every 10 ml of 50% glucose that is added to a litre of dialyzing fluid concentrations in the dialysis fluid will increase the volume of fluid removed.
- Balsol® fluid with added glucose ('home-made bicarbonate dialysis') can be used instead of Dianeal® if high lactate is a problem. Remember, there is potassium 4 mmol/l in Balsol®.
- Higher glucose concentrations in the dialysis fluid will increase the volume of fluid removed. Importantly, significant fluid shifts can occur with strong solutions.
- Dialyzing cycles consist of the following periods:
- Fill: 10 minutes, dwell: 30–60 minutes, drain: 10–20 minutes. More rapid cycles remove more electrolytes.
  - Removal of potassium can be facilitated by increasing the cycle volume and by increasing the number of cycles (shorter dwell times).
  - Additives:
    1. Heparin 500 – 1 000 U/l
    2. Potassium chloride: 4 mmol/l if required
    3. Antibiotics: cefotaxime 125 mg/l and vancomycin 15 mg/l pending sensitivities.
       - Send fluid for culture before adding antibiotics.

24 Burns

S. Cox, H. Rode

Paediatric burns

Burn injuries pose a major threat to children and remain a devastating injury resulting in severe physical scarring and psycho-social implications.

Burns in children differ from those in adults for the following reasons: children have thinner skin with fewer layers, the extent and depth of the burn are often more severe, the child's body proportions differ resulting in greater evaporative water and heat loss, and fluid requirements are greater in children.

Causes

The causes of burns in children range from scalds and flame burns to contact, electrical and chemical burns in descending order of frequency, with infants and toddlers being burned more often. Approximately 4% of burns are due to non-accidental injury. About 90% of childhood burns are preventable.

Pathophysiology of the burn wound

The depth of a burn is determined by the amount of energy delivered to the site, the contact time and skin thickness.

The release of inflammatory mediators results in isotonic fluid shifts from the intravascular space to the burned area. These fluid losses are maximal 3–12 hours post-injury in small burns and 24–48 hours in larger burns. In burns larger than 25% this fluid loss involves the whole body in a generalised systemic inflammatory response. Effective circulating fluid volume is decreased and hypovolaemia and shock may develop.

Management

First aid

- The patient and treating team must be free from all flame, electrical or chemical hazards.
- Remove hot, smouldering, or chemical-soaked clothes.

- Wash away chemicals with copious amounts of water.
- Cooling the burn with tap water (16–18° C) for 20–30 minutes is effective up to 3 hours post burn. Ice or iced water may increase the depth of the burn.
- Prevent hypothermia in larger burns.
- Cover with plastic wrap, gauze or a moist towel to reduce pain and contamination.

Evaluation by medical professionals
- Follow the ABCs of resuscitation with the ATLS surveys.
- Fire burns often have an inhalational and airway component. Suspected inhalational burns and smoke inhalation require 100% oxygen via face mask.
- Hot fluid burns to the face may cause oral or pharyngeal burns resulting in airway compromise.
- Intubation is preferred (uncuffed tube in children under 10) before airway closure. Stridor is a late sign.
- Catheterise bladder if burns exceed 20%.
- Address concurrent injuries.
- Give analgesia (see p. 567) and tetanus prophylaxis.
- Completion of the primary survey should result in a patient with a secured airway and restored circulatory volume.

If there is any doubt regarding assessment, resuscitation or management, a burns unit should be contacted telephonically for advice.

Assessment of burn depths
- Superficial burns will heal spontaneously.
- Deep burns need surgery.
- Wound evolution occurs – depth can be established more accurately in 3 to 4 days.

Table 1 Characteristics of burn wounds at different depths

Depth	Etiology	Sensation	Appearance	Healing
Superficial	Sunburn	Painful	Red, moist, oedematous, soft, blanches, superficial blisters	± 7 days
Superficial dermal	Scalds, flash burns, weak chemical	Painful, sensitive to air/temperature changes	Erythematous, blisters, serous exudate, moist	7–14 days

Depth	Etiology	Sensation	Appearance	Healing
Deep dermal	Prolonged heat contact, chemical	Painful	Mottled red to pale, blanches on pressure and refills slowly	14-21 days
Full thickness	Immersion, flame, electrical, chemical	Painless to touch and pinprick, may hurt at deep pressure	No blanching, pale, white, charred, hard, dry, leathery, hair absent	No spontaneous healing

Assessing body surface area involved

- *Palmar surface*: The surface area of the patient's hand (including fingers) is about 1% of total body surface area.
- *Rule of nines*: This is a good, quick way to estimate medium to large burns in patients older than 10 years. In Figure 1 the child figure represents an infant up to 1 year. For every year thereafter the head decreases in relative size by approximately 1% and each leg gains 0.5%.

Figure 1 Rule of nines in adult and child

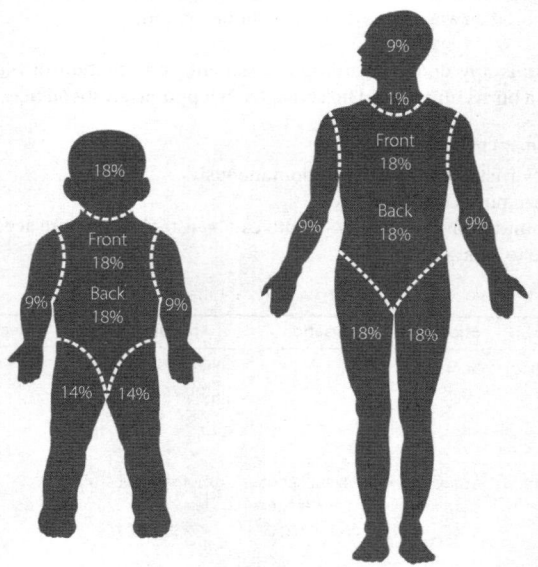

Referral criteria

- All burns in patients < 1 year of age
- 1 to 2-year-olds with > 5% total body surface area (TBSA) burns
- All ages with > 10% TBSA burns
- Full thickness burns
- Electrical, chemical burns
- Circumferential burns
- Associated inhalational burns
- Burns to face, flexures, perineum, hands and feet
- Infected burns
- Where child abuse is suspected
- Concomitant trauma or pre-existing medical conditions.

Prior to transfer, all patients need an established airway, adequate intravenous access and fluid resuscitation in progress, burn wounds covered, preferably with a sterile, waterproof dressing or Melaleuca Alternifolia Hydrogel (*Burnshield*®), potential hypothermia addressed, and adequate analgesia in the form of an opiate.

Fluid requirements

- Intravenous fluids should not be delayed until arrival in a definitive burns facility.
- Children under 2 with > 5% and any patient with > 10% TBSA burns will require intravenous fluid therapy.
- Shocked patients need a bolus of Ringer's lactate at 20 ml/kg.
- Fluid therapy thereafter consists of 2 components – replacement of ongoing losses and maintenance requirements (see Table 2).
- Resuscitation formulae should be used as a guide titrated to urine output, specific gravity (< 1.020), pulse, blood pressure, respiration and sensorium.
- Urine output should be 1–1.5 ml/kg/hr in the child.
- Inhalational injuries require additional fluid.
- Children require maintenance fluid, with 5% dextrose in addition to resuscitation fluids. Use modified Ringer's lactate (Hartmann's solution) for ongoing losses, and paediatric maintenance fluid for maintenance.

Table 2 Suggested formulae for fluid calculation

Fluid calculation for the first 24 hours:
3 ml/kg in weight / % TBSA 50% given in first 8 hours 50% given in next 16 hours Children receive maintenance fluid in addition, at hourly rate of 4 ml/kg for first 10 kg of body weight *plus* 2 ml/kg for second 10 kg of body weight *plus* 1 ml/kg for > 20 kg of body weight
Fluid calculation for the second 24 hours:
1.5 ml/kg in weight / % TBSA – total Divide by 24 for an hourly rate Maintenance fluid in addition as above

Escharotomies

- Deep dermal or full thickness burns are inelastic.
- Circumferential full thickness burns require escharotomy to enable adequate peripheral perfusion and prevent limb loss (see Figure 2).
- Any escharotomies required should ideally be performed prior to transfer.

Figure 2 Escharotomy sites

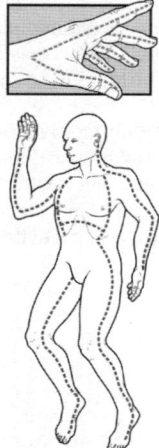

Analgesia

Burns are exceptionally painful and require regular analgesia.

- Analgesia should be tailored to specific requirements such as acute pain, procedural pain relief and chronic pain.
- In the acute setting, the following agents are suggested:
- Morphine: 10-40 mcg/kg/hr infusion IVI
- Tilidine HCl (Valoron®): 0.5-1 mg/kg/dose
- Paracetamol: 20 mg/kg/dose

Enteral feeding

- Energy and protein demands must be met as soon as possible, usually by enteral feeding, to negate the excessive metabolic response to the injury.
- Children with small wounds can usually tolerate oral or nasogastric feeds. Contraindications include clinical shock, ileus and burns greater than 20% TBSA.
- Naso-jejunal feeding is a suitable alternative in major burns with gastric stasis.

Wound care

- The area is cleaned (showered) with a water-based disinfectant (chlorhexidine soap).
- Blisters larger than 2% TBSA and loose skin should be removed and smaller blisters should be punctured.
- Swab wounds for bacteriology on admission and repeat twice a week.
- Small superficial or partial thickness wounds can be treated on an outpatient basis. Examples of topical agents include silver sulfadiazine *(Flamazine®)*, povidone-iodine *(Betadine®)*, mupirocin *(Bactroban®)* and chlorhexidine *(Hibitane®)*. All require daily changes of dressings. Agents such as nanocrystalline silver *(Acticoat®)* can be left for two to three days.
- Use a sterile dressing tecÿique.
- No single agent is totally effective against all burn-wound microbes. Treatment should be guided by the results of bacteriology cultures and the sensitivity of organisms.
- Large or deep burns with any of the admission criteria listed above require referral to a burns centre.

Surgery

The single most important principle is to achieve wound closure as expeditiously as possible. This reduces the risk of sepsis, decreases morbidity, and restores function.

- All full-thickness fire burns should be tangentially excised and grafted electively as soon as resuscitation is complete.
- This entails sequential excision of thin layers of eschar until bleeding dermis has been exposed, after which there should be immediate grafting.
- No more than 15–20% surface area should be excised at any one time.
- Spontaneous separation of eschar: Ideally suited for burns of the perineum. Daily debridement by means of hydrotherapy, and washing with antiseptic soap solutions.
- A burn wound is ready for skin grafting when there is a uniform bed of healthy granulation tissue or immediately after excision of all non-viable tissue if the resulting bed is not infected.
- A split skin graft (Thiersch) is preferable.
- Split skin grafts are usually meshed 1 : 1.5. Sheet grafts should be used where possible for cosmetically sensitive areas and hands.
- Topically applied adrenaline 1 : 30 000 or Kaltostat may reduce capillary bleeding from donor and recipient areas.
- A group B streptococcal infection of the wound is a contraindication for grafting.
- Low-grade infection with other organisms does not necessarily preclude skin grafting.
- A cephalosporin antibiotic should be given as prophylaxis with all large skin-grafting procedures.
- In larger burns, where there is limited donor site available, temporary closure can be achieved by donor allograft or a temporary synthetic skin substitute.

Wound infection

Indications for systemic antibiotic therapy are:
- Proven wound sepsis
- Septicaemia
- Thermal injury with a respiratory tract infection
- Early tangential excision.

Re-evaluate therapy every five days according to bacteriology results.

Ongoing care

Therapists involved in the burns team maintain joint mobility, and apply and construct splints, which are crucial to the long-term functional outcome of a patient. Early splinting of involved flexures in combination with pressure garments after healing and continued goal-directed physiotherapy help to prevent joint contractures and minimise scarring that may limit rehabilitation.

Healed burn wounds need to be regularly moisturized. Itching should be treated by moisturisers and occasionally oral medication. Sunscreen is vital to prevent increased pigmentation. Hypertrophic scars as well as any late blistering need to be referred.

Rehabilitation is an ongoing process continuing well beyond initial wound closure, and involves a team of psychologists, physical and occupational therapists and reconstructive surgeons.

Conclusion

The management of burns in children and adults follows the same basic principles (see Figure 3). While smaller and more superficial burns can be adequately treated on an outpatient basis, the successful management of severe larger burns requires a dedicated multi-disciplinary team within the framework of a dedicated burns unit. If the principles of early resuscitation, adequate nutrition, maximum tissue preservation, early wound coverage, psychological and social support are adhered to, there will ultimately be a successful outcome for patients with these potentially devastating injuries.

Figure 3 Treatment algorithm for burns adapted from Alsbjorn et al.

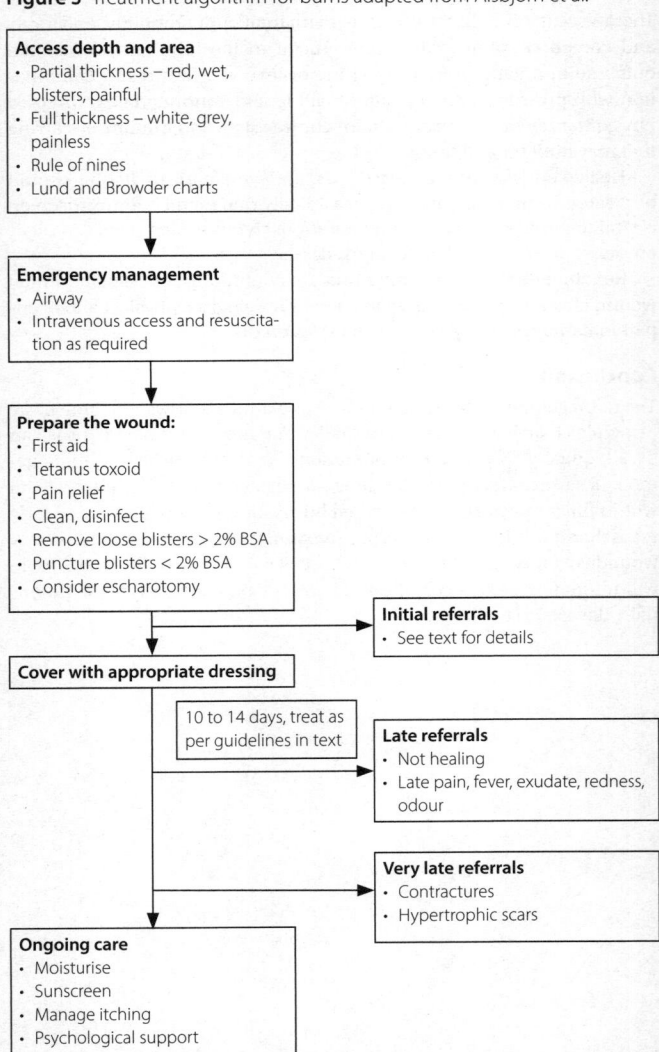

Recommended reading

1. Alsbjorn, B. et al. Guidelines for the management of partial-thickness burns in a general hospital or community setting – recommendations of a European working party. *Burns*. 2007; 33(2):155-160.
2. *Emergency management of the severe burn: course manual.* 11th ed. Education committee of The Australian and New Zealand Burn Association Limited. 2008.
3. Karpelowsky, JS and Rode, H. Basic principles in the management of thermal injury. *SA Fam Pract*. 2008; 50(3):24-31.
4. Niekerk, A, Rode, H. and Laflamme L. Incidence and patterns of childhood burn injuries in the Western Cape, South Africa. *Burns*. 2004; 30(4):314-317.
5. Venter, M, et al. Enteral resuscitation and early enteral feeding in children with major burns. *Burns*. 2007; 33(4):464-471.
6. Venter, TH, Karpelowsky, JS and Rode, H. Cooling of the burn wound: the ideal temperature of the coolant. *Burns*. 2007; 33(7):917-922.

Appendix A

These charts can be downloaded from the World Health Organization website:
http://www.who.int/childgrowth/standards/chart catalogue/en/index.html

Weight-for-age boys: birth to 10 years (z-scores)	546–547
Length/height-for-age boys: birth to 19 years (z-scores)	548–549
Weight-for-length boys: birth to 2 years (z-scores)	550
Weight-for-height boys: 2 to 5 years (z-scores)	551
Head circumference-for-age boys: birth to 5 years (z-scores)	552
BMI-for-age boys: 5 to 19 years (z-scores)	553
Weight-for-age girls: birth to 10 years (z-scores)	554–555
Length/height-for-age girls: birth to 19 years (z-scores)	556–557
Weight-for-length girls: birth to 2 years (z-scores)	558
Weight-for-height girls: 2 to 5 years (z-scores)	559
Head circumference-for-age girls: birth to 5 years (z-scores)	560
BMI-for-age girls: 5 to 19 years (z-scores)	561

Handbook of Paediatrics

Weight-for-age BOYS
Birth to 5 years (z-scores)

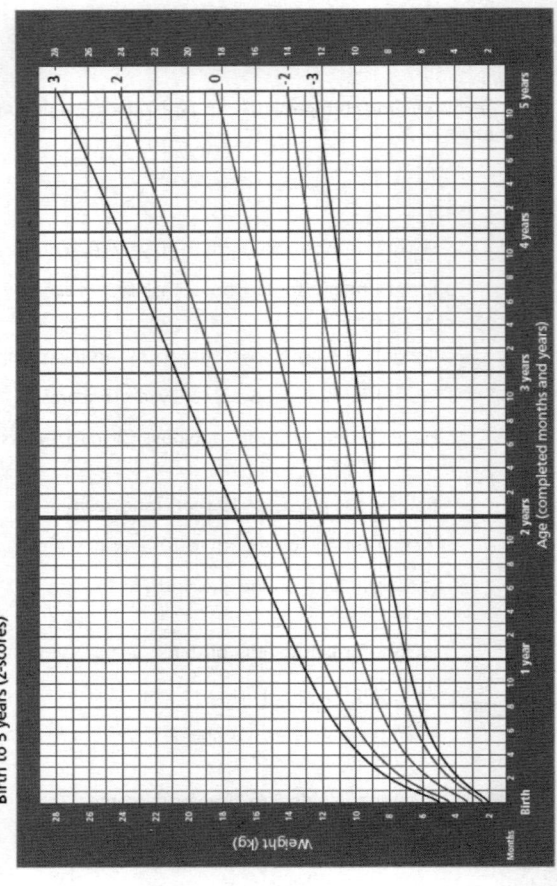

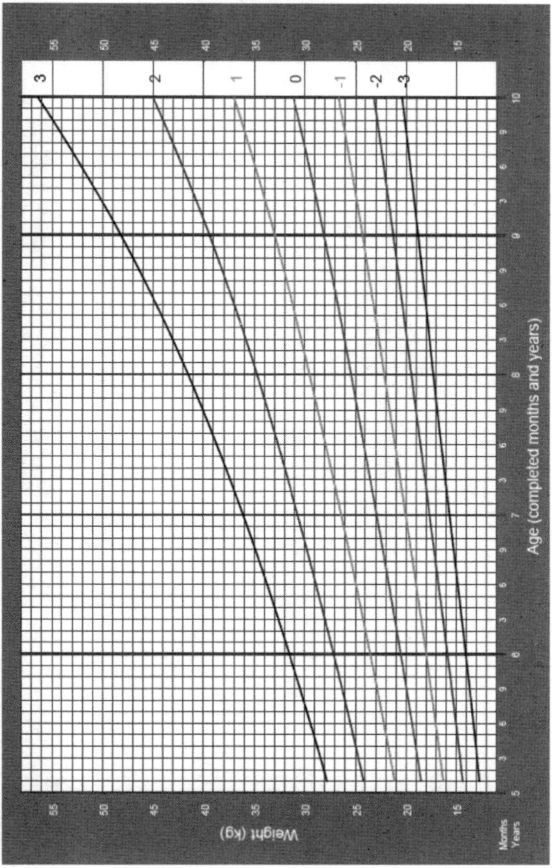

Appendix A

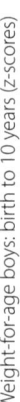

Weight-for-age boys: birth to 10 years (z-scores)

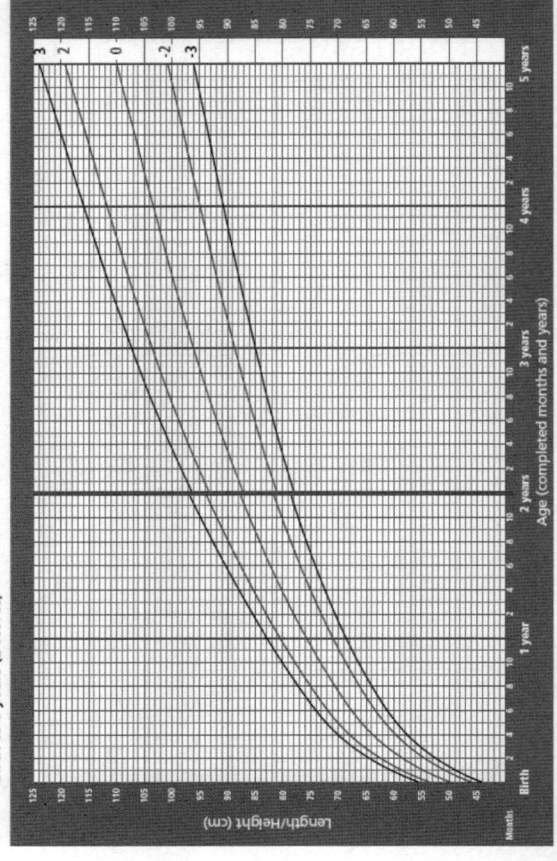

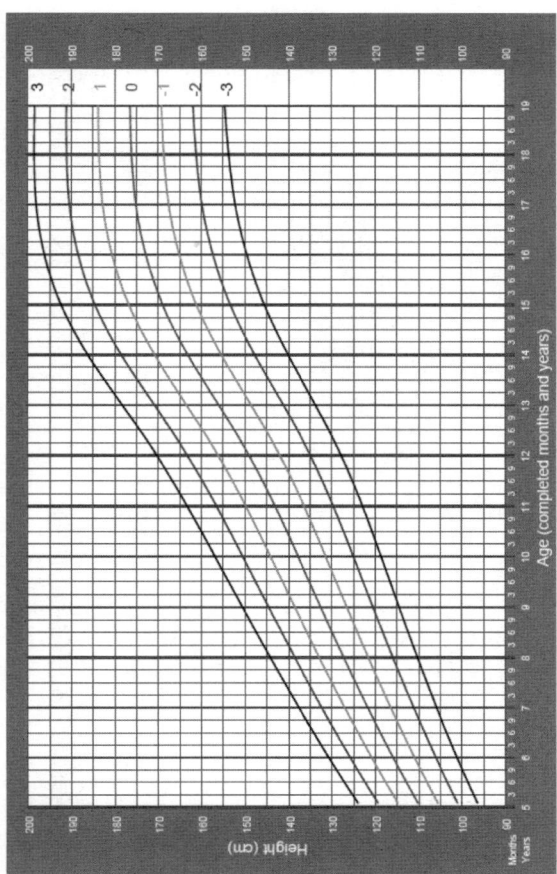

Length/height-for-age boys: birth to 19 years (z-scores)

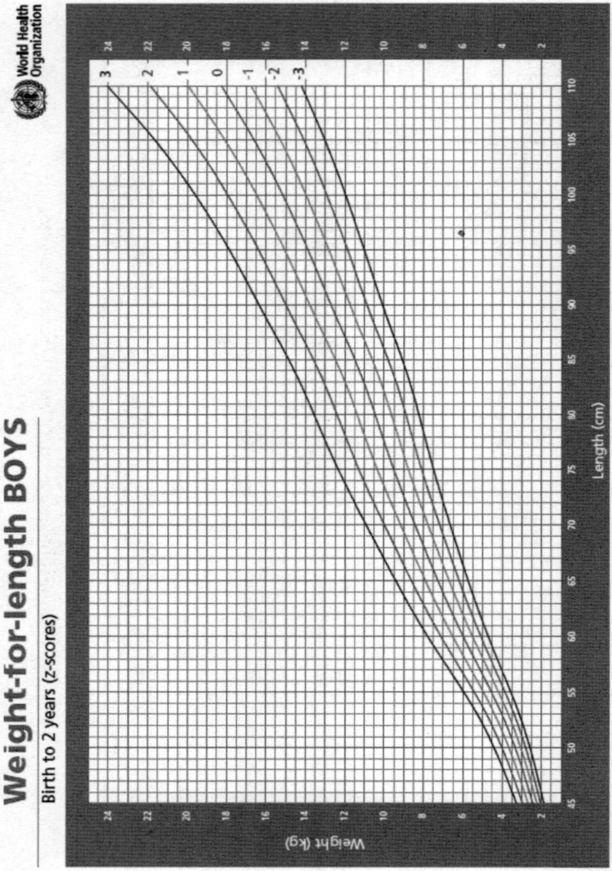

Weight-for-length boys: birth to 2 years (z-scores)

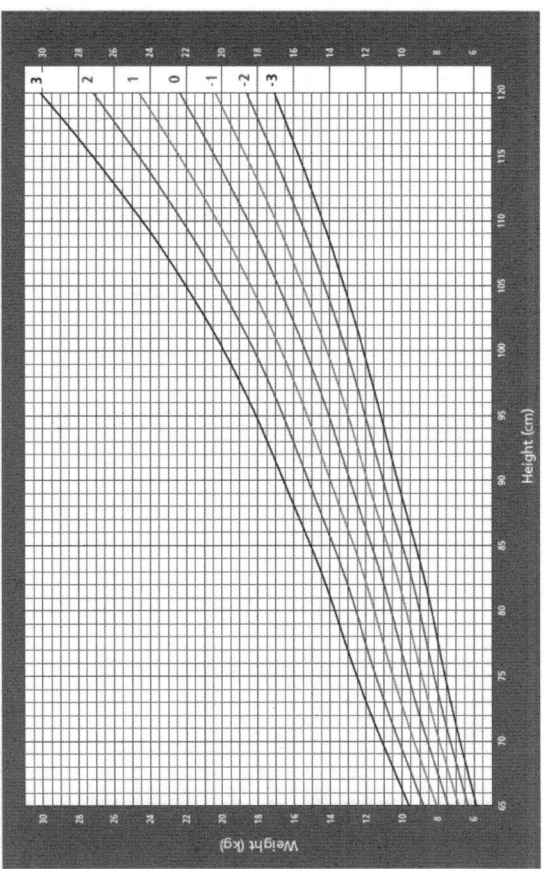

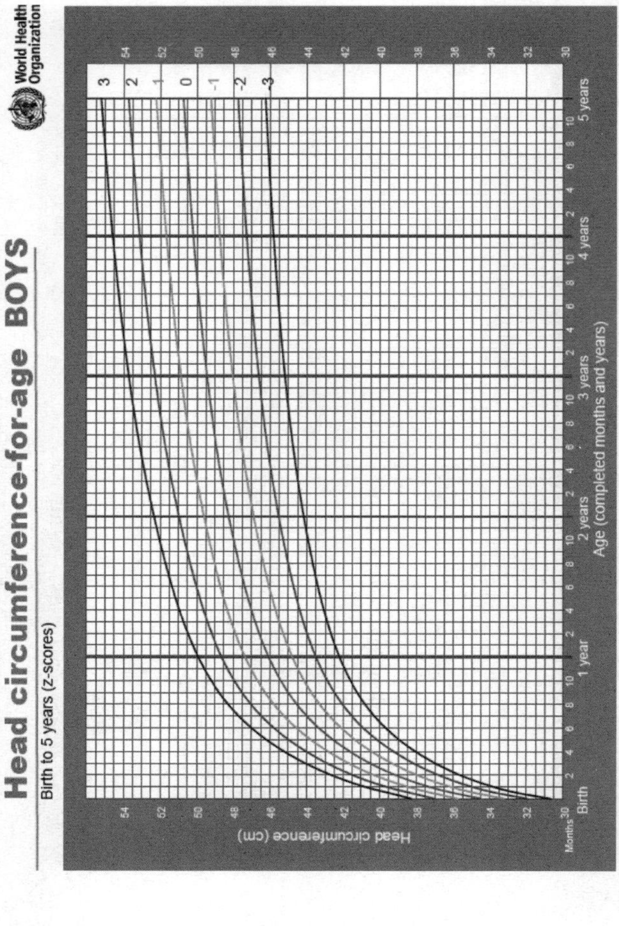

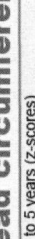

Head circumference-for-age boys: birth to 5 years (z-scores)

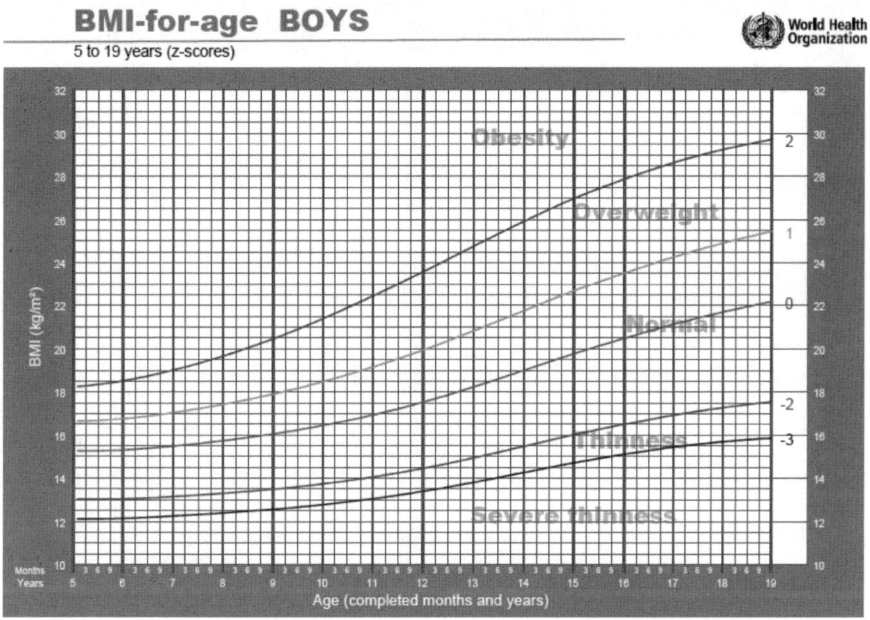

Appendix A 563

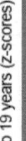

BMI-for-age boys: 5 to 19 years (z-scores)

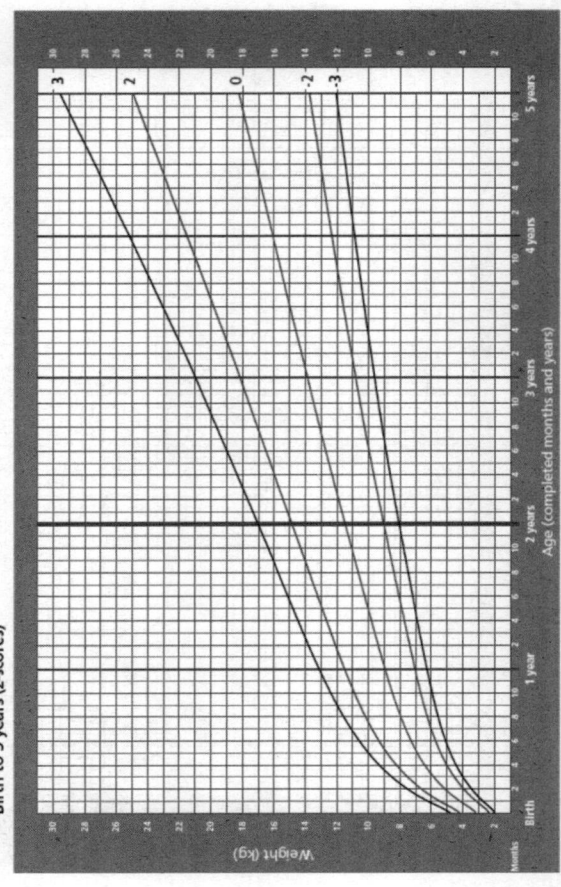

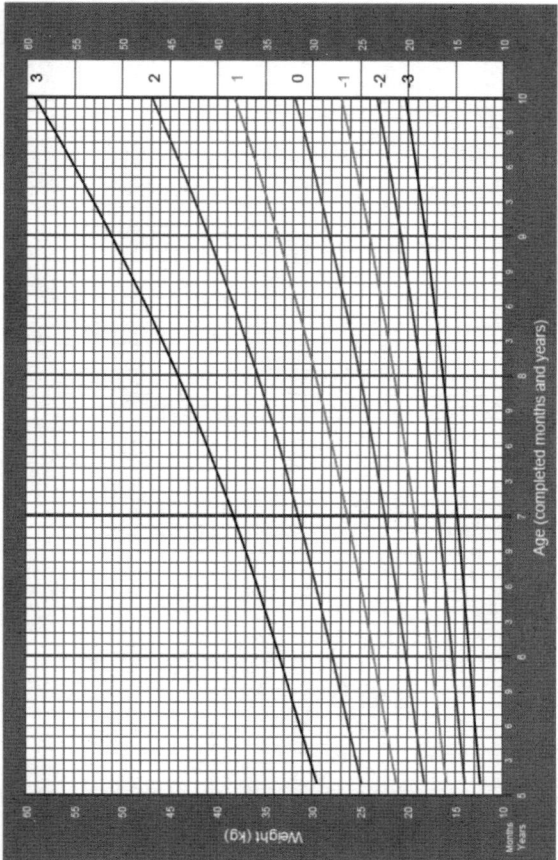

566 Handbook of Paediatrics

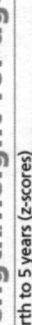

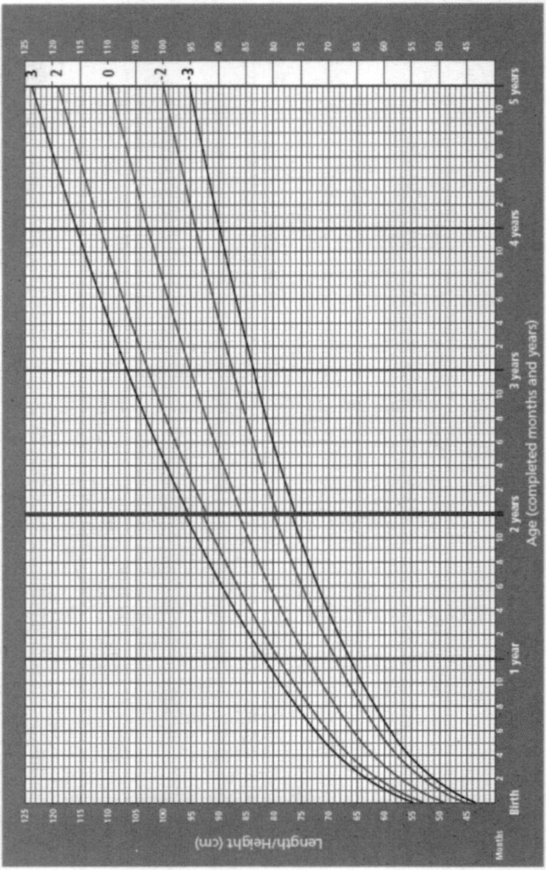

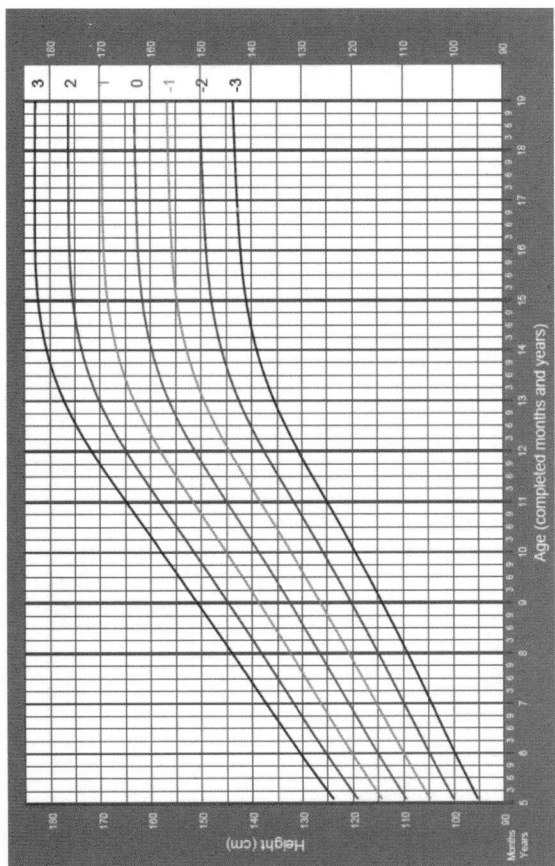

Length/height-for-age girls: birth to 19 years (z-scores)

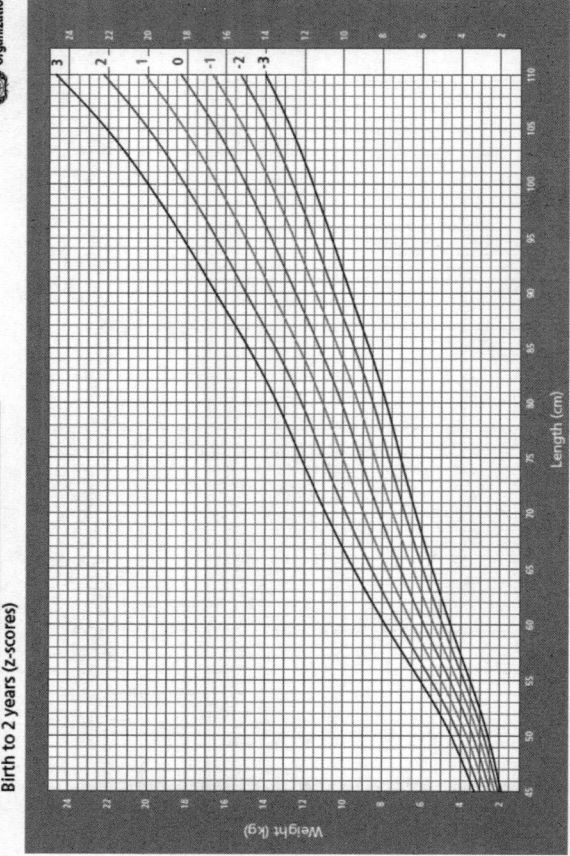

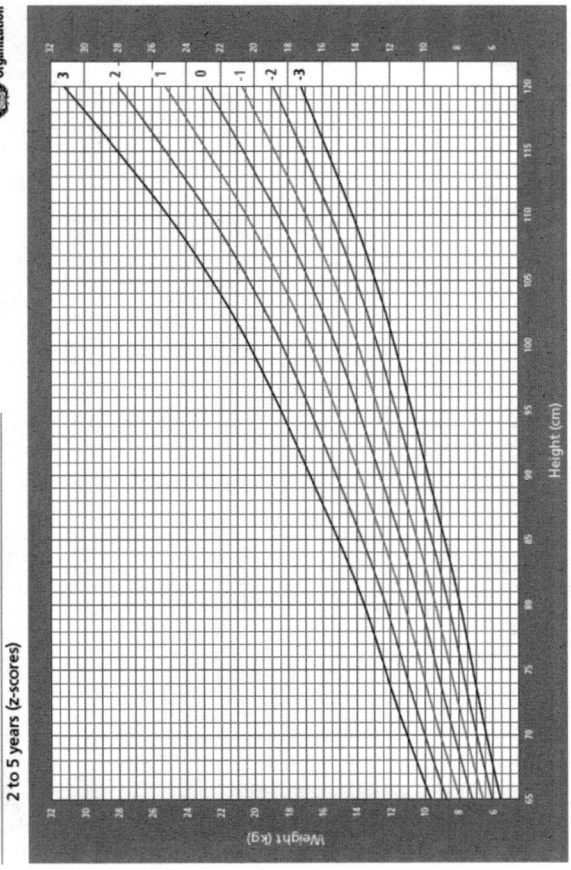

Weight-for-height girls: 2 to 5 years (z-scores)

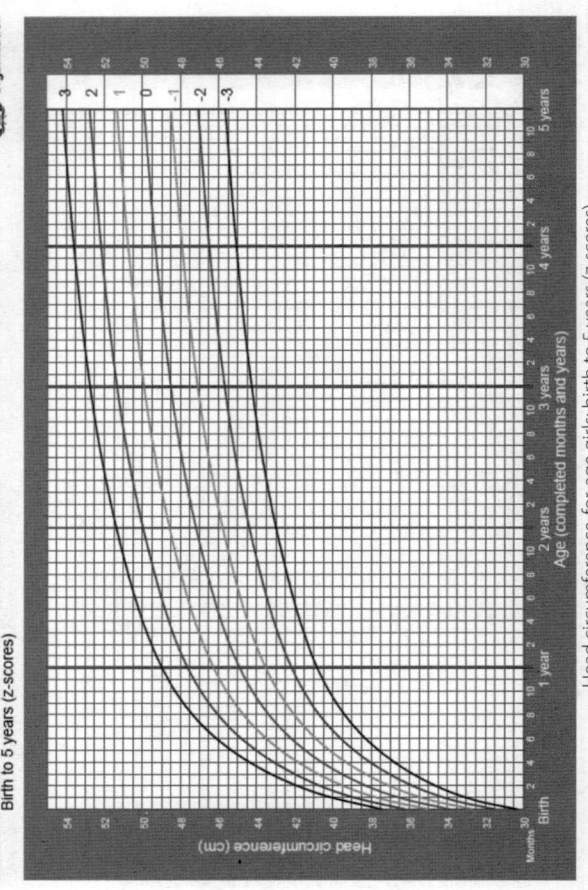

Head circumference-for-age girls: birth to 5 years (z-scores)

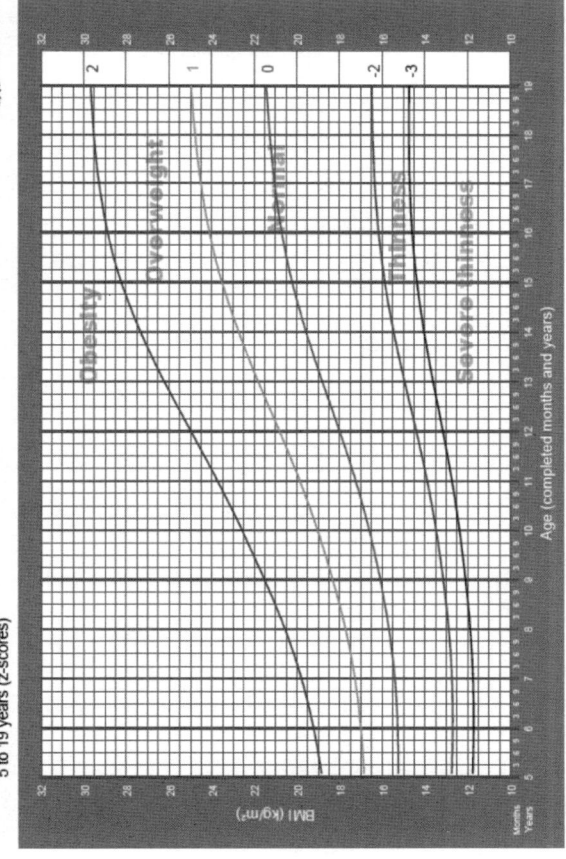

BMI-for-age girls: 5 to 19 years (z-scores)

Index

Page numbers in bold refer to figures and tables.

A

α-1-antitrypsin
  clearance 127
  deficiency **134**, **135**
abdomen injuries 26
abdominal paracentesis 522–525
  anatomy of the femoral triangle **525**
  arterial puncture 525
  dangers 522
  sites **522**
  vascular anatomy of the neck **523**
  venipuncture 523–524
ABO incompatibility **75**, 76
  [see also haemolytic disease of the newborn]
  treatment 78
abscess 106, **144**, 187, 189, 204, **250**, 421, 449, 494–496, 530
  abdominal wall 495
  amoebic 495
  brain 185, 203, 214, 453
  breast 85, 495
  cold **269**
  deep external iliac nodes 497
  epidural 206
  lacrimal 443
  liver 279, 495, 497
  organ **334**
  peri-anal 496
  peritonsilar **99**, 102, 458
  psoas muscle 495
  pyogenic 495
  retropharyngeal **99**, 102, **185**, 459
  subperiosteal 452
acid-base disturbances 468–472, **469**
acidosis 79, **81**, 170, 171, 282, 285, **364**, **365**, 402, 468, 471
  cerebral 368
  hyperchloraemic 471
  lactic 51, 313, **314**, **469**, 471
  metabolic **40**, 65, 73, 89, 126, 139, 236, 239, 240, 262, 282, 285, **373**, **468**, **469**, **470**, 470–471
  renal tubular (RTA) **163**, 377, 389, 390, **470**, 471, **482**, 484
  respiratory **468**, **469**, 472
acquired bleeding disorders 402–403
  disseminated intravascular coagulation (DIC) **401**, 402
  thrombocytopenia 402–403
acquired heart disease 175–180, **176**, **179**
  infective endocarditis 177–179, **179**
  pericardial disease 180
  previous heart valve replacement 179
  rheumatic fever 175–177, **176**
acute adrenal insufficiency 373

clinical features **373**, 373
definition and management 373
acute disseminated encephalomyelitis (ADEM) 210
acute haematogenous osteomyelitis (AHO) 431–432
acute liver failure (ALF) 137–139
  diagnosis, investigations and prognosis 138
  treatment 138–139
acute post-streptococcal glomerulonephritis (APGSN) 230–232
  clinical presentation 230–231
  indications for referral 232
  investigations 231
  management 231
  pulmonary oedema 232
acute renal failure 236–241, 284
  anaemia 239
  causes and clinical presentation 236
  choice of renal replacement therapy 240–241
  dialysis 42, 138, 228, 232, 238, 240, 241, 393, **481**, **483**,**485**, 542–543
  diet and caloric intake 238
  fluid and electrolyte balance 238–239
  investigations 237
  management 238
  medications and indications for dialysis 240
  post-renal failure 238
  pre-renal failure 238
  renal parenchymal failure 238
  seizures 240
acute scrotum 506
adenoids, enlarged 457, 460
  clinical features and treatment 457
  indications for adenoidectomy 457
adenopathy **255–256**, 402
  cervical 458
  tuberculous 119
adenovirus **92**, 112, **213**, 227, 259, 444
adequate physiology 1
aerophagia 22, **23**, 26
agammaglobulinaemia 112
AIDS 37, 180, 292, 318, 359, 504
  HIV/ 37
airway 1, **2**, **3**, **4**, 6–9
  assessment 7
  obstruction 1, 7, 89, **90**, 102, 107, 275, 302, 319, **319**, 355, 457, 458, 459, 472, 503, 511
  treatment 7–9, **8**
airway obstruction 1, 7, 89, **90**, 102, 107, 275, 302, 319, **319**, 355, 457, 458, 459, 472, 503, 511
  clinical signs 7

extrathoracic sites **91**
grading **100**, 100–101
identification of site **91**
intrathoracic sites **91**
peripheral **90**, **91**, 92–94, 96, 110, 112, **112**, 113, 119
severe 95, 99, 100, 107
total 90
Alagille's syndrome **134**, **135**
alkalosis **482**
hypochloraemic metabolic 141
metabolic **468**, **469**, 472, 504
respiratory 139, **468**, **469**, 472
allergic conjunctivitis 444
allergic disorders 325–333
angio-oedema **329**, 332–333
allergic rhinitis 325–328, **326**
anaphylaxis 251, 252, 328, **329**, 330–332
urticaria **329**, 332–333
food allergy 328–330, **329**
allergic rhinitis (AR) 325–328
classification **326**
diagnosis 326
differential diagnosis 327
treatment 327–328, **327**
Alport's syndrome 230, 454
altered states of consciousness 191
agitation and confusion 191
lethargy and coma 191
ambiguous genitalia 371, 374–375
definition 374
dos and don'ts **375**
management 375
sexual determination and differentiation in the foetus 374
Amblyomma hebraeum 266
amblyopia (lazy eye) 440–441, 442
squint (strabismus) 440, 441, 447
amoebiasis **143**, 495
anaemia 14, 26, 50, **54**, 65, 76, 131, 142, 151, **153**, 156, 159, 160, **164**, 171, 178, 217, 236, 239, 242, 282, 285, 291, 292, **297**, 302, **306**, **314**, 316, 360, 387, 394–398, 399, 402
diagnosis 394–395
folate deficiency 396
haemolytic **143**, **255**, 396–398, **397**
iron deficiency **154**, 171, 200, 279, 293, 396
management 395
normocytic 428
severe 78, 79, 89, 282, 285
sickle cell 142, **397**, **398**, 398–400
anal fissure 130, 131, 148, 149, 496
anaphylaxis 251, 252, 328, **329**, 330–332
definition 330–331
initial investigation and management 331
management of hypotension 331
post-treatment steps 332
angio-oedema **329**, 332–333
classification 332
clinical evaluation 332–333
definition 332
hereditary (C1 esterase inhibitor deficiency) 333
investigations 333
treatment 333
ano-rectal malformations/imperforate anus 487, **489**, 493
anthropometric indices 154–155
percentiles and Z scores 154–155
anti-D globulin 77
anti-hypertensive drugs **245–246**
anticonvulsant drugs 41, 52, 73, 165, 197, 200, 216, 285, 289, 303, 360, **389**, 396, 516, **519**
apathy **100**, **154**, 156, 404
Apgar score 45, **45**
aphonia 99
apnoea 2, **49**, **54**, 55, 58, 61, 63, 69, 72, 96, 170, 211, 263, 473, **480**
sleep 190
[*see also* obstructive sleep apnoea]
appendicitis **150**, 496, 497
arthritis 127, 228, **256**, **269**, 332, 419, 425–430
approach to child with limp **430**
clinical assessment 426–428
definition 425
diagnosis 425
differential diagnosis: mono-arthritis, acute onset **427**
differential diagnosis: mono-arthritis, gradual onset **427**
differential diagnosis: polyarthritis **428**
examination 426–427
history 426, **426**
inflammatory causes **425**
investigations 428
juvenile idiopathic arthritis (JIA) **164**, 425
management of JIA 429–430
newer therapy 430
non-inflammatory causes **426**
prognosis in JIA 428
reactive **256**, 269
septic (SA) 27, 431–432
surgery 430
ascariasis 496–497
ascites 66, **140**, 232, 235, **272**
aseptic tecÿique 543
aspergillosis 141
asphyxia
birth 44, **54**, 72, **81**, 402
sleep-disordered breathing **108**, 108
aspiration lung disease 110–112
causes 110
gastro-oesophageal reflux disease (GORD) **91**, 110
laryngeal incompetence 95, 110, 111
asthma **91**, **92**, 93, 94, 98, 190, **245**, 252, 319–325, 329, **355**, **377**, **379**, 410, 455, 456, 517, 530
acute/severe (*status asthmaticus*) **324**, 324–325

adjusting therapy based on control 323
choice of inhaler **322**
diagnosis 94, 319–320, **319**, **320**
dosage 321
education and review 322
leukotriene receptor antagonists (LTRAs) 321, 323
levels of control **322**
long-acting β-agonists (LABAs) 321, 323
treatment 320–322
asthma, allergic problems and immunodeficiencies 319–338
ataxia **41**, 185, 187, 196, 201–202, 343, **349**, 405
atelectasis 25, 70, 112, 115, 263
athetosis 203
atresia
bile duct **75**, 79
biliary 132, 133, **134**, **135**, 164, 497–498
choanal 454
colon **489**, 491
duodenal **150**, **489**, 491
ileal **150**
intestinal 487
oesophageal 112, **150**, 487, **489**, 490–491
pulmonary **168**
small-bowel **489**, 491
attention deficit hyperactivity disorder (ADHD) 355–357
common comorbidities 355
definition and diagnosis 354
hyperactivity 355
impulsivity 355
inattention 354–355
other potential causes 355
pharmacological treatment 356–357
psychosocial treatment 356
rating scales 356
auscultation 93, 96, 174
autistic-like conditions and autism 353–354
clinical features 353–354
definition 353
diagnosis and treatment 354
AVPU score 18

B

back pain 186
balanoposthitis 499
Bardet-Biedl syndrome **379**
barium
enema 132, 490, 491, 492, 493
swallow 95, 111, **112**, 151, 166, 460
BCG vaccine **247**, 250, 251, 252, 269, 270, 271, 305
adverse reactions **250**, 250, 305
bilharzia **143**, 290
cercarial dermatitis 290
clinical features, diagnosis and treatment 290
Katayama fever 290
biliary tract obstruction **143**

bilirubin 55, 76, 77, **80**, **81**, 132, **395**
conjugated 75, 79, **135**, **398**
defective excretion 132
defective metabolism 132
encephalopathy 74, 78, 79
total **135**, **398**
unconjugated 74–75, 76, 79
birthmarks 409
pigmented (melanocytic) naevi 409
vascular naevi and malformations 409
Bitot's spots **153**
bleeding disorders 204, **229**, 400–404
acquired 402–403
congenital 403
inherited 403–404
blood gas 99, 169
analysis **4**, 9, 11, 169, 170, 191, 468
arterial (ABG) 22, 23, 25, **469**, 471
arterial cord/infant 44
interpretation of parameters **468**
monitoring 50, 51
TCO_2 **163**, **390**
venous **365**, 471
blood in stool 130–132
diagnosis 130–132
special investigations 131
treatment 132
blood pressure **3**, **14**, **192**, 239, 243, 245, 261, 463
automated measurement **4**
diastolic 242
effect of anaesthesia **8**, **245**
low/decreased 22, 24, 122, 241, 244, 261, 479
monitoring/assessment 14, 15, 39, 50, 73, 191, **198**, 207, 223, 228, 231, **234**, 239, 242, 244, 245, 261, 284, 356, 357
raised/increased 188, 356, 513
systolic **3**, 242
Blount's disease **379**, 435, 436
bone and joint problems 425–438
bone marrow failure 51
Bordetella
parapertussis 263
pertussis 263
bradycardia **3**, **14**, 47, 61, 182, **466**, **480**, **483**, **484**, **485**
brain activity monitoring **4**
branchial arch and cleft remnants 498
breastfeeding 44, 54, 55, 56, 57, 82–86, 124, 252, 295, 296, 297, **299**, 316, **317**, 494, 517
breast abscess 85
breast engorgement 85
demand feeding 85
expressing milk 84
jaundice 74–82
mastitis 83, 85
milk storage 84–85
tecŸique 83–84
breastmilk 51, 56, 57, 77, 82, 86, 295
heat-treating/pasteurization 55, 84

jaundice 74–82
breathing 1, **4**, **5**, 6, 9–13
  assessment 9
  fast 89
  monitoring 11–12
  noisy 89–91, 95, 99, 109, 119
  therapy 9–11, **10–11**
  ventilation 7, **8**, 12–13, 25, **46**, 62, 71, 73, 173, **192**, 232, 452, **469**, 472, 488
bronchiectasis 112–113, 141, **297**, 302, **306**, 334
  classification 112–113, **112**
  clinical features, diagnosis, and treatment 113
bronchiolitis **91**, **92**, 93, 96–99, 113, 119, 173, 301
  clinical features 96–97
  diagnosis 97
  discharge and follow-up 98–99
  obliterans 319
  prevention 96
  treatment 97–98
bronchodilator response test (BRT) 94, 97, 98
bronchography 113
bronchopneumonia **91**, **92**
bronchopulmonary dysplasia (BPD) 110, **164**, **320**
bronchoscopy 111, **112**, 114, 115, 120
Budd Chiari **143**
burns 32, **32**, **397**, 402, **461**, 462, 532
  chemical 447
  corrosive oesophageal 29

C

calcium homeostasis 477, 486
  [*see also* hypercalcaemia and hypocalcaemia]
Candida spp 68, **99**, 267, **307**, 410, 411, 413–414, **S5**
  [*see also* thrush]
carbon monoxide poisoning 11, **13**, **40**, **41**, **470**
cardiac
  arrest 1, 2, **3**, 239, 477, **480**, **481**
  arrhythmia 1, **14**, 15, **108**, 125, **192**, 200, 222, 356, **484**
  congenital lesions **13**, 172, 179, 204
  contusion 22
  disease 1, **13**, 142, **167**, 170, 202, 203, 205, 231, 355, **379**, 466, 488
  dullness 92
  examination 167
  failure 73, 74, 78, 97, **154**, 160, 161, 167, 168, **167–169**, 177, 181, 230, 243, **245**, 245, 257, 282, 285, 394, 462, **464**, 464, 465, 472, **478**
  function **13**
  hypertension **40**, 189, 204, 227, 230, 231, 232, 236, 239, 240, 242–246, **244**, 264, **379**, **393**
  injury 25
  iso-enzymes 25
  monitoring 205, 238, 244
  monitors **4**, 15, 331
  murmur 174
  output 11, 16, 177
  pulsation 92
  rhythm disorders 180–182
  shunts 89
  surgery 174, 179, **397**
  tamponade 25, 117
  ultrasonography 109
  ultrasound **272**
cardiac failure 73, 74, 78, 97, **154**, 160, 161, 167, 168, **167–169**, 177, 181, 230, 243, **245**, 245, 257, 282, 285, 394, 462, **464**, 464, 465, 472, **478**
  acute severe 173
  congestive **108**, **143**, 168, 173–174, 464, 465, 500
  less severe 173
cardiac rhythm disorders 180–182
  complete heart block 180–181
  tachycardia **3**, **14**, **17**, **40**, 62, 73, 101, 122, 177, 180, 181–182, **245**, **246**, 260, 328, 496
cardiomegaly 73, **168–169**, 181, 231
cardiovascular collapse 172, 330
cardiovascular problems 167–182
carditis 175, 176, 177, **177**
  rheumatic 176, **176**
cerebral palsy 52, 79, 111, 162, **164**, 165, 197, **199**, 203, 214, 252, 338, 339, 340, **340**, 341–344, 438
  ataxic 201
  classification 343
  definition and prevalence 341
  management 343–344
cervical spine **4**, 6–9, 23
  deformity 506
  injury 6, 7, 9
cheilosis **154**
chicken pox **255**, 256–257
  incubation period **254**
child abuse 29–38
  evaluation **35–36**
  management 37–38
  physical 31–36, **32**, **33**, **34**, **35**
  predisposing factors 30
  reporting suspected abuse and court testimony 38
  sexual assault 36–37
  types of abuse 30–31
childhood cancer 404–407
  approach to suspected malignancy 405–407
  blood product transfusion 406–407
  febrile neutropaenia 405–406
  infection 405
  warning signs 404–405
childhood poisoning 39–43
  antidotes 42–43
  drug elimination procedures 42

identification of poison 39–42, **40–41**
laboratory support 43
management 39–43
poison information centres 43
child psychiatry 353–362
Chlamydia
spp 62, **106**, 107, 444
trachomatis **106**, 107, 444
choking **21**, 114, 115, 534
cholangitis 497
sclerosing **134**
choledochal cyst **75**, **134**, **135**
cholera 125, 253, 257, 294
incubation period **254**
treatment 257
chordee 502
chorea 175, 202, 203
rheumatic **176**
Sydenham's 202
chorioamnionitis 51, 61, 62, 71
chronic hepatic disease 141–142, **359**
chronic renal failure 241–242
management principles 241–242
risk factors 241
chronic weakness 208–209
Charcot-Marie-Tooth (CMT) 209
chronic inflammatory demyelinating polyradiculoneuropathy (CIDP) 209
distal 209
Duchenne muscular dystrophy 209
myopathies 206, 209
proximal 208–209
spinal muscular atrophy 206, 208
circulation 1, **4**, **5**, 6, 13–18
assessment 14–15
monitoring 15–16
shock 22, 25, 260
treatment 16
vaso-active drugs 17–18, **17–18**
volume administration 16–17
circumcision 227, 498–499, 502, 503
cirrhosis 136, 141, **164**, **478**, 498
cleft lip 494
cleft palate **164**, 165, 494
management 494
cliteromegaly **383**
Clostridium
difficile 127
tetani 265
clotting abnormalities **401**
clotting factors 132, 400, 402
club foot 434
coarctation 168, **168**, 172, **243**
colic
biliary 497
infantile 145–146, **329**, 503
renal (calculus) 227, **392**, 496
colitis 127, 278, 328
colonic bleeding 130
computerized tomography (CT) scan [*see* CT scan]

conduct disorder 355
congenital
abnormalities/anomalies 62,64, 186, **320**, **340**, **342**, **382**, 441, 487, 491
adrenal hyperplasia (CAH) with acute adrenal insufficiency 374
bilateral choanal atresia 454
bone disease 26
cardiac lesions **13**, 181
cataracts 445
cleft lip and palate 494
cysts **119**, 185, 459
deformities 433, 434
disorders **386**
hearing loss 453
heart block **14**, 180, 181
heart disease 96, 165, 167–174, 181, 203, 206, **320**, **377**
hepatic fibrosis **134**
infections **75**, **76**, **143**, 165, 205, 280
laryngeal cleft **111**
myasthaenia gravis 206
naevi 409
neutropaenia 337
ptosis 442
renal anomalies 236, 241
retinal disease 440
sepsis 44
squint 444
stenosis **99**, 459
vertical talus 438
congenital heart disease 96, 165, 167–174, 181, 203, 206, **320**, **377**
approach 167–169, **167**
common heart conditions in babies **168–169**
cyanosis 167, **168–169**, 170–172
congestion
lung 89
nasal 96, 326, 327
pulmonary venous **169**, 173, 231
systemic venous 142, **143**, 173
congestive cardiac/heart failure 173–174
conjugated hyperbilirubinaemia 75, **75–76**, 82, 132, 133–134, **398**, 497
causes **133–134**
diagnostic approach 133
evaluation of infants with **135**
conjugation 75
conjunctivitis 63, 6, **255**, **256**, 326, 426
acute rhino- 444
allergic 444
follicular 444, 445
phlyctenular 269, 445
purulent 443
vernal 445
viral (epidemic pink eye) 444
constipation 130, 146, 147–149, 219, 220, 223, 224, 227, 277, 343, **386**, **392**, 492, 496, 504, 505
chronic 147

clinical features and diagnosis 148
definitions 147
treatment 148-149
conversion disorder 357-358
   definition, clinical features and diagnosis 357
   treatment 358
convulsions 3, 4, 79, 88, 157, 192, 215, 236, 240, 252, 260, 263, 265, **269**, 282, 285, 286, 293, 344, 345, **369, 370, 372, 392**, **475**, 515
   acute 192-193
   afebrile 197
   febrile **193**, 194, 196, **256**
   generalized 193, 194, 264
   management 39
co-oximetry 11
cor pulmonale 107
corrosive oesophageal burns 29
corticosteroids 100, 104, 106, 120, 275, 289, 324, 331, 360
   inhaled 98, 320, 321
   intranasal 327
   oral 98
   topical **412**
Corynebacterium diphtheria 257
cough 94, 98, 99, 104, 111, 113, 114, 115, 117, **118, 150, 256**, 259, 263, 269, 270, 281, 290, 292, 300, 304, 319, 326, 343, **427**, 458, 534
   approach to 88
   inability to 88
   psychogenic 88
   whooping 294, 505
coughs and colds 93-94
   treatment 93-94
cow milk protein allergy (CMPA) 145, 146
crackles 92, 96, 97, 9, 165, 173, 463
craniotabes 154
crichothyroidotomy 7
Crigler-Najjar syndrome 133
critically ill child 1-20
   approach 2-3
   clinical priorities 6-19
   drugs 19
   equipment 3-5, **3-5, 10**
   fluid administration 19-20
   management priorities 1
CroŸ's disease 130, 131, **377**
croup **91**, 93, 99-102, 111, **256**, 259, 260, 538
   clinical features 99, **99**
   diagnosis 100
   discharge and follow-up 102
   grades of obstruction **100**, 100-101
   treatment 100
Cryptosporidium parvum 126, 127, 278
   clinical features, diagnosis and treatment 278
CT scan 18, 24, **33, 35**, 113, 116, 120, 128, 184, 188, 190, 191, 194, 202, 204, 206, 211, 213, 214, 215, 216, 243, 244, **272**, 272, 279, 289, **342**, 343

Cushing's syndrome 243, **376, 377**
cutaneous vascular lesions 500-501
cyanosis 2, 24, **41**, 45, 70, 71, 72, **101**, 109, 167, **168-169**, 170-172, 263, **482**, 534
   absent 168
   central **46**, 47, 69, 169-170, **324**
   older child 170-172
   present 168
cyanotic heart disease 2
cyst
   branchial arch 504
   congenital 185, 459
   duplication 131, 488, 503
   erythematous 408
   lung 117, **119**
   meibomian 442
   procedure 536, 542
   pseudocyst 117
   sublingual 505
cystic adenomatoid malformation 488
cysticercosis 289
cystic fibrosis (CF) **75, 91, 92**, 93, 98, 110, 112, 113, **134**, 140-142, **144, 164, 165**, **320**, 472, **479**, 492, 493, 505
   clinical features and diagnosis 141
   treatment 141-142
cystic hygroma 499
cytomegalovirus (CMV) 62, 105, **133, 143**, 301, **307**, 334, **340**, 453, 454

D

daytime incontinence 222-224
   assessment 223
   classification **222**
   evaluation 222-224
   management of dysfunctional voiding 224
   management of overactive bladder 223-224
death, causes of in children 1-2
dehydration 39, 74, 78, 121-126, 127, 136, 190, 204, 206, 236, 257, 363, **364**, 393, 462, 466, 467, **482**, 504, 511
   assessment **364**
   cellular 474
   correction 125, 128, 238, 285
   hypernatraemic 466
   mild to moderate 123-124
   prevention 124, 158, 467
   severe 124, 125, 126, **341**, 466
   signs 122, **466**
delirium 215, 358-359
   definition 358
   clinical features, diagnosis and treatment 359
dermatology 408-424
   acne 408-409, **S1**
   birthmarks 409
   drug reactions 413
   eczema 410-412
   fungal infections 413-417

ichthyosis 417, **S8**
molluscum contagiosum **306**, 417, **S9**
papular urticaria 418, **S9**
pediculosis 418-419
pityriasis rosea 419
psoriasis 417, 419-420, **S10**
scabies 420-421, **S11**
streptococcal and staphylococcal infections 421-422, **S12**
warts **306**, 422-424
dermomyositis 208, 425
development 338-352
developmental delay **108**, 165, 210, 218, 302, 338, 355, **387**
  approach 341, **342**
  global 340
  static 210
developmental disabilities 338-339
  aetiology **340**
  definitions 338
  focal 339
  global 339
  prevalence 338
developmental dysplasia of the hip (DDH) 434-435
developmental milestones and warning signs **344-351**
  areas to consider 344
diabetes 249, 370, 416, 530
  holistic management **368**
  insipidus 219, 474, **475**
  mellitus **164**, 219, 360
diabetes insipidus 219, 474, **475**
diabetes mellitus **164**, 219, 360
  insulin dependent (IDDM) 141, 223
  type 1 369, **369**
  uncontrolled (Mauriac syndrome) **144**
diabetic hypoglycaemia 363, **367**, 369-371
  clinical features **369**
  definition 369
  high blood glucose **371**
  management **370**
  normal or low blood glucose **371**
  sick day management 370-371
  symptoms and signs in type 1 diabetes **369**
diabetic ketoacidosis (DKA) **150**, 363-368, **371**, 461, **469**, **470**, **471**, **482**, **484**
  definition 363
  management 363, **364-367**, 368
dialysis 42, 138, 228, 232, 238, 240, 241, 393, **481**, **483**, **485**
  acute intermittent haemodialysis 241
  acute peritoneal 241, 542-543
  continuous veno-venous haemofiltration and dialysis 241
diaphragmatic hernia (congenital) 69, 487, 488
  clinical presentation, diagnosis and management 488
diarrhoea 39, **40**, 98, 123, 124, 126, 130, 149, 161, 162, 171, 238, 252, **255-256**, 259, 277, 278, 281, 289, 291, **307**, **329**, 370, **371**, **469**, **470**, **475**, 477, **483**, 515
  acute 121, 123, 124, 126, **129**
  bloody mucoid 290, 293
  chronic 124, 126, 127, 128, **129**, 141, 148, 279, **482**, **484**
  infectious 125
  mild/parenteral 121
  osmotic 127
  persistent 123, 126-129, **129**, 161, 162, **297**, **306**, 486
  recurrent 125, **297**
  secretory 125, 127
  severe 162, 278, 467
  treatment 128, **129**
  watery 158, 170, 257, 278, 279
diathesis 138, 139
diphtheria 257-258, 294, 336, 459
  complications 257
  immunization 99, **99**, **247**, 248
  incubation period **254**
  treatment 258
diplopia 441, 447, **480**
direct Coombs test 76, **395**, **398**
disability (D) **4**, 6, 18-19
drooling 29, 41, **99**, 165, **198**, 348, 460, 490
Dubin-Joÿson syndrome **134**
dysentery 121, 123,125, 126
dysphagia 41, 95, **99**, 151, 413
  febrile 102-107
dyspnoea 24, 173, 174, **400**, 510, 511
  progressive 25
dystonia **185**, 202

E

early warning systems 2-3, **2-3**
ear, nose and throat problems 448-460
  ear 448-454
  nose 454-457
  throat 458-460
echocardiogram (ECHO) 73, 176, 178, 243, 244, 259
ectopia vesicae (bladder exstrophy) 499
eczema (dermatitis) 410-412
  atopic 410, 411, 417
  contact 410, 412
  general measures 412
  herpeticum **255**
  napkin 410, 499
  nummular 410, 411
  pityriasis alba 411, **S2**, **S3**
  seborrhoeic dermatitis 411
  treatment 410-412
egg allergy and vaccines 251
electrocardiogram (ECG) 25, 39, 109, 158, 175, 181, 202, 231, 239, 243, 244, 284, 356, **365**, **480**, **481**, **482-483**, **484**
electroencephalogram 52, 53, 108, **193**, 194, 195, 196, 201, 215, 272, **342**, 343, 359
  amplitude integrated (aEEG) cerebral function monitor 49, 50, 52

non-urgent 197
urgent 197
electrolyte abnormalities 474–486
  daily electrolyte requirement 474
elliptocytosis **75**, **397**
emergencies and trauma 1–43
empyema 106, 115, **116**, 116–118, 187, 213, 214–215, 453
encephalitis 126, 190, **193**, 203, 204, 210, 215–216, **255–256**, 267, 280, 292, 359, 360, **479**
  acute 259
  aetiology 215
  clinical presentation 215
  diagnosis 215
  herpes 215
  management 215–216
  meningo- 1, 462
  post infectious 215
  primary 215
  viral 216, 303
encephalopathy 45, 51, 138, **140**, 201, 206, 217, 249, 252, 263, **341**, 466, **482**
  bilirubin 74, 78, 79, **81**
  haemorrhagic 474, **475**
  HIV 210, 302, **307**
  hypertensive 231, 243, 359
  hypoxic ischaemic (HIE) 44, 48–52, **54**, 58, **164**, 203, 205, **341**
  moderate 50
  neonatal (NE) 44, 48
  severe 50
encopresis 147
end-tidal pCO$_2$ monitoring 12
endocrinology 363–393
endoscopy 29, 108, 109, 119, 128, 132, 151, 330
Entamoeba histolytica 278–279
  clinical features 278–279
  diagnosis and treatment 279
Enterococcus spp 62, 278
enterocolitis 132
  food-induced 328
  necrotizing (NEC) 51, 56, 64, 65, 131, 132
entero-hepatic circulation 74
enterovirus 206, **213**, **255**, 256
enuresis **108**, 218, 223, 224, 457
  alarm 221
  causes of secondary enuresis 219
  contributing factors 218–219
  classification 219
  definition and prevalence 218
  evaluation 219–220
  management 220–221
  mono-symptomatic (MNE) 219, 221
  nocturnal 218, 221
  non-mono-symptomatic (NMNE) 219
  primary 219, 221
  secondary 219
  treatment 221–222
  treatment-resistant 222

epiglottitis **99**, 102–104
  diagnosis 102–103
  management 103–104
  symptoms and differential diagnosis 102
epilepsy 194–200
  antitretroviral therapy 200
  focal 194–195
  generalized 195–196, **198**
  syndromes 196–197
  treatment 197–200, **198–200**
epilepsy syndromes 196–197
  infantile spasms 196, 197, **199**, **200**
  Landau-Kleffner syndrome 197
  Lennox-Gastaut syndrome 196, **198**, **199**
  management 196
  severe myoclonic epilepsy 196
epistaxis 130, 400, 402, 457, 534
Epstein Barr virus (EBV) **143**, **213**, **255**, **397**
equipment 3–5, **3–5**
  monitoring **3–4**
  resuscitation 4–5, **4–5**, **10**
erythema 36, **99**, 249, 258, 260, 332, 410, 415, 419, **S10**, **S14**
  gingival **306**, **S5**
  infectiosum **255**
  marginatum 175
  multiforme 413
  nodosum **250**, 269
  papules, nodules, pustules, cysts and scale 408, 415, 421, **S1**, **S4**, **S8**
  punctate **256**
Escherichia coli 126, **213**, 225, **397**, 406
exchange transfusion 76, 78
  guidelines chart 78, **81**
exomphalos 499
  ruptured 489
  unruptured 488–489
eyelids (congenital defects)
  defective eyelids 441
  lid lumps 442
  ptosis (blepharoptosis, drooping eyelid) 207, 405, 440, 442
eyes and vision 439–447
eyes (congenital defects)
  big (enlarging) 442
  [*see also* glaucoma, congenital; oedema, corneal]
  watering (epiphora) 442–443, 444
eye/visual assessment 439–440
  fix-and-follow test 439–440
  milestones 439
  probable causes of poor responses 440
  signs suggesting poor vision 440

F

faecal impaction 147–149
  clinical features and diagnosis 148
  definitions 147
  treatment 148–149
faecal incontinence (soiling) 147, 148, 149
failure to thrive (FTT) 30, 65, 86, 95, **108**, 141,

162–166, 173, 174, 224, 259, 269, 281, **297**, 304, **334**
 aetiology 164–166, **164**
 definition 162–164
 investigations 166
 management 166
familial dysautonomia 111
familial intrahepatic cholestasis **134**, **135**
fast breathing 89
 approach to 89
 causes 89
 respiratory rate limits 89, **89**
febrile dysphagia syndrome 102–107
fetal alcohol syndrome **340**, **342**, 355
fine needle aspiration biopsy 535–537
fingertip injuries 28
fistula
 arteriovenous 524
 broncho-oesophageal 110, 112
 coronal 499
 palatal 494
 peri-anal 496
 rectourethral 493
 rectovaginal **297**, **307**, 493
 rectovesical **297**
 tracheo-oesophageal (TOF) 110, 112, **150**, 335, 487, 491
flexible or postural flat foot 438
floppy infant 205–206
 central hypotonia 205–206
 lower motor neuron (LMN) 205, 264
 peripheral hypotonia 205, 206
 upper motor neuron (UMN) 205
fluids, electrolytes and acid-base 461–486
fluids
 extracellular (ECF) **461**
 Holliday-Segar calculator 462
 intracellular (ICF) **461**
 maintenance 461–463, **461**, **463**
 replacement 463–467
folate deficiency 396
follicular conjunctivitis 444, 445
food allergy 328–330
 definition 328
 diagnosis and investigations 329–330
 manifestations 328, **329**
 treatment 330
foreign body (FB) inhalation 21, 28, **91**, **99**, 104, 114–115, 119, **150**, **320**, 457, 459
 diagnosis 114–115
 treatment 115
foreign body (FB) 28, **28**
 embedded **383**, 446, 456
 in ear canal 448
 obstruction 112, 335
fragile X syndrome **340**, **342**, 355
functional gastrointestinal disorders 146–147
 definition and causes 146
 recurrent abdominal pain syndrome(RAPS) 146–147
fungal infections of the skin 413–417

Candida spp 68, **99**, 267, **307**, 410, 411, 413–414, **S5**
 pityriasis versicolor 414, **S6**
 tinea infections 415–417, **S6**, **S7**, **S8**
fused labia 499–500

G

G6PD 76
 deficiency **75**, 286, **287**, **397**, **398**
galactosaemia **75**, 79, **134**, **135**, **144**, 164, 165, 446
gamma-globulin, intravenous 78
Gardner's syndrome 131
Gardnerella vaginalis 267, **268**
gastric dilatation 22, **23**, 264
gastritis 146, **150**, 505
gastroenteritis 111, 121–126, **150**, 171, 328, 370, 462, 465, **479**
 complications 125–126
 dehydration 121–122
 [*see also* the main entry for dehydration]
 diagnosis 122–123
 shock 121–122
 [*see also* the main entry for shock]
 treatment 123–125
gastrointestinal problems 121–152
gastro-oesophageal reflux (GOR) 93, 95, 98, 110, 111, 141, **150**, 151–152, **164**, 166, **320**, 320, 335, 343
 diagnosis 151–152
 disease (GORD) **91**, 110, 151, 152
 treatment 152
gastroschisis 487, 489
 clinical presentation and management 489
Gauchers disease 142, **144**
generalized epilepsy 195–196, **198**
 absence epilepsy 195, **198**
 atypical absences 195
 childhood absence epilepsy (CAE) 195
 drop attacks 196, **198**
 generalized tonic clonic seizures (GTCS) 195, 196, **199**
 juvenile myoclonic epilepsy (JME) 195
 myoclonic seizures 196, **199**
 tonic seizures 195
genu varum and genu vulgum 435–436
Giardia intestinalis (ex *G. lamblia*) 279
 clinical features, diagnosis and treatment 279
Gilbert's syndrome 133
Glasgow Coma scale (GCS) 18, 24, 183, 191, **191**, **193**
glaucoma
 congenital 442, 443
 secondary 446
glossitis **154**
glucocorticosteroids 263, 270
 inhaled **321**
glucuronidase 74, 75
glycogen storage disease **144**
goitre **154**, 388

gonadal failure
　primary **385**
　secondary **385**
growth and development 375–385
growth and nutrition 153–166
growth failure **140**, 154, 160, 162, 429
Guedel airway **4**, 7
Guillain-Barrè syndrome 1, **118**, 207, 264, 357

H

haemangioma 131, 187, 459, 500, 503, 504, 536, 542
　capillary 501
　cutaneous 131
　eyelid 442
　intestinal 131
　liver 501
haematology and oncology 394–407
haematoma 185, 206, 524
　deep-seated 400
　extradural 33
　intracranial 24, **75**, 187
　local 524, 538
　orbital 447
　retinal 35
　scalp 24
　subdural 33, 184
haematuria 227–230
　glomerular 229–230
　history and examination 227–228, **228**
　macroscopic 227
　microscopic 227
　non-glomerular **229**
haemoglobin 11, 55, 76, 172, 239, 284, 394, 396, 399
　average volume **394**
　degradation 32
　fetal 74
　in sickle cell anemia 398
haemoglobinopathies **143**, 255, **395**, **397**, **426**
haemoglobinuria 228
haemolysis 75, **81**, 132, 133, 282, **395**, **481**, **482**
　auto-immune **395**, 396
　brisk 396, 400
　indolent 396
　investigation **398**
　severe 239
haemolytic
　anaemia **143**, **255**, 396–398, **397**
　crisis 398
　disease of the newborn (ABO, Rh) **76**, 76, 77, 79
haemolytic anaemia **143**, **255**, 396–398, **397**
　acquired 396
　congenital 142, 396, 398–400
　[see also sickle cell anaemia]
　investigations **398**
haemolytic uraemic syndrome (HUS) 116, 230, 236, 237
haemophilia 136, 204, **426**, **427**, 433
　A 403
　B 403–404
Haemophilus
　influenzae 113, 116, 117, 180, 203, 212, **213**, 431, 432, 449
　influenzae type b 102, 247, 294, 300
　spp 178, 398, 443
haemoptysis 130
haemorrhage **13**, 26, 403, 500
　antepartum 77
　concealed 22
　control of 13–18
　corneal 446
　gastrointestinal 130
　intra-abdominal 22
　intracranial 49, 52, **54**, **75**
　intraventricular 205
　peptic ulcer 131
　pulmonary 61
　retinal 33, 447
　splinter 178
　subarachnoid 185
　variceal 131
　vitreous 446–447
hand, foot and mouth disease **255**
Harrison's sulcus 92, **389**
HCO_3 468, 469, **469**, 470, 471, 472
head and neck injuries 23–24
headache **108**, 147, 149, 183, 185, 187, 189–191, 211, 212, 215, 221, **256**, 264, 266, 281, 336, 356, 361, **365**, **369**, **372**, **392**, 404, 405, 455, 474, **477**, 515
　management and differentials 190
　migraine 190
　pathological 189
　severe 215
hearing loss in children 449, 450, 452, 453–454, 457
　clinical features and investigation 454
　risk factors 453
hemiplegia 183, 203–205
　acute/sub-acute 203–205
　chronic 205
　congenital 205
　differential diagnosis 203–204
　management 204–205
Henoch-Schönlein syndrome 131, 230, **234**, 441
hepatic excretion 74
hepatic failure 51, 137, 313
hepatic fibrosis (congenital) **134**
hepatitis 79, **150**, **255**–256, 258,9, 313, 314, 336, 413
　A (HAV) 133, 134–136, 138, **254**, 294
　acute 253
　autoimmune 134, **143**
　B (HBV) 62, **133**, 136–137, **137**, 138, **143**, 234, **247**, 254, **254**, 294, 318
　C (HCV) 336

chronic 136, **137**, 137, 353
fulminant 134
idiopathic neonatal **135**
neonatal **135**, 141, 497
non-A, non-B 294, 336
hepatitis A virus (HAV) **133**, 134–136, 138, 294
  clinical features and diagnosis 134
  incubation period **254**
  management and prevention 136
  vaccine 248
hepatitis B virus (HBV) 62, **133**, 136–137, 138, **143**, 234, 254, 294, 318
  diagnosis 136
  immunoglobulin (HBIG) 253
  incubation period **254**
  markers 136, **137**
  nephropathy 231
  treatment 137
  vaccine **247**
hepatocellular
  carcinoma 136
  injury **75**
hepatomegaly 142, **154**, 173, 290, 292, **464**, 495
  causes 142
hepatosplenomegaly 62, 63, 66, **135**, 165, 280, **296**, **306**, 394, 402, 428, **430**
  'apparent' 142
  approach to child with 142–144
  causes 142, **143–144**
  pathological mechanisms 142
  pseudo 96–97
hernia **164**, 187, 501–502, 507
  cerebellar **185**
  diaphragmatic 69, 487, 488
  fluid 501
  hiatal 151
  hydrocoele 501
  inguinal **150**, **489**, 502, 506
  para-umbilical 502
  strangulated 145
  supra-umbilical 502
  tonsillar 185
  umbilical **386**, 502
herpes 68, **213**, 215, 259, 260, 453
  encephalitis 215
  gingivostomatitis **255**
  HHV6 **256**
  simplex 62, 64, **133**, **143**, **203**, **215**, **255**, **307**, 406, 410, 444, 445
  stomatitis 260
  zoster **255**, **296**, **297**, **306**
Hirschsprung's disease 148, **489**, 492, 493
  presentation, diagnosis and management 492
histoplasmosis **143**
HIV antiretroviral therapy 307–316
  and anti-TB therapy 309, 312, **312**
  drug doses 309, **310–311**
  drug toxicity 313, **314**

indications 307–308, **308**
indications for changing therapy 314–315
monitoring 313
preparation 308
recommended first-line treatment regimens **309**
resistance testing 315–316
second-line treatment **316**
HIV infection 295–318
  antiretroviral therapy 307–316
  bacterial pneumonia 301, **306–307**, 444
  chronic lung disease 302
  clinical manifestations 296
  clinical staging **306–307**
  CNS infections 303
  diagnosis 296–300
  encephalopathy 303
  haematological conditions [see anaemia; thrombocytopenia]
  immunological assessment 307
  lymphoid interstitial pneumonitis (LIP) **297**, 302, **306**, **320**
  malignancy 302
  Pneumocystis jiroveci (PCP) 105, 106, **297**, 301, **307**, 405
  post exposure prophylaxis (PEP) 316–318, **317**
  prevention of vertical transmission 295–296
  prophylaxis 303–305, **304**, **305**
  seizures 303
  testing 297–300, **298–299**
  tuberculosis 302
  viral pneumonia 110, 112, 301, **306–307**
Hoover's sign 91, 92, 96
Human papilloma virus (HPV) 422
hyaline membrane disease (HMD) **54**, 69, 73
  definition, clinical features, diagnosis, and treatment 69
hydatid cysts **143**, 185, 206, 289
hydrocephalus 184, 185, 186, 187, 189, 201, 213, 214, **272**, 280, 289
hyperalimentation **144**
hyperbilirubinaemia
  causes of neonatal **75–76**
  conjugated 75, **75–76**, 82, 132, 133–134, **133–134**, **398**, 497
  management 77
  obstructive **497**
  physiological 77
  unconjugated 75, **75–76**, 79, 132, 133
hypercalcaemia 148, **164**, **391**, 392–393, **482**
  clinical features **392–393**
  definition 392
  hypocalciuric **391**
  management 393
  normal values 392
hypercapnoea 12
hypergammaglobulinaemia 293
hyperkalaemia 231, 238, 239, 240, **373**, 477
  management **481**

hypermagnesaemia **484**, 486
hypernatraemia 52, 123, 125, 126, 467,
474–475
management 475
hyperparathyroidism 162, **391**
hyperphosphataemia 239, **482**
hypersplenism **140**, 402
hypertension **40**, 189, 204, 227, 230, 231, 232,
236, 239, 240, 242–246, 264, **379**, **393**
acute 244–245, **244**
adolescent essential 243, 245
benign intracranial (BIH) 190
chronic 245
intracranial **8**, 11, 12
investigation 243–244
management 244–245
persistent **234**
persistent pulmonary **54**, 72–73, **234**
portal (PHT) 131, **140**, 141, 142, **143–144**,
290
proven 242–243
pulmonary 12, 54, **108**, 109, 290
secondary **243**
severe 244–245, **244–245**
systemic **108**
hypertensive crisis 244
hyperthyroidism **164**, 165, 203, 355, 356,
388, **391**
causes **388**
clinical manifestation and treatment 388
primary **385**, 437
hyperventilation **49**, 195, **319**, 472
hypocalcaemia 51, 52, 125, 126, 139, 162,
236, 239, 242, 262, **389**, **482**, **483**, **484**,
486
hypogammaglobulinaemia 335, 336, 337
hypoglycaemia 51, 52, **54**, 57–60, 61, **75**, 125,
126, 136, 139, 153, 170, 213, 217, 240,
282, 285, 286, 372–373, **373**, 465, 473,
477, 489, 513
clinical features 58, 372, **372**
complications 60
definition 57, 372
diagnosis 58
in diabetics 363, **367**, 369–371, **369**, **370**,
371
investigations **373**
neonatal 44, 57
overt causes **372**
severe 57
treatment/management 39, 47, 51, 55, 58,
59, 60, 157, 158, 283, 285, 372, 373, **464**,
473
hypokalaemia 1, 125, 126, 139, 173, 262, 368,
477, **485**, 486, 504
management **480**
hypomagnesaemia 51, 52, 126, 139, **482**,
484, 486
hyponatraemia 51, 52, **54**, 125, 126, 141, 213,
221, 240, 262, 282, **373**, 462, 465, 476, 504
management **478–479**

hypoparathyroidism **391**, **392**, 482
hypophosphataemia 162, **482**
hypopituitarism **134**
hypoplastic left heart syndrome **168**, 172
hypospadias 499, 502
hypotension **3**, 6, 26, 139, 203, 241, **256**, 260,
261, 264, **373**, **484**
management 331
hypothermia 31, 44, 47, 48, 50, 53, **54**, 58,
60–61, 65, 153, 157, 158, 170, **386**, 402,
515
complications 61
prevention 60, 157
treatment 61
hypothyroidism **75**, 79, 82, **134**, **135**, 148,
376, **377**, **479**, 493, 503
acquired 387–388
causes **386**, 387
congenital 386, **386–387**, 387
management 387
primary **382**, **385**, 437
secondary (pituitary) 381, **385**, 388
subclinical **385**
tertiary (hypothalamic) **385**, 388
hypotonia **118**, 125, 165, 202, 343, **345**, **379**,
386, 389
central 205
peripheral 205, 206
hypoventilation 190, 264, 472
hypoxaemia 1, **2**, 9, 12, 65, **75**, 79, 263, **400**
clinical assessment 9
systemic arterial 72
hypoxic ischaemic encephalopathy (HIE) 44,
48–52, **54**, 58, **164**, 203, 205, **341**
clinical assessment 48–50
definitions 48
HIE score 48, **49**
management 50–52
Sarnat classification of encephalopathy 48

I

ileus 15, 123, 126, **480**, 496
meconium 141, **150**, 487, 489, 492
paralytic 125, 262
immune deficiency 128, **320**
immune thrombocytopaenic purpura
(ITP) 402–403
immunization and infections 247–294
immunization
adverse events 249
missed opportunities 251
practical points 253–254
precautions and contra-indications 251–
253
schedule **247**
immunodeficiency diseases 334–337
primary (PIDs) 250, 270, 334, **335**
secondary (SIDs) 334, 335
immunosuppression and vaccines 252
impacted wax 448
inborn errors of metabolism 52, **75**, 150,

240, 470
infantile colic 145-146, **329**, 503
  clinical features and diagnosis 145
  treatment 145-146
infection in newborns 61-68
  clinical presentation 62-63
  clinical signs and risk factors 62
  definitions **61**
  diagnosis 63-64
  important infections 64-67
  less serious infections 67-68
  local infections 63
  sources 61-62
  systemic infections 63
infections of the CNS 210-217
  cerebral malaria 216-217
  encephalitis 126, 190, **193**, 203, 204, 210, 215-216, **255-256**, 267, 280, 292, 359, 360, **479**
  meningitis 1, 52, 64, 65, 126, 185, 187, 188, 190, 191, **193**, 203, 204, 210-214, 217, **255, 256**, 261, 277, 285, **307, 334, 341, 342**, 359, 453, **479**
  neurocysticercosis 214, 216, 289
  TB meningitis (TBM) 204, 211, 212, **213**, 214, **269**, 269, **272, 273, 274**, 303
infectious mononucleosis 255
infective endocarditis 177-179, 214, 230
  clinical presentation 177-178
  investigations 178
  prophylaxis 179, **179**
  treatment 178-179
inflammatory bowel syndrome 131
influenza **213**, 370
  immunization 142, 248, 251, 253, 305, 399
  incubation period **254**
  virus **213**
inherited bleeding disorders 403-404
  haemophilia A 403
  haemophilia B 403-404
  indications for transfusion of clotting factor 404
  Von Willebrand disease (vWD) 403
injections 529-532
  injection sites 530-532, **531, 532**
injured child 20-38
  background 20
  classification 20, **20**
  management 21, 27-38
  primary survey and resuscitation 21-23
  secondary survey and management 23-27
  statistics 20, **21**
injured eye 446-447
  chemical burns 447
  lacerations 446
  orbit 447
  vitreous haemorrhage 446-447
intellectual disability 52, 214, 339-341, 343
  definitions 339-340
  prevalence 340
intestinal obstruction **164**, 477, 487, 489-490, 492, 503
  clinical presentation, investigations and management 490
  common causes **489**
intrahepatic cholestasis 135
  familial **134**
intrapartum fetal hypoxia 44, 45, 48, 51
intravenous (IV) line placement 526-529
  cut-down tecȲique 528, **529**
  indications and placement 526-527
  intraosseous route 527, **528**
intubation 3, 24, 39, **46**, 71, 73, 173, 182, 189, **192**, 232, 262, 511, 539
  emergency 540
  endotracheal 7, **8, 11**, 11, 25, 42, 101, 103, 109, 111, 539-541, **541**
  equipment 103
  nasal 540-541, **541**
  nasogastric 534
  oral 540, **541**
  tecȲique 103, **103**
intussusception 131, 132, 145, **150**, 497, 502-503, 505
  clinical presentation, investigation and management 503
iron deficiency anaemia **154**, 171, 200, 242, 279, 293, 355, 358, **395**, 396, 502
Isospora belli 279
  clinical features, diagnosis and treatment 279

J

jaundice 44, **54**, 63, 65, 66, **80, 135**, 136, 138, 142, 146, 224, 253, **254**, 277, 280, 282, 313, 394, **398, 400**, 497, 504
  approach 132-134
  cholestatic 497
  haemolytic 79
  [*see also* haemolytic disease of the newborn]
  neonatal 74-82
  obstructive 141
  [*see also* neonatal jaundice]
  prolonged 79-82, **386**
  recurrent 394, 399

K

kala azar 142
kangaroo mother care (KMC) 44, 54, 56-57, 60
  advantages 57
  forms 57
Kawasaki syndrome **255**, 258-259, **441**
  diagnosis and clinical features 258
  treatment 259
keratomalacia **153**
Klebsiella spp 62, 406
Kleihauer test for fetal cells 50
kwashiorkor 142, **155**, 270

L

lacerations
  simple 27
  tongue 28
lactose intolerance 127, 145, 146, **164**
Landau response **346**, **347**
Langerhans cell histiocytosis (LCH) 142, **144**
laryngeal cleft 110, 111
laryngeal incompetence 95, 110, 111
  diagnosis and treatment 111
laryngitis 99, **99**, 151
laryngomalacia **91**, 95–96, 459
  congenital 95
  complex 95, 96
  diagnosis and investigations 95
  management 95–96
  simple 95
leishmaniasis 142
leukaemia **143**, 185, 204, 271, **397**, 402, 404, 405, **430**, 459
  chronic myeloid (CML) 142, **143**
level of consciousness (LOC) 23, **49**, 183, 284
  abnormal 48
  altered 189, **364–365**, **370**, **392**
  assessment 18
  depressed 12, 15, 42, 122, 188, 215, 282, 285, **464**, 472
  deteriorating 24, 188, 213
  disturbed 236, 240
limb and bone injuries 26–27
lipid storage disease 142
lipodystrophy 204
Listeria monocytogenes 212, **213**
liver failure 51, 313, **372**
  acute (ALF) 137–139
  chronic, complications and management **140**
low birthweight infants 44, 53–57, **54**, 62, 66, 70, 85, **377**
  definitions 53–54
  fluids and feeding 55–56
  kangaroo mother care (KMC) 44, 54, 56–57, 60
  problems and care 54–55
lumbar puncture 52, 64, 190, 191, 194, 210, 214, 272, 285, 515, 521, 527
  contra-indications 188, **191**, 261
  technique 532–533, **533**
lymphadenopathy 156, 165, 280, 290, 394, 426, 428, **430**
  cervical 258, 498
  generalized **296**, **305**
  localized 405
  mediastinal 275
  regional 266
  tuberculous 263

M

macrocephaly 184
macroglossia 489, 503
magnesium homeostasis 477, 486

[*see also* hypermagnesaemia; hypomagnesaemia]

magnetic resonance imaging (MRI) 50, 206, 210, 214, 215, 216, 223, 243, 244, 289, **342**, 343, 493, 497
major depressive disorder (MDD) 360–361
  definition and symptoms 360
  diagnosis 360–361
  treatment 361
malabsorption 126, 127, **163**, **164**, 165, 279, 292, **377**, **389**, **390**, 396, **484**
malaria 142, 162, 281–288, 294, **372**, **397**
  cerebral 216–217
  clinical features 281–282
  definition and diagnosis 281
  management of complications 285–286
  prevention 287–28, **288**
  rapid antigen test 216, 281
  recurrent **143**
  severe 281, 282, 283, 284, 286, 288
  treatment 282–284, **286–287**
  uncomplicated 281, 282, 283
Malassezia furfur 414
malnutrition 126, 127, **140**, 142, **144**, 153–161, 162, 252, 269, 270, 340, **341**, **372**
  acute 155
  chronic 155, **482**
  classification 154–155, **155**
  familial **342**
  moderate 155–156, **155**, **306**
  nutritional assessment 153–154, **153–154**
  oedematous 155, 156
  protein-energy 334
  severe 122, 123, 125, 141, 156–161, **153–154**, **155**, 161, 162, 166, **307**, 466, **482**, **484**
malrotation 128, **150**, 151, **164**, **489**, 491
Mantoux method [*see* tuberculin (Mantoux) test]
mastoiditis 450, 452–453
  acute 453
  acute-on-chronic 452
mean corpuscular volume **394**
measles 161, **213**, 215, **256**, 259–260, 269, 270, 294, 334, 406
  clinical features and diagnosis 259
  immunisation **247**, 253
  immunoglobulin 260
  incubation period **254**
  treatment and prophylaxis 260
  vaccine 159, 248, 251, 252, 253
Meckel's diverticulum 131, 132, 503
meconium aspiration syndrome (MAS) 54, 69, 70–71, **341**
  definition, clinical features, and diagnosis 70
  treatment and prevention 71
meconium ileus 141, **150**, 487, **489**, 492
  management 492
meconium plug syndrome **489**, 493
meningeal irritation 211

meningism 260
meningitis 1, 52, 64, 65, 126, 185, 187, 188, 190, 191, **193**, 203, 204, 210–214, 217, **255**, 256, 261, 277, 285, **307**, 334, **341**, **342**, 359, 453, **479**
  aseptic 211, **255**
  bacterial 63, 211, 212, **213**, 216, 285, 303
  causes **213**
  meningococcal 212, **254**, **256**, 303
  treatment **67**, 189, 212, 216
  tuberculous (TBM) 204, 211, 212, **213**, 214, **269**, 269, **272**, **273**, **274**, 303
  viral 211, 212, **213**, 215, 262
meningococcal
  meningitis 212, **254**, **256**, 303
  disease treatment **262**
  infection 294
  septicaemia **191**, 260–262, **262**
  vaccine 248–249
meningococcal septicaemia (meningococcaemia) **191**, 260–262
  clinical features 260
  diagnosis 261
  prophylaxis 262, **262**
  treatment 261–262
meningomyelocele 64, 186, 434, 438
mesangiocapillary GN (MCGN) 230
metabolic acidosis **40**, 65, 73, 89, 126, 139, 236, 239, 240, 262, 282, 285, **373**, **468**, **469**, 470, 470–471
  high anion gap 470
  normal anion gap 470
methaemoglobinaemia 11, **41**, 43
microcephaly 165, 184, 280, **379**
micronutrient deficiency 127, 159, 302
middle ear cleft 450, 451
Miller Fisher syndrome 202
mitochondrial disorders 201, 204, 210, **470**
monitoring equipment 3–4
  automated blood pressure monitor **4**
  blood gas analyzer **4**
  brain activity monitor **4**
  cardiac monitor **4**
  end-tidal CO$_2$ monitor **3**
  glucometer **4**
  invasive pressure monitoring facility **4**
  radiology services **3**
  saturation monitor **4**
monkeypox **255**
mood disorder 355
movement disorders 201–203
mucopolysaccharidosis 144
multi-organ failure 51, 116
mumps **213**, 215, 504
  incubation period **254**
  vaccine 248, 251, 254
Mycoplasma 204, 215, **397**
  pneumoniae **106**, 107
myoclonus 48, 195, 196, **198**, 203
myositis 111

N

Nail-patella syndrome 230
nasal obstruction in the neonate 454
nasal prong oxygen 13, 24, 70, 71, 72, 97, **97**, 324
natal cleft 187, 415
neck stiffness 185, 211
Neisseria
  gonorrhoeae (gonococcus) 62, 267, 443, 444
  meningitidis (diplococcus) **213**, **256**, 260, 261, 443
nematodes 290–293
  Ancylostoma caninum/braziliense 290–291
  Ancylostoma duodenale 291, 292, 293
  Ascaris lumbricoides 291
  Enterobius vermicularis 292
  Necator americanus 291, 292, 293
  Strongyloides stercoralis 292
  Toxocariasis (visceral larva migrans) 292–293
  Trichuris trichiura 293
neonatal jaundice 74–82
  assessment and management 76–77
  breastfeeding 74, 75, 76
  breastmilk 74–75
  early onset 76
  onset after 24 hours 76–77
  pathological 75–76
  physiological 74
  treatment 77–79
neonatal problems 44–87
neonatal seizures 52–53, **199**
  causes and diagnosis 52
  clinical presentation 52
  definition 52
  treatment 53
nephritis 243, **256**, 259, 413
  acute 229, **255**
  interstitial 230
nephropathy
  hepatitis B-associated 231
  HIV-associated **307**
  IgA (Berger's disease) 229
  reflux 241, **243**
nephrotic syndrome 230, 232–236, **478**
  definition and clinical presentation 232
  investigation **233**
  management of oedema 235
  minimal change (MCNS) 232, **234**
  relapses 235–236
  treatment **234**
nervous system and neuromuscular disorders 183–217
neuroblastoma **143**, 404
neurocysticercosis 204, 216, 289
  clinical presentation 216
  diagnosis 216, 289
  management 216
neurological disease/disorders 1, **185**, 186, 217, 218, 264, **377**

focal signs 24, 189, **191**, 1914, 210, 211, 215
general signs 64, 142, 184, 236, **365**, **405**, **442**
localized and progressive signs 24, 214
infections 1
[see also meningitis; meningoencephalitis]
static 252
neurological
  assessment/examination 18, 5, 52, 148, 183, 220, 441
  deterioration 186, 259, **365**
  emergency 196
  equipment **5**
  intoxication 1
  management 19
  manifestations in HIV 302–303
  monitoring 18, 244, **365**
  status/function, change in **3**, 286
  weakness 1
neuromuscular
  disease 1, 339, 460
  dysfunction 111
  irritability **484**
neuro-regression 183, 195, 196, 210
Niemann Pick disease **144**
night blindness **153**
noisy breathing 89–91, 95, 99, 109, 119
  approach to 89–91
  relationship between noise and obstruction **90**
  site of obstruction 89–91, **90**, **91**
  [see also airway obstruction]
nosocomial infections 2, 12, 105, 286
nutrient deficiency 56, 153, 161–162, 164, **164**
  [see also vitamin deficiency]
  clinical features **153**–**154**
  micronutrient 127, 159, 302
  zinc 162

O

obesity 243, 375, 376, 379
  causes **376**
  clinical features suggesting a possible genetic syndrome **379**
  consequences **379**
  definition 376
  management 379
obstructive sleep apnoea 219, 220, **379**, 457, 458
  syndrome (OSA/OSAS) 107
occult spinal dysraphism 186–187
oedema 20, 65, 67, 173, 231, 291, **478**, **479**, 502
  abdominal/gut 174, 227, 231, 489, 495, 496
  angio-oedema **329**, 332–333
  cerebral 33, 42, 49, 138, 213, 215, 216, 260, 261, 262, 289, 363, **365**, 474, 476, **479**, 511
  conjunctival 444
  corneal 442, 443
  endotracheal 540

eyelid 444
facial 413
generalized 232
laryngeal **329**
lymphoedema 421
malnutrition 141, 153, **154**, **155**, 156, 158, 159, 160, 467
myxoedema **387**
palms and soles 258, 513
papilloedema 187, 190, 472, 533
post-operatic 503
pulmonary 42, 89, 96, **108**, 172, 177, 231, 232, 235, 236, 239, 243, 285, 536
renal 235, 236
scrotal 506
symmetrical 153, **155**
tissue, 19, 499
oedematous malnutrition 141, 153, **154**, **155**, 156, 158, 159, 160, 467
oesophagitis 146, **150**, 151, 505
  eosinophilic 152, 328
  gastro-oesophageal reflux-induced 111
  reflux 145
oligohydramnios 490
omphalitis 63, 67, 507
oppositional defiant disorder 355
organisation of work environment 2
organomegaly 205
osteomyelitis 65, **334**, 524
  acute haematogenous (AHO) 431–432
  chronic 431
otitis
  externa (diffuse, 'swimmer's ear') 449
  externa (furunculosis) 449
  media **193**, 259, **306**, 494, 515, 534
otitis media **193**, 259, **306**, 494, 515, 534
  active chronic 450–452
  acute 449–450
  cholesteatoma 451
  inactive chronic 451
  with effusion (glue ear) 452
outflow tract obstruction
  left ventricular **168–169**
  right ventricular 168, **168–169**, 170, 171
oxygen therapy 9, **10–11**, 15, 41
  [see also resuscitation equipment]
  positive pressure ventilation **11**
  T-piece ventilation **10**

P

pain management in children 512–519
  assessment and measurement of pain 513
  drugs **518–519**
  FLACC scale 513
  non-pharmacological treatment 517
  principles of treatment 514–516
  pharmacological treatment 516–517
  weaning from opioids and benzodiazepines 517–518
palliative care 508–512, **508**
  definition 508–509

goals 509
good practice 510–512
withholding/withdrawal of life-saving care 509–510
palliative care and pain management 508–520
palpation 7, 92, 223
pancreatitis 141, **150**, 313, **314**, **392**, 497
panic attacks **319**
pansinusitis 214
papillomatosis
laryngeal **99**
respiratory 459
parathyroid hormone 27, 242, 391–392
management of disorders **391**
treatment of disorders **392**
paratyphoid fever 294
parenteral
diarrhoea 121
nutrition 55, **75**, **129**, **134**, 166, 477
steroids 101
transmission of hepatitis 136
treatment 284, **287**, **370**, 422
vaccination 249
parotid enlargement **306**, 504
paroxysms 93, 94, 183, 200–201, **254**, 263
benign paroxysmal vertigo 201
pseudoseizures 201
reflex anoxic attacks 200
syncope (fainting) 174, 181, 201, 522, 536
parvovirus B19 **255**, **395**, **400**
patent ductus arteriosus (PDA) **54**, 73–74, 89, **168–169**
definition, clinical features and diagnosis 73
treatment 73–74
pathogens 93, 105, **108**, 113, 117, 126, 127, **129**, 300, 406, 414, 450
pCO$_2$ 50, 189, 468, **468**, 471, 472
end-tidal monitor 3
end-tidal monitoring 11
suitable levels 12
percussion 92, 96, 110, 536
pericardial disease 180
clinical presentation, investigation and management 180
periodontitis **306**
peripheral airway obstruction (PAO) **90**, **91**, 92–94, 96, 110, 112, **112**, 113, 119
acute 92
bilateral air trapping (BAT) 92–93, **92**, 96, 110
chronic 92
coughs and colds 93–94
GORD-associated [see gastro-oesophageal reflux disease (GORD)]
persistent/recurrent **92**, 93, 110, 111
peritonitis 26, 67, 131, **233**, **269**, 291, 292, 492, 496, 503, 522, 538
persistent diarrhoea (PD) 123, 126–129, **129**, 161, 162, **297**, **306**, 486

definitions 126–127
diagnosis 127–128
treatment 128–129, **129**
persistent pulmonary hypertension **54**, 72–73, **234**
definition and clinical features 72
diagnosis and treatment 73
Perthes' disease **427**, 430, 436–437, **436**
pertussis 93, 263, 270
clinical features, diagnosis and treatment 263
incubation period **254**
treatment 94
vaccine **247**, 249, 252
Peutz-Jeghers syndrome 131
phimosis 499
phosphate homeostasis 477, 486
[see also hyperphosphataemia and hypophosphataemia]
phototherapy 75, 76, 77–78, 79, **81**, 420
guidelines **80**
Pierre Robin syndrome 109, 494
Plasmodium
falciparum 281, 282, 286
knowlesi 281
malariae 281, **287**
ovale 281, 286, **287**
vivax 281, 286, **287**
platyhelminths and cestodes 289–290
cysticercosis 289
Echinococcus spp 289–290
Hymenolepis spp 289
Taenia solium 216, 289
pleural collections 115–118
aseptic **116**, 117
classification **116**
diagnosis 115
empyema 106, 115, **116**, 116–118
management **116**, 117–118
pyopneumothorax 115, **116**, 116–118
treatment **116**, 116–117
pleural drainage 535
pneumatosis intestinalis 64, 65
Pneumococcus spp (ex: *Streptococcus pneumoniae*) **398**, 431, 432, 443, 496
pneumonia 64, 69, 89, 93, 104–107, 111, 127, **255**, **256**, 259, 263, 277, 285, 292, **297**, 301, 302, **334**, 360, 413, 462, 466, 472, **479**, 491
antibiotic therapy 105–107, **106**
aspiration **108**, 151, 286
bacterial 300–301, **306–307**, 444
bronchopneumonia **91**, **92**
clinical features 104, **105**
community acquired (CAP) 104
congenital 71
diagnosis 104
necrotizing 114
of the newborn 71
treatment 105
viral 110, 112, 301, **306–307**

pneumonitis 70, 267, 280, 291, 292
  acute transient (Loeffler's syndrome) 291
  chemical **40**
  lymphoid interstitial (LIP) **297**, 302, **306**, **320**
pneumothorax 16, 69, 71–72, 115, 488, 536
  clinical features, diagnosis, and treatment 72
  definition 71
  drain **13**
pO_2 189
poliomyelitis 206, 264, 294
  abortive 264
  clinical features, diagnosis and treatment 264
  incubation period **254**
  non-paralytic 264
  paralytic 248, 264
  vaccine **247**
polyarthritis 255, **430**
  differential diagnosis **428**
  migrating 175
  rheumatoid-factor negative **428**
  rheumatoid-factor positive **428**
polycystic ovary syndrome 379
polycythaemia 54, 58, 73, **75**, 76, 109
polyhydramnios 490, 491
polyps
  'cherry tumour' 507
  distal 130
  intestinal 131
  nasal 327
  rectal 505
  suspected 132
portal hypertensive gastropathy 131
Prader-Willi syndrome 376, **377**
precocious puberty 382–384
  aetiology of gonadotrophin-dependent **382**
  aetiology of gonadotrophin-independent **382**
  approach **383, 384**
  classification **385**
  definition 382
primary ciliary dyskinesia syndrome **320**
primary immunodeficiency diseases (PIDs) 250, 270, 334, 335
  common manifestations **334**
  diagnosis 337, **338**
  treatment 336–337
procedures 521–544
  general principles 521
  restraints 521
proctocolitis 505
  allergic 123, 130, 132, 328
progressive multifocal leukoencephalopathy (PML) 307
protein losing enteropathy (PLE) 127
protein sensitization 130
prothrombin ratio (INR) 136, 138, 159, 179, 401, **401**

pruritis 291, 336
  ani 292
  vulvovaginal 280
pseudoataxia 201
pseudohypoparathyroidism **391, 392, 482**
Pseudomonas
  aeruginosa 113, 141, 406
  spp 443, 450
puberty 379–385
  abnormal 382–385
  delayed 382, 385, **385**
  physical changes 379, **380–381**
  precocious 382–384
pulse oximetry 9, 97, 104, 167, **324**
pulsus paradoxus 100, **100**, **324**
purpura 66, **256**, 260, 332, 394, 404
  conjunctival 260
  fulminans 402
  immune thrombocytopaenic (ITP) 402–403
  Henoch-Schönlein 131, 230, **234**, **441**
  skin 260
pustules 421, **S1**
  satellite 413, **S5**
  scalp 415, **S7**
  skin 63, 68, 408, 415
  superficial **S12**
pyloric stenosis **150**, **164**, **469**, 472, **489**, 504
  clinical presentation 504
  complications 504–505
  diagnosis and management 505
pyogenic
  abscess 495
  infection 115, **116**, 117, **211**, **430**, 504
  spondylitis 433
pyopneumothorax 115, **116**, 116–118

R

rabies 28, 264–265
  clinical features 264
  passive immunisation 253
  post-exposure prophylaxis and treatment 265
  vaccine 249
raised intracranial pressure 187–189
  causes 187
  clinical features 187–188
  investigations 188
  management 188–189
rectal prolapse 141, 293, 505
recurrent abdominal pain syndrome (RAPS) 146–147
  clinical features 146–147
  treatment 147
red cell abnormalities
  congenital **397**
  microenvironment **397**
red eye (unilateral) 445
  herpes simplex 444
  phlyctenular conjunctivitis 269, 445
red eyes with purulent discharge 443–444

purulent conjunctivitis 443
  ophthalmia neonatorum 444–445
red eyes with watery discharge 444
  viral conjunctivitis (epidemic pink eye) 444
red itchy eyes 444–445
  acute rhinoconjunctivitis (allergic conjunctivitis) 444
  vernal conjunctivitis 445
regurgitation 95, 110, 149, 176
  aortic 176, 177
  mitral 176, 177, **177**
renal failure **41**, 126, 139, 158, 228, 231, 232, **234**, 237, **256**, 262, 267, 282, 285, 461, 462, **469**, **470**, 478, **482**, **484**
  acute 236–241, 284
  chronic 219, 241–242, 543
  intrinsic 51
  oligo-anuric 230
replacement fluids 463–467
  ongoing losses 467
  rehydration 465–467
  resuscitation 463–465
respiratory 19, 43, 114, 115, **140**, 142, 151, 162, 171, **192**, **255**, 301, 328, **329**, 330, 331, 332, **377**, **387**, 460, 468, 488, 514, 516, 544
  acidosis **468**, **469**, 472
  alkalosis 139, **468**, **469**, 472
  arrest 2, **3**
  decompensation 22
  disease 1, 44, 170, 180
  distress 2, 12, **40**, 63, 65, 66, 68, 69, 70, 71, 72, 160, 167, 169, 363, **400**, 402, 487, 488
  drive **8**, 9
  effort 12, **45**, 47, 50, 107, 109, 454, 472
  failure 25, 39, 68, 141, 257, 264, **469**
  function **15**, 117
  infection 88, 93, 96, 104, 121, 142, 158, 162, 171, 236, 252, 257, 301, 302, **306**, **320**, 335, 449, 450, 451, 455, 456, 458, 459
  muscle dysfunction 118, **118**
  rate 9, 12, 18, 57, 89, **89**, 94, 104, 158, 160, 284, 465
  secretions **8**, 104, 301, 511
  surgery **179**
  system 50, 92, 165, 207, 257
respiratory disease 1, 44, 170, 180
  of the newborn 68–74
respiratory distress **2**, 12, **40**, 63, 65, 66, 68, 69, 70, 71, 72, 160, 167, 169, 363, **400**, 402, 487, 488
  acute respiratory distress disorder (ARDS) 282
respiratory muscle dysfunction 118
  assessment **118**
respiratory problems 88–120
respiratory syncytial virus (RSV) 96, 98
resuscitation 1, 2, **5**, 5, 9, 19, 21, 25, 26, 39, 44, 60, 71, 130, **140**, 172, 182, 191, **234**, 261, 262, 329, 332, **364**, **365**, **400**, 406, 471, **479**, 490, 496, 497, 503, 514, 526
  area **3**, **4**
  at birth 44–47
  cardiopulmonary (CPR) 510
  'do not resuscitate' orders 510
  equipment 4–5, **4–5**
  fluid **5**, 14, 17, 22, 122, 285, 463–465, 469
  primary survey and 21–23
resuscitation at birth 44–47
  Apgar score 45, **45**
  birth asphyxia 44, **54**, 72, **81**, 402
  clinical features and treatment 45–47
  intrapartum fetal hypoxia 44, 45, 48, 51
  neonatal resuscitation algorithm **46**
resuscitation equipment 4–5, **4–5**
  3-way taps and syringes **5**
  bag-mask ventilation **5**, **10**
  buretrols **5**
  cannulae **5**, **10**
  endotracheal tubes **4**
  facemasks **5**, **10**
  fluid **5**
  Guedel airway **4**, 7
  hard collars **4**
  head boxes **5**, **10**
  head locks **4**
  intra-osseous needles **5**
  laryngoscope **4**
  McGill's forceps **4**
  paediatric 2, **3**, **4**, 4, 5
  opthalmoscope **5**
  refrigerator with O-negative blood **5**
  spinal boards **4**
  suctioning equipment **4**
  surgical airway equipment **4**
  tubing and connections **5**
reticuloendothelial hyperplasia 142, **143**
retinoblastoma 441, 446
Reye's syndrome 138, **144**, 150
Rhesus disease 58, **75**
  prevention 77, 79
rheumatic carditis 176, **176**, 179
rheumatic chorea **176**
rheumatic fever (RF) 175–177, 202, **256**, 294, **425**, 428, **430**, 458
  acute **428**
  diagnosis 175–176, **176**
  Duckett-Jones criteria 175, **176**
  prevention 177, **177**
  treatment 176–177
rhinitis 252, 323, **329**
  allergic (AR) 325–328
  medicamentosa 327
  non-allergic with eosinophilia syndrome (NARES) 327
  vasomotor 327
rhinosinusitis 455–456, 457
rhinovirus 96
rickets 92, 162, 236, 389–390, **391**, **426**, 435, 436
  approach and treatment **163**, 390, **390**

causes **389**
clinical features **389**
definition 389
hypophosphataemic **163**, **389**
renal 437
vitamin D deficiency 162, **482**
Rickettsia africae 266
rickety rosary **154**
roseola infantum **256**
rotational variations in children: in-toeing and out-toeing 435
rotatory subluxation **185**
rotor syndrome **134**
rubella 62, 64, **133**, **143**, **213**, 215, **256**, **340**, 453
congenital 446, 454
incubation period **254**
vaccine 248, 251, 252

S

Salmonella
spp 286, **297**
typhi 249277
saturation
acceptable levels 11–12
discharge 167
mixed venous (central) 6, **15**, 15, 16
monitoring of **11**, 15, 69, 108, **192**
normal 167
oxygen 9, 15, 25, 50, 55, 73, 97, 98, 99, 100, 105, 169, 172, 262, 543
transcutaneous 170, 172
scarlet fever **256**
incubation period **254**
Schistosoma
haematobium 290
mansoni 290
sclerema 61, 65
scleroderma 111, **425**
seizures 18, 39, 42, 44, 45, 48, 58, 64, 123, 126, 183, 191, **191**, 192–194, 195, 197, 200, 201, 210, 211, 213, 231, 239, 240, 280, 285, 289, 303, 341, **342**, 343, 344, 356, **373**, **389**, 470, 473, 474, **479**, **482**
absence [*see* epilepsy]
acute convulsions 192, **193**
apyrexial **193**
clonic [*see* epilepsy]
documentation 18
epilepsy [*see* epilepsy]
febrile 126, 194
focal 24, 52, 214
generalized 24, 52, 194
intractable 53, **199**
monitoring 19
myoclonic [*see* epilepsy]
neonatal 52–53, **199**
partial 194, 195, 197, **199**, **200**, 216
pyrexial **193**
recurrent and persistent 50, 53, 216
status epilepticus 52, 192, **199**

subclinical 49
tonic clonic [*see* epilepsy]
treatment 24, 188, 198, **199**, 216, 217, **475**
sepsis 16, 28, 43, 51, 52, 53, 79, **81**, 112, 115, 200, 205, 206, **341**, **365**, **372**, **464**, **469**, 493, 505
abdominal 496
chronic ear 214
congenital 44
dental 214
Gram negative 212
intracranial 452, 453, 455
non-specific 64
orbital 455
salicylate **469**
skin 68, **191**
venous 16
septicaemia 58, 65, 67, 132, **133**, 139, **143**, **226**, 236, 286, **334**, 402, 431, 432, 471, **482**
meningococcal **191**, 260–262
severe malnutrition 122, 123, 125, 141, 157–161, **153–154**, **155**, 161, 162, 166, **307**, 466, **482**, 484
definition, clinical presentation and investigations 156
treatment 156–161
sexually transmitted infections 267–268
diagnosis 267
treatment **268**
Shigella spp 121, 125, 126, 130
shingles **255**
Shirodkar suture 62
shock 1, 13–18, 26, 39, 71, 126, 167, **168**, 172, 182, **191**, 217, 236, 238, 252, **256**, 257, 261, 262, 285, **364**, **373**, 465, **466**, 467, **469**, 470, **470**, 497, 522, 527, 535
anaphylactic **13**
and dehydration 121–126
assessment 121–122, **364**
cardiogenic **13**, 181, 468
cardiovascular 65
cardiovascular signs 14
circulatory 22, 25, 260
clinical signs **14–15**
dissociative **13**
hypovolaemic **13**, 122, 132, 257, 260, 285, 463, **464**, 464, 468
management priorities 16
neurogenic (spinal) **13**, 24
obstructive **13**
oxygen therapy 9
septic **13**, 172, 277, 462, 471
severe **4**, 26
treatment **4**, 6, 16, 39, 65, 122, 124, 158, 261, 262, 373, **465**
types and causes **13**
short stature 375–376
definition 375
differential diagnosis 375, **377**
management 378
target heights 375

sickle cell anaemia 142, **397**, **398**, 398–400
  crises 398
  diagnosis 399
  management 399–400
sickle cell disease 204, 220, 228
single gene defects **376**
sinusitis 190, **306**, 320, 323, 327, 335, 534
skeletal tuberculosis 433–434
  spinal tuberculosis 433
  tuberculous arthritis 433–434
sleep-disordered breathing (SDB) 107–109
  adverse effects **108**
  diagnosis, treatment, and emergency airway relief 109
  examination 108–109
  history 108
slipped upper femoral epiphysis (SUFE) 437–438
small-bowel obstruction
  distal 491
  proximal 491
spherocytosis 75, **397**
spider naevi 131
spina bifida 186–187, **222**, 223, 505
splenomegaly 142, 156, 178, **255**, 277
  causes 142
spO₂ **2**
squint (strabismus) 184, **185**, 189, 346, 405, 440, 441, 447, 506
  acquired deviations 441
  congenital deviations 441
  constant 441
  non-paralytic (concomitant) 441
  paralytic 441
Staphylococcus
  aureus 62, 68, 106, **116**, 117, 141, 178, 300, 406, 410, 431
  epidermidis 406
  resistant 432
  spp 255, 449, 450
status epilepticus **4**, 52, 192
  management **192**, **198–199**
statutory notifiable diseases 293–294
steatohepatitis 379
steatorrhoea 127, 141
stenosis 119, 499
  anal 493
  aortic 168, 172
  congenital subglottic **99**
  duodenal **489**, 491
  intestinal 487
  laryngeal 459
  meatal 503–504
  mitral 168, **176**, 177
  oesophageal **119**
  pulmonary 168, 171
  pyloric **150**, 164, **469**, 472, **489**, 504–505
  renal artery **246**
  small bowel **489**
  tracheal **119**, 459
stertor 7

Stills disease (RA) **143**
Streptococcus
  group A β-haemolytic 175, 202, **256**, 431, 458
  group B (GBS) 62, 63, 71, 212
  pneumoniae (see also *Pneumococcus* spp) **116**, 117, 212, **213**, 300, 449
  pyogenes 410
  spp 62, 255, 431, 432
  viridans 178, 406
stridor 7, 89, **90**, 100, 104, 151, 269, 270, **482**
  acute 459
  chronic 459–460
  inspiratory 99, 100
  laryngeal 459
Sturge-Weber syndrome 204
sudden infant death syndrome (SIDS) **108**, 152, 249
surgical problems 487–507
syphilis 37, 62, 64, 66–67, 82, **133**, 267, 318
  congenital 66, **66**, 75, 79, 294
  conjugated hyperbilirubinaemia 133
  conjunctivitis **67**
  hepatosplenomegaly **143**
  secondary 419
  treatment **268**
  VDRL 37, 66, **135**, **233**, 419, 424
systemic lupus erythematosis (SLE) **143**, 181, 204, 230, 231, **234**, **250**, **397**, 415, **428**, 428

T

tachycardia 3, **14**, **17**, **40**, 62, 73, 101, 122, 180, **245**, **246**, 260, 328, 496
  broad complex 182
  narrow complex 181–182
  persistent resting 177
  supraventricular (SVT) 181
  ventricular 181
tachypnoea 3, 24, **40**, 70, 73, 92, 96, 97, 98, 104, **105**, 115, 118, 169, 171, 172, 173, 236, 282
  persistent 68
  'quiet' 70
  transient (TTN) 69, 70
Takayasu's disease/arteritis 204, **243**, 243, 425
tall stature 376
  definition and management 376
  differential diagnosis 376, **378**
Tay Sachs disease 144
TB
  chest radiography 271
  clinical features 269, **269**
  culture 271
  diagnosis 270–271
  [see also tuberculin (Mantoux) test]
  diagnostic certainty 272
  drug-susceptible 275
  drug-resistant 276
  extensively drug resistant (XDR) 268

extrapulmonary 268
interferon-gamma release assays 271
investigation **272**
isoniazid 277
meningitis (TBM) 204, 211, 212, **213**, 214, **269**, 269, **272**, **273**, **274**, 303
multi-drug resistant (MDR) 268
Mycobacterium tuberculosis complex 180, **213**, 250, 268, 269, 272
nodal compression 118, 120
pre-XDR 269
pulmonary 268
rifampicin 277
skeletal 433–434
treatment and prophylaxis **273–274**, **275**
tension pneumothorax 13, 21, 22, 25, 71–72, 116, 117, 535
clinical features, diagnosis, and treatment 72
definition 71
tetanus 265–266, 294, **336**
cephalic 265
clinical features 265
immunization **247**, 253
immunoglobulin (HTIG) 265, 266
incubation period **254**
local 265
neonatorum 294
prevention 266
prophylaxis 27
toxoid vaccine 27, 28, 266
treatment 265–266
tetany 126, 472, **482**
thoracentesis 537
thorax injuries 24–25
thrombocytopaenia 51, 65, **255**, 256, 267, 302, 400, 402–403, 500
chronic **306**
idiopathic 204, 403
thrombocytosis 428
thrush 29, 63, 68, **99**, 334, 413–414
thyroid function 79, **135**, 148, 387
thyroid gland disorders **154**, 360, 385–388
laboratory values **385**
thyroiditis 388
tick bite fever 266–267
clinical features 266–267
definition 266
diagnosis and treatment 267
tics 203, 356, 357
tinea (dermatophyte) infections 415–417
tinea capitis 415, **S6**, **S7**
tinea corporis 415, 419, **S8**
tinea cruris 415
tinea faciei 415
tinea manuum 415
tinea pedis 415
tinea unguium (onchomycosis) 415
tinea versicolor 414, **S6**
treatment 415–417
Todd's paresis 204

tongue tie 506–507
tonsillectomy 403, 458
tonsillitis 102, 370, 458, 515
acute pseudomembranous 459
clinical features, treatment 458
torsion
testicular appendage 506
testis 145, 506, 507
tibial 435
torticollis ('wry neck') 185, **185**, 506
totally obstructed episodes (TOES) 107, 109
Tourette syndrome 203, 355
toxic shock syndrome **256**
Toxoplasma gondii 280, **340**
clinical features, diagnosis and treatment 280
tracheo-bronchial obstruction 93, 119–120
causes **119**
diagnosis 119–120
TB nodal compression 118, 120
tracheomalacia **119**, **320**
tracheostomy 7, 96, 109, 265, 538
transient synovitis of the hip 432–433
transient tachypnoea of the newborn (TTN) 69, 70
definition, clinical features, diagnosis, and treatment 70
trauma 1
traumatic stress 361–362
clinical features and diagnosis 361–362
post-traumatic stress disorder (PTSD) 362
treatment 362
trematodes 290
schistosomiasis (bilharzia) **143**, 290
tremor 203, 208, **349**, 388, **482**
triage 2, 124
systems 2
Trichomonas vaginalis 267, **268**, 280
clinical features, diagnosis and treatment 280
tuberculin (Mantoux) test (TST) 104, **116**, 117, 120, 156, 180, **233**, 243, 270–271, 304, **430**, **433**, 434, 445, 498, 530
causes of false negative 470–471
causes of false positive 271
tuberculoma 185, 216, **269**
tuberculosis [see TB]
tumour
bony 131
brain 184, 185, 187, 189, 204, 206, 243, **377**, **382**, **383**, 404
'cherry' 507
infancy 500
intra-abdominal 128
kidney **229**
lysis syndrome **482**
necrosis factor a 430
parotid 504
pituitary 437
posterior fossa 185, 201
primary 185

pseudotumour cerebri **379**
pyloric/'olive' 505
soft tissue 131
solid **397**
spinal 405
sternomastoid **185**, 506
thyroid **388**
Wilm's **243**
typhoid **143**, 270
 incubation period **254**
 vaccine 249, 253
typhoid fever 277–278, 294
 diagnosis 277–278
 rose spots 277
 treatment 278
tyrosinaemia **144**
 type 1 **134**

U

ulcer 250, 445
 duodenal **150**
 gastric **150**
 meatal 503
 peptic 131, 146
ulcerative
 colitis 130
 gingivitis/periodontitis **306**
ultrasound
 abdominal 128, 132, **135**, 147, **272**, 279, 495, 497, 503, 505
 antenatal 488, 490, 491
 appendix 496
 cardiac 180, **272**
 cranial 49, 50, 52, 184, 289
 hip 434, 435
 kidneys **233**, 236, 237, 243
 liver 138, 495, 497
 pleural 116
 retinal 447
 thoracic 536
 thyroid 387
 urinary tract 66, 223, **226**, 227, 237, 493
umbilicus 507
unconjugated hyperbilirubinaemia 75, **75–76**, 79, 132, 133
 complications 79
undescended testis 507
urinary
 catecholamines 243
 incontinence **40**
 output 173, 238
 reducing substances 166
urinary incontinence **40**, 222–224
 daytime 222–224
 in children 218–224
urinary tract
 abnormalities 186, 335, 493
 abscess 279
 infections [see the main entry for urinary tract infections]
 injury 26
 obstruction 237, 238
urinary tract infections 62, 65–66, 79, 127, **164**, 219, 223, 224–227, 231, 496, 405, 537
 clinical presentation 224
 diagnosis 224, **225**
 investigation **226**
 lower (LUT) 219, 220
 management **225**
 prophylaxis 66, **67**, 158–159
 recurrent 220, 227
urine collection 538–539
 'clean catch' and bladder catheterization 538
 suprapubic aspiration 538–539
urticaria **329**, 332–333
 acute ordinary 332
 chronic 332, 333
 classification 332
 clinical evaluation 332–333
 contact 333
 definition 332
 episodic 332
 investigations 333
 physical 332–333
 treatment 333
 urticarial vasculitis 332

V

variceal haemorrhage 131, 132
varicella 201, **213**, 215, 257, 270, 406
varicella zoster 204, 253, **255**
 immune globulin (VZIG) 257, 406
 vaccination status **233**
 vaccine 248, 257
varices
 acute bleeding **140**
 gastric 131, **150**
 oesophageal 130, 131, **150**
vaso-active drugs 17, **17–18**
ventilation 7, **8**, 12–13, 25, **46**, 62, 71, 73, 173, **192**, 232, 452, **469**, 472, 488
 adequate 24, 47, 53
 assisted 22, 24, 25, 71, 96, 98, **118**, 170, 207, 262, 263
 bag mask **5**, **10**
 baseline assessment 11
 challenges 12
 equipment **5**
 high frequency oscillatory (HFOV) 69, 73
 impaired 21, 107
 inadequate **8**, 45, 472
 indications 12
 intermittent positive pressure (IPPV) 69, 73
 monitoring **3**
 nasal CPAP 13
 support 12–13
Vibrio cholerae 257
viral exanthema **256**
visceromegaly 146
vitamin deficiency

A 125, **153**, 161, **161**
B **154**, 202
C **154**
D **154**, 162, **163**, **389**, **482**
[*see also* rickets]
K 401
vitamins/multivitamins 141, 156, 159, 311
  A 125, **129**, **140**, 156, 260
  C 396
  D 56, **140**, 420, 477, **482**
  E **140**
  K 42, 65, 139, **140**, 159, 505
vocal cords 103, 538, 539
  papules 423
vocal cord paralysis 95, **118**, 319
  bilateral **118**, 118
  unilateral **118**
volvulus 145, **150**, **489**, 491, 492, 497
vomiting 21, 39, **40**, 56, 63, 65, 95, 110, 121, 123, 145, 149–150, **150**, 152, 184, 187, 189, 190, 201, 211, 213, 215, 224, **225**, 236, 239, 243, **245**, 278, 279, 281, 283, 284, 315, 324, **329**, 330, **364**, 370, **371**, **373**, **392**, 405, **461**, **464**, 466, 467, 474, **479**, **482**, 491, 492, 496, 503, 515, 534
  bile-stained 149, 490, 491
  cyclical **150**
  definitions 149
  differential diagnosis **150**
  persistent 21, 136, 138, 275, 472, 490, 504

W

Waardenburg's syndrome 454
warts **306**, 422–424
  common 422, **S14**
  condylomata accuminata 423, **S16**
  mosaic 423
  mucosal 423, **S16**
  paint 423, 424
  plane 422, **S15**
  plantar 422, **S15**
  treatment of common warts 423
  treatment of genital warts 423–424
  treatment of plantar warts 424
wasting **154**, 155, 209
  adrenal salt **479**
  cerebral salt 213, **479**
  distal hand and foot muscles 156
  moderate **155**
  severe 153, **155**, 156
weak child 206–209
  acute weakness 206
  anterior horn cell 206
  botulism 206, 208
  chronic weakness 208–209
  dermatomyositis 208, 425
  muscle 208
  myasthaenia gravis **40**, 206, 207
  neuromuscular junction 207–208
  organophosphate poisoning 208
  peripheral nerve 207
  [*see also* Guillain-Barré syndrome]
wheezing 7, 89, **90**, 92, 93, 94, 96, 98, 114, 115, 165, 173, 269, 270, 319, 320, 323
  exercise-induced 319
  intensity **324**
  multiple triggers 94
  post-bronchiolitic 98–99
  recurrent 94, 319, 320
  responsive to bronchodilator 94
  single trigger 94
white pupil (leococoria) 405, 445–446
  acquired 445
  cataracts 165, 440, 445–446, 454
World Health Organization (WHO) 20, 44, 82, 86, 155, 157, 159, 162, 176, 250, 257, 264, 266, 277, 285, 303, 307, 465, 508, 516
  antiretroviral therapy in children **308**
  Baby Friendly Hospital Initiative (BFHI) 82
  classification of injuries **20**
  classification of malnutrition **155**
  clinical staging of HIV for infants and children **305–307**
  dosing schedule for children **304**
  duration of secondary prophylaxis **177**
  diagnostic criteria for rheumatic fever **176**
  list of causes of child and adolescent death 20, **21**
  palliative care 508–509
  step ladder approach 516
  ten step programmes 82, 157, 465
Williams syndrome 355, **391**, **482**
Wilm's tumour **243**
Wilson's disease **134**, **135**, 144

X

xerosis
  conjunctivae **153**
  corneae **153**

Y

yellow fever 294
  vaccine 249, 251, 253